CAR T-Cell

Editors

CARON A. JACOBSON
PARTH S. SHAH

HEMATOLOGY/ONCOLOGY
CLINICS OF NORTH AMERICA

www.hemonc.theclinics.com

Consulting Editors
GEORGE P. CANELLOS
EDWARD J. BENZ JR.

December 2023 • Volume 37 • Number 6

ELSEVIER

1600 John F. Kennedy Boulevard • Suite 1800 • Philadelphia, Pennsylvania, 19103-2899

http://www.theclinics.com

HEMATOLOGY/ONCOLOGY CLINICS OF NORTH AMERICA Volume 37, Number 6
December 2023 ISSN 0889-8588, ISBN 13: 978-0-443-18300-3

Editor: Stacy Eastman
Developmental Editor: Shivank Joshi

Hematology/Oncology Clinics (ISSN 0889-8588) is published bimonthly by Elsevier Inc., 360 Park Avenue South, New York, NY 10010-1710. Months of issue are February, April, June, August, October, and December. Business and Editorial Offices: 1600 John F. Kennedy Blvd., Ste. 1800, Philadelphia, PA 19103–2899. Customer Service Office: 3251 Riverport Lane, Maryland Heights, MO 63043. Periodicals postage paid at New York, NY and at additional mailing offices. Subscription prices are $484.00 per year (domestic individuals), $1190.00 per year (domestic institutions), $100.00 per year (domestic students/residents), $510.00 per year (Canadian individuals), $100.00 per year (Canadian students/residents), $1232.00 per year (Canadian institutions) $580.00 per year (international individuals), $1232.00 per year (international institutions), and $255.00 per year (international students/residents). International air speed delivery is included in all *Clinics* subscription prices. All prices are subject to change without notice. **POSTMASTER:** Send address changes to *Hematology/Oncology Clinics of North America*, Elsevier Health Sciences Division, Subscription Customer Service, 3251 Riverport Lane, Maryland Heights, MO 63043. Customer Service (orders, claims, online, change of address): Elsevier Health Sciences Division, Subscription **Customer Service, 3251 Riverport Lane, Maryland Heights, MO 63043. Tel: 1-800-654-2452 (U.S. and Canada); 314-447-8871 (outside U.S. and Canada). Fax: 314-447-8029. E-mail: journalscustomerservice-usa@elsevier.com (for print support); journalsonlinesupport-usa@elsevier.com (for online support).**

Reprints. For copies of 100 or more, of articles in this publication, please contact the Commercial Reprints Department, Elsevier Inc., 360 Park Avenue South, New York, New York 10010-1710; Tel.: 212-633-3874, Fax: 212-633-3820, E-mail: reprints@elsevier.com.

Hematology/Oncology Clinics of North America is covered in *MEDLINE/PubMed (Index Medicus), EMBASE/ Excerpta Medica, and BIOSIS.*

Contributors

CONSULTING EDITORS

GEORGE P. CANELLOS, MD
William Rosenberg Professor of Medicine, Department of Medical Oncology, Dana-Farber Cancer Institute, Boston, Massachusetts, USA

EDWARD J. BENZ Jr, MD
President and CEO Emeritus, Dana-Farber Cancer Institute, Director Emeritus, Dana-Farber/Harvard Cancer Center, Richard and Susan Smith Distinguished Professor of Medicine, Professor of Pediatrics, Professor of Genetics, Harvard Medical School, Boston, Massachusetts, USA

EDITORS

CARON A. JACOBSON, MD
Associate Professor of Medicine, Harvard Medical School, Dana-Farber Cancer Institute, Boston, Massachusetts, USA

PARTH S. SHAH, MD
Assistant Professor of Medicine, Dartmouth Geisel School of Medicine, Department of Hematology, Dartmouth Cancer Center, Lebanon, New Hampshire, USA; Medical Oncology, Dana-Farber Cancer Institute, Boston, Massachusetts, USA

AUTHORS

KATHERINE CUMMINS, MBBS, PhD, FRACP, FRCPA
Peter MacCallum Cancer Centre, University of Melbourne, Melbourne, Australia

REBECCA EPPERLY, MD
Department of Bone Marrow Transplantation and Cellular Therapy, St. Jude Children's Research Hospital, Memphis, Tennessee, USA

SAAR GILL, MBBS, PhD, FRACP
Division of Hematology-Oncology, University of Pennsylvania Perelman School of Medicine, Philadelphia, Pennsylvania, USA

VICTORIA M. GIORDANI, MD
Pediatric Oncology Branch, Center for Cancer Research (CCR), National Cancer Institute (NCI), National Institutes of Health, Pediatric Hematology/Oncology, Johns Hopkins Hospital, Baltimore, Maryland, USA

MARK P. HAMILTON, MD, PhD
Center for Cancer Cell Therapy, Stanford Cancer Institute, Division of Blood and Marrow Transplantation and Cellular Therapy, Division of Hematology, Department of Medicine, Stanford University School of Medicine, Stanford, California, USA

GLENN J. HANNA, MD
Dana-Farber Cancer Institute, Boston, Massachusetts, USA

LAQUISA C. HILL, MD
Assistant Professor, Section of Hematology and Oncology, Department of Medicine, Center for Cell and Gene Therapy, Texas Children's Hospital and Houston Methodist Hospital, Dan L. Duncan Comprehensive Cancer Center, Baylor College of Medicine, Houston, Texas, USA

CARON A. JACOBSON, MD
Associate Professor of Medicine, Harvard Medical School, Dana-Farber Cancer Institute, Boston, Massachusetts, USA

GRACE A. JOHNSON, BS
University of South Florida Morsani College of Medicine, Tampa, Florida, USA

FREDERICK L. LOCKE, MD
Department of Blood and Marrow Transplant and Cellular Immunotherapy, H. Lee Moffitt Cancer Center, Tampa, Florida, USA

SHAM MAILANKODY, MD
Cellular Therapy Service, Myeloma Service, Department of Medicine, Memorial Sloan Kettering Cancer Center, Department of Medicine, Weill Cornell Medical College, New York, New York, USA

SHANNON L. MAUDE, MD, PhD
Associate Professor of Pediatrics, Division of Oncology, Cancer Immunotherapy Program, The Children's Hospital of Philadelphia, Department of Pediatrics, Perelman School of Medicine, University of Pennsylvania, Philadelphia, Pennsylvania, USA

SUSAN E. MCCLORY, MD, PhD
Instructor, Division of Oncology, Cancer Immunotherapy Program, The Children's Hospital of Philadelphia, Department of Pediatrics, Perelman School of Medicine, University of Pennsylvania, Philadelphia, Pennsylvania, USA

LEKHA MIKKILINENI, MD, MA
Blood and Marrow Transplantation and Cellular Therapy, Stanford University, Palo Alto, California, USA; Stanford School of Medicine, Stanford, California, USA

DAVID B. MIKLOS, MD, PhD
Center for Cancer Cell Therapy, Stanford Cancer Institute, Division of Blood and Marrow Transplantation and Cellular Therapy, Department of Medicine, Stanford University School of Medicine, Stanford, California, USA

IBRAHIM N. MUHSEN, MD
Fellow, Section of Hematology and Oncology, Department of Medicine, Center for Cell and Gene Therapy, Texas Children's Hospital and Houston Methodist Hospital, Dan L. Duncan Comprehensive Cancer Center, Baylor College of Medicine, Houston, Texas, USA

KARTHIK NATH, MD
Cellular Therapy Service, Department of Medicine, Memorial Sloan Kettering Cancer Center, New York, New York, USA

CARLOS A. RAMOS, MD
Professor, Section of Hematology and Oncology, Department of Medicine, Center for Cell and Gene Therapy, Texas Children's Hospital and Houston Methodist Hospital, Dan L. Duncan Comprehensive Cancer Center, Baylor College of Medicine, Houston, Texas, USA

NIRALI N. SHAH, MD, MHSc
Pediatric Oncology Branch, Center for Cancer Research (CCR), National Cancer Institute (NCI), National Institutes of Health, Bethesda, Maryland, USA

PARTH S. SHAH, MD
Assistant Professor of Medicine, Dartmouth Geisel School of Medicine, Department of Hematology, Dartmouth Cancer Center, Lebanon, New Hampshire, USA; Medical Oncology, Dana-Farber Cancer Institute, Boston, Massachusetts, USA

ERIC L. SMITH, MD, PhD
Director of Translational Research, Immune Effector Cell Therapies, Assistant Professor, Harvard Medical School, Dana-Farber Cancer Institute, Boston, Massachusetts, USA

ADAM S. SPERLING, MD, PhD
Medical Oncology, Dana-Farber Cancer Institute, Division of Hematology, Brigham and Women's Hospital, Boston, Massachusetts, USA

SAAD Z. USMANI, MD, MBA, FACP
Cellular Therapy Service, Myeloma Service, Department of Medicine, Adult Bone Marrow Transplant Service, Memorial Sloan Kettering Cancer Center, Department of Medicine, Weill Cornell Medical College, New York, New York, USA

JEREMIAH A. WALA, MD, PhD
Dana-Farber Cancer Institute, Boston, Massachusetts, USA

Contents

Over the past decade, CAR T cell therapy has transformed the treatment of
relapsed or refractory B-ALL in children and adults. CD19-directed CAR
T cells can induce complete remissions in a large majority of patients with
B-ALL, and up to half of these patients will go on to maintain durable remissions. However, significant challenges remain for patients who relapse or
do not respond. This review will discuss the history of CAR T cell therapy
for B-ALL, the treatment considerations for CAR T cell recipients, and current clinical trials and future directions for CAR T cell therapy in B-ALL.

Chimeric antigen receptor (CAR) T-cell therapy is a revolutionary therapy
increasingly used in the treatment of non-Hodgkin B-cell lymphoma.
This review focuses on the use of CAR T-cell therapy in aggressive B-
cell lymphoma including clinical indications, known short- and long-term
toxicity, mechanisms of CAR T-cell efficacy and tumor resistance, and future directions in the treatment of aggressive lymphoma with CAR T-cell
therapy.

The advent of chimeric antigen receptor (CAR)-T cell therapy has revolutionized the treatment of several hematological malignancies. Although
the initial benefit was mainly observed in aggressive leukemias and lymphomas, recent data have resulted in the approval of multiple CAR-T
therapies in indolent lymphomas, with ongoing research showing great
promise for further improvements and therapeutic optimizations. In this article, we review the published data and approved therapies for CAR-T cell
therapy for indolent lymphomas focusing on mantle cell lymphoma and follicular lymphoma while describing the work in chronic lymphocytic leukemia and future strategies.

Multiple myeloma is the second most common hematological malignancy
with an approximate incidence of up to 8.5 cases per 100,000 persons per

year. Over the last decade, therapy for multiple myeloma has undergone a revolutionary change. Chimeric antigen receptor (CAR) T-cell therapy has played a major role in this evolution. In this review, we discuss the existing state of CAR T-cell therapy in myeloma while evaluating several newer therapies and targets expected in the near future.

The authors review the current use of chimeric antigen receptor (CAR)-transduced T cells (CAR-T) in Hodgkin lymphoma (HL) and T-cell lymphomas (TCL) and discuss the data on CD30-targeting CAR-T cells, which seem to be safe and effective in HL. In addition, the authors examine the use of CAR-T cells targeting CD30, CD5, or CD7 in TCL, while highlighting the unique challenges of their use in this subset of lymphomas. Furthermore, the authors present future directions and ongoing trials investigating the use of CAR-T cells in TCL and HL.

Up to 30% of patients with acute myeloid leukemia (AML) who undergo chimeric antigen receptor (CAR) T-cell therapy have evidence of response, although trials are highly heterogeneous. These responses are rarely deep or durable. CD123, CD33, and CLL-1 have emerged as the most common targets for CAR T cells in AML. CAR T cells against myeloid antigens cause myeloablation as well as cytokine release syndrome, although neurotoxicity is rarely seen. Future efforts should focus on AML-specific antigen discovery or engineering, and on further enhancing the activity of CAR T cells.

We review chimeric antigen receptor (CAR) T-cell therapy for solid tumors. We discuss patient selection factors and aspects of clinical management. We describe challenges including physical and molecular barriers to trafficking CAR-Ts, an immunosuppressive tumor microenvironment, and difficulty finding cell surface target antigens. The application of new approaches in synthetic biology and cellular engineering toward solid tumor CAR-Ts is described. Finally, we summarize reported and ongoing clinical trials of CAR-T therapies for select disease sites such as head and neck (including thyroid cancer), lung, central nervous system (glioblastoma, neuroblastoma, glioma), sarcoma, genitourinary (prostate, renal, bladder, kidney), breast and ovarian cancer.

As chimeric antigen receptor (CAR) T-cell therapy is increasingly integrated into clinical practice across a range of malignancies, identifying and treating inflammatory toxicities will be vital to success. Early experiences with CD19-targeted CAR T-cell therapy identified cytokine release syndrome and neurotoxicity as key acute toxicities and led to unified initiatives to mitigate the influence of these complications. In this section, we provide an update on the current state of CAR T-cell-related toxicities, with an emphasis on emerging acute toxicities affecting additional organ systems and considerations for delayed toxicities and late effects.

Grace A. Johnson and Frederick L. Locke

CAR T cell therapy has significantly shaped the treatment landscape for refractory hematologic malignancies including large B-cell lymphomas, multiple myeloma, and leukemias. While response rates for a previously dismal prognosis have improved, certain obstacles still remain to achieving CAR T infallibility. In this article, we review the data surrounding proposed resistance mechanisms of tumors to CAR T, including the implications of target loss, exhausted T cells as effete effectors, the necessity of maximal CAR T expansion to durable response, the negative impact of an inflammatory milieu and a suppressive tumor microenvironment, and the optimal tumor-to-effector ratio that associates with best outcomes. The future of CAR T should aim to mitigate these weaknesses in order to bolster the efficacy of this revolutionary therapy.

Karthik Nath, Sham Mailankody, and Saad Z. Usmani

Chimeric antigen receptor (CAR) T-cell therapy and bispecific antibodies are a class of T-cell engaging immunotherapies that have demonstrated considerable promise for patients with blood cancers. In comparison with traditional cancer therapeutics, T-cell engaging therapies harness the power of the host immune system to attack malignant cells expressing a target antigen of interest. Although these therapies are altering the natural history of blood cancers, the availability of several products has created uncertainty regarding treatment selection. In this review, we discuss the role of CAR T-cell therapy in the emerging era of bispecific antibodies with a particular focus on multiple myeloma.

Eric L. Smith

Over the last 10 years CAR T cell therapies have been shown to be transformative for B- and plasma-cell malignancies, however the field is only beginning to realize the potential benefit to patients of such therapies. Over the next 10 years it is expected that advances will be made in durable response rates for patients with B/plasma cell malignancies; expansion to T-cell, myeloid, and solid malignancies; and in delivery and manufacturing to transform the field.

HEMATOLOGY/ONCOLOGY CLINICS OF NORTH AMERICA

SERIES OF RELATED INTEREST

Surgical Oncology Clinics
https://www.surgonc.theclinics.com
Advances in Oncology
https://www.advances-oncology.com

THE CLINICS ARE AVAILABLE ONLINE!
Access your subscription at:
www.theclinics.com

Preface

CAR T Cells: Past Successes, Current Limitations, and Future Opportunities

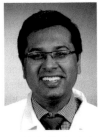 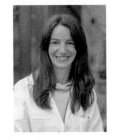

Parth S. Shah, MD   Caron A. Jacobson, MD
Editors

Second-generation chimeric antigen receptor (CAR) T cells targeting CD19 made a huge splash around 2010 when the first reports of durable complete responses in B-cell leukemias and lymphomas began to emerge. Since that time, single-institution first-in-human studies led to multicenter, phase 2 studies where similarly impressive results were recapitulated and garnered regulatory approvals across the globe for B-cell acute lymphoblastic leukemia and large B-cell lymphoma (LBCL). Following these approvals, we have seen results in large, multicenter "real-world" series demonstrate nearly identical overall response rates, complete response rates, duration of response, progression-free survival, and overall survival despite the majority of patients being ineligible for the pivotal clinical trials. In these post–commercial experiences, despite competing medical comorbidities, baseline organ dysfunction, and poor performance status, toxicities remain relatively even to slightly improved. This is likely owing to an improved understanding on how to manage these toxicities, such as cytokine release syndrome (CRS) and immune effector cell–associated neurologic syndrome (ICANS), more aggressively without sacrificing efficacy. This success has expanded use beyond these aggressive and highly refractory B-cell malignancies, and successful studies in mantle cell lymphoma and follicular lymphoma have led to label expansions in these diseases. On the heels of the success of CD19 CAR T-cell therapies, CAR T-cells targeting B-cell maturation antigen (BCMA) yielded similarly promising results in multiple myeloma (MM), resulting in 1 to 2 years off therapy for over half of patients in the advanced setting, many of whom had seen continuous therapy since the time of their diagnosis. Studies exploring earlier use of these therapies in high-risk patients, randomized against current standards of care, in both LBCL and MM, have demonstrated superiority of CAR T cells—in some cases with prolonged survival–over decades-long established therapies, and have moved, or will invariably move, CAR T cells up into earlier lines of therapy for the patients who need it, and might benefit from it, most This has not been the slow, incremental progress we have become used to in oncology clinical investigation—this has been revolutionary for some of the most highly refractory and hardest to treat blood cancers, many of which previously had no promising treatment options.

Despite these remarkable successes, there is considerable room for improvement with these therapies in order to fully realize their potential. Within blood cancers, over half of patients will either not respond or will relapse within 1 to 2 years, and these relapsing or refractory diseases after CAR T-cell therapy have become the new unmet need. In addition, these therapies are cumbersome, logistically challenging in their involvement of a multidisciplinary approach, extraordinarily expensive, and carry a unique toxicity profile requiring specialized expertise. As a result, they are offered only in select centers that can support the infrastructure necessary for this compli-cated patient and billing journey as well as the clinical expertise required to manage the patients medically. The result is that many patients who need these therapies live hundreds of miles away from a treatment center requiring moving far from home for a month or longer for their CAR T-cell episode. This is impossible for some due to social and economic reasons, and thus access and equity issues remain major concerns regarding these therapies. Finally, effective CAR T-cell and other cellular therapies have eluded many of our more common solid tumors, where thera-pies such as these could have an even larger impact.

In this issue of *Hematology/Oncology Clinics of North America*, we explore in detail the successes of CAR T cells in B-cell leukemias and lymphomas and MM, but also the limitations in terms of toxicity risks as well as resistance mechanisms, the uncovering of which is a necessary step to improve these therapies and enhance safety and ac-tivity in even more patients. We take what we have learned from the CAR experience in these diseases and apply that knowledge to other blood cancers, like chronic lympho-cytic leukemia, acute myelogenous leukemia, and T-cell and Hodgkin lymphoma, as well as solid tumors. We explore issues related to cost and access, and how these therapies fit within the new landscape of therapies that include bispecific antibodies and other drugs that target CD19 and BCMA. And finally, we leave you with a vision for the future and a message of hope grounded in the next generation of products and trials to enter the clinic.

Parth S. Shah, MD
Dartmouth Cancer Center
1 Medical Center Drive
Lebanon, NH 03766, USA

Caron A. Jacobson, MD
Dana-Farber Cancer Institute
DFCI 450 Brookline Avenue
Boston, MA 02494, USA

E-mail addresses:
parth.s.shah@hitchcock.org (P.S. Shah)
caron_jacobson@dfci.harvard.edu (C.A. Jacobson)

The Current State of Chimeric Antigen Receptor T Cell Therapy for B Lymphoblastic Leukemia

Susan E. McClory, MD, PhD[a,b], Shannon L. Maude, MD, PhD[a,b,*]

KEYWORDS

- Chimeric antigen receptor • CAR T cell • B lymphoblastic leukemia • B-ALL

KEY POINTS

- CAR T cell therapy for relapsed/refractory B-ALL has transformed the treatment landscape.
- CD19-directed CAR T cell therapy can induce remission in 60-90% of patients with B-ALL and can successfully promote durable remission in many patients.
- Treatment of relapse following CAR T cell therapy remains a challenge.
- Novel investigational CAR T cell therapies directed at alternative B cell targets or with improved engineering or manufacturing processes are currently in clinical trials to address this challenge.

INTRODUCTION AND BACKGROUND

Significant improvements in the treatment of pediatric and young adult B cell acute lymphoblastic leukemia (B-ALL) have yielded an overall survival rate of >90%, yet 10-20% of patients will experience relapse or refractory disease with significantly reduced survival.[1] Thus, relapsed/refractory B-ALL remains the most common cause of pediatric cancer morbidity and mortality.[1] Further, B-ALL in adults carries an overall survival of 11-65%, with age heavily impacting outcomes[2] and relapsed or refractory B-ALL remains difficult to treat with poor survival.[3] However, cellular therapies and specifically chimeric antigen receptor (CAR) T cell therapy have offered significant promise in treating both adult and pediatric B-ALL. More than 11 years ago, the first pediatric patient with B-ALL was infused with autologous CD19-directed CAR

[a] Division of Oncology, Cancer Immunotherapy Program, The Children's Hospital of Philadelphia, Philadelphia, PA, USA; [b] Department of Pediatrics, Perelman School of Medicine at the University of Pennsylvania, Philadelphia, PA, USA
* Corresponding author. Division of Oncology, The Children's Hospital of Philadelphia, 3012 CTRB, 3501 Civic Center Boulevard, Philadelphia, PA 19104.
E-mail address: maude@chop.edu

Hematol Oncol Clin N Am 37 (2023) 1041–1052
https://doi.org/10.1016/j.hoc.2023.06.003
0889-8588/23/© 2023 Elsevier Inc. All rights reserved.

T cells at the Children's Hospital of Philadelphia (CHOP),[4,5] and since then thousands of children and adults have been infused with CAR T cells for refractory or relapsed B-ALL, either as part of a clinical trial or as recipients of one of the 2 current FDA-approved commercial CAR T cell products for B-ALL, tisagenlecleucel and brexucabtagene autoleucel.

CAR T cells are T cells that are genetically engineered to express a chimeric antigen receptor that targets antigens on the surface of cancer cells. This antigen specificity is generated by fusing an antibody-binding domain to signaling domains responsible for down-stream T cell activation. The use of an antibody-binding domain (scFv), rather than a T cell receptor, allows CAR T cells to recognize the antigen directly on the surface of a tumor cell in the absence of an MHC molecule, which are frequently down-regulated on cancer cells.[6,7] Most CAR T cells developed to date combine activating and co-stimulatory domains directly into the CAR construct. Most commonly, this has been a combination of CD3-ς with either 4-1BB or CD28.[6-11] The first CAR T cells developed, including the two FDA-approved products for B-ALL, are directed to the B cell antigen CD19, which is expressed widely on multiple B cell malignancies, including B-ALL.[4,12-14] However, multiple CAR T cell products targeting CD22, CD20, and other B-ALL antigens are now in clinical trials or development.[15-24] In this review, we will discuss the history of CAR T cell therapy for B-ALL, the current recommendations for its use, and its future directions.

DISCUSSION
The Road to FDA Approval of the First CAR T Cell Therapies for B-ALL

Over the past 2 decades, multiple trials have found CD19-directed CAR T cells to be highly successful at inducing an initial remission in both pediatric and adult B-ALL,[4,5,13,25-30] and this has resulted in the FDA approval of two CD19-CAR T cell products to date: tisagenlecleucel for pediatric and young adult patients with multiply relapsed or refractory B-ALL in 2017[31] and brexucabtagene autoleucel for relapsed or refractory adult B-ALL in 2021.[32]

CTL019, which ultimately became known as tisagenlecleucel, is an autologous CD19-directed CAR T cell product with CD3-ς and 4-1BB activating and co-stimulatory domains. The first in-human trials used CTL019 in adult patients with CLL, demonstrating feasibility[12-14] but soon after, clinical trials investigating CTL019 for children and adults with B-ALL began.[4,25,27] Of the first 30 pediatric and young adult patients treated with CTL019 in a phase I/II single-institution trial, 90% experienced a complete morphologic remission at the 1-month timepoint and 22 of these 30 achieved MRD negativity.[4] The event free survival rate (EFS) was 67% and overall survival (OS) rate was 78% at 6 months, suggesting for the first time that CAR T cells could be incredibly successful at inducing and maintaining remission.[4] ELIANA, a global phase I/II trial of the use of tisagenlecleucel in pediatric relapsed/refractory B-ALL across 25 centers, similarly reported an 81% MRD-negative remission rate within the first 3 months following infusion and 12-month relapse-free survival (RFS) of 59%.[5] Importantly, these two trials demonstrated CTL019 persistence for as long as 39 months, that durable remission could be achieved without consolidative hematopoietic stem cell transplant (HSCT), and that CTL019 could induce remissions in patients with a wide range of leukemic burden pre-infusion.[4,5] ELIANA was also the first trial to demonstrate feasibility of centralized CAR T cell manufacturing, paving the way towards a scalable CAR T cell therapy that could be accessible at sites throughout the world. The early success of CTL019 in the first single-center trial, and subsequently in ELIANA, ultimately led to the 2017 FDA approval of tisagenlecleucel for patients up to age 25 years with B-ALL in its second or greater relapse or for chemotherapy-refractory disease in the same patient population,[31] marking the first FDA approval of both a gene therapy product and CAR T cell in the US. Tisagenlecleucel is now also approved for use in adult patients with relapsed/refractory diffuse large B cell lymphoma and follicular lymphoma.

Since its approval, additional studies have continued to assess tisagenlecleucel's efficacy, safety, and durability. Recently, the 3-year update of ELIANA demonstrated that of 79 patients enrolled, EFS at 3 years was 44%, OS was 63%, and RFS was estimated at 52%, demonstrating durable long-term remissions in nearly 50% of these pediatric and young adult patients.[33] Of these, 11 patients underwent consolidative allogeneic hematopoietic stem cell transplant (alloHSCT) while still in remission following tisagenlecleucel treatment.[33] These data further suggest that CD19-directed CAR T cell therapy can offer the potential for long-term remission and cure. Furthermore, the feasibility and efficacy of tisagenlecleucel as a commercially available CAR T cell therapy has now been assessed by multiple studies looking at real-world experiences in centers within the US.[34–36] A 2020 report from the Center for International Blood and Marrow Transplant Research (CIBMTR) detailed the experience of 255 patients with B-ALL from 73 centers and found an initial complete remission rate of 85.5%, with one year EFS 52.4% and OS 77.2%, similar to the first 2 CTL019 trials.[34] A Pediatric Real World CART Consortium report in 2022 reported that of 185 infused pediatric and young adult patients at 15 centers, tisagenlecleucel was associated with an 85% CR rate, a 12-month OS of 72% and EFS of 50%,[35] again strikingly similar to prior studies overall.

Simultaneously, clinical trials for adult B-ALL were underway.[26–28,37] KTE-X19 is a CD19-directed CAR T cell that incorporates a CD3-ς and CD28 costimulatory domain initially developed at the National Cancer Institute.[37,38] Additionally, it involves a modified manufacturing process that specifically removes malignant cells from the leukapheresis product to improve CAR T cell production even in the setting of high peripheral blast counts.[39] In 2021, results from ZUMA-3, a multicenter phase 2 trial of KTE-X19, demonstrated a 71% overall complete remission rate (OCR) with 52% achieving complete remission at the 3-month mark and 97% of responders achieving MRD negativity.[40] Based on the findings of the ZUMA-3 trial, KTE-X19 was approved by the FDA for relapsed/refractory B-ALL under the name brexucabtagene autoleucel in 2021.[32] It had been approved for adults with relapsed/refractory mantle cell lymphoma the year prior.[32] In 2022, updated ZUMA-3 outcomes demonstrated that after 26.8-months median follow-up, median duration of remission was 14.6 months and duration of overall survival was 25.4 months.[41] Of the 71 patients, 12 patients underwent alloHSCT after KTE-X19 treatment while either in a CR, a CR with incomplete recovery, or an aplastic bone marrow without blasts and without having received any additional anti-leukemic therapy.[41]

Currently, patients aged 18-25 years old with relapsed or refractory B-ALL may be candidates for either tisagenlecleucel or brexucabtagene autoleucel, but there are no head-to-head trials comparing the two therapies.[42] ZUMA-4, assessing the efficacy and safety of KTE-X19 for pediatric relapsed/refractory B-ALL (NCT02625480), is ongoing.

Treatment Considerations

How to incorporate CAR T cell therapy into a treatment regimen for B-ALL is an active area of study and discussion. Further, how to factor in the likelihood of toxicity, the impact of prior treatments on CAR T cell success, how to best predict long-term response, and how to approach stem cell transplant after CAR T cell therapy for

B-ALL all remain important considerations and are discussed later in discussion. For additional discussion, Myers and colleagues[42] recently reviewed current recommendations for how to approach risk factors for CAR T cell success or failure in children and young adults.

Toxicity of CAR T cells for B-ALL

Cytokine release syndrome (CRS) and Immune effector cell-associated neurotoxicity syndrome (ICANS) were recognized within the first trials of CAR T cells in humans[4,25,26,29,43] and remain the most pervasive toxicities associated with CAR T therapy. Each represents a spectrum of immunopathology associated with CAR T cell activation and expansion, and consensus definitions have now been established.[44,45] Within the clinical trials leading up to FDA approval for both tisagenlecleucel and brexucabtagene autoleucel, grade 3 or higher CRS rates ranged from 24 to 49% and grade 3 or higher ICANS ranged from 13 to 14%,[40,46] whereas lower rates have been reported in multi-center real-world scenarios following FDA approval, likely reflecting a lower disease burden in many of the patients treated off study.[34,35] How to mitigate, prevent, and treat CRS and ICANS has evolved over the last decade of CAR T cell experience and now includes a spectrum of treatment options including the IL-6 blocking antibodies tocilizumab and siltuximab, corticosteroids, and additional targeted cytokine blockade with anti-IL-1 and IFNy antibodies.[44] Please see the full discussion of CAR T cell toxicities and their management as covered in a separate article in this issue.

Pre-infusion factors impacting CAR T cell success

Disease burden at the time of CAR T cell infusion should be considered in any patient undergoing CAR T cell therapy as it may impact response, survival, and toxicities. Both ELIANA and ZUMA-3, which led to the FDA approval of CAR T cells for B-ALL, required >5% morphologic disease within the bone marrow at the time of enrollment.[40,46] However, both tisagenlecleucel and brexucabtagene autoleucel are approved for any relapsed or refractory B-ALL in their respective patient populations, regardless of disease burden. Multiple studies have now clearly established that higher disease burden is associated with an increased risk of CAR T cell treatment failure compared to low disease burden. A CHOP-based trial of tisagenlecleucel found that patients with >40% bone marrow involvement had worse EFS (34% vs 78%) and OS (60% vs 92%) compared with lower disease at the time of infusion.[47] Further, multiple studies have established that any disease burden >5% of the bone marrow is associated with decreased OS, EFS, RFS, and toxicities including CRS and ICANS.[35,48–51] Similarly, the presence of active non-CNS extra-medullary disease at the time of CAR T therapy is associated with lower EFS,[42,49,50] but prior CNS or other EMD was not associated with worse outcomes.[42,52] Thus, while patients with high disease burden can and do respond to CAR T cell therapy and may experience durable remission, they remain at higher risk of relapse or toxicity.

Second, how prior therapy may impact CAR T cell success may also be considered. Blinatumomab is a bispecific T cell engager (BiTE) which targets CD19 on leukemia cells and engages with CD3 on endogenous T cells to increase T cell activation and cytotoxicity. As its use for B-ALL has expanded in both adults and children, there has been concern that its prior use could impact the efficacy of CD19-directed CAR T cells by downregulating CD19 or impacting the ability of CD19-specific CAR T cells to target CD19,[3,42] and case studies described CD19 CAR T cell failure in patients who had previously received blinatumomab.[53] Indeed, several studies did suggest that prior blinatumomab use was associated with worse outcomes, including decreased rate of CR[40,54]; however, in ZUMA-3 it did not affect relapse-free survival or OS.[40] Furthermore, in a multicenter study of 420 children and young adults who received CD19-directed CAR T cell therapy, prior blinatumomab failure was directly associated with lower CR rates (65% vs 93%), and shorter EFS, RFS, and OS, whereas blinatumomab exposure alone was not,[49] suggesting that the association of prior blinatumomab treatment to lower CR may be more directly due to either sensitivity to CD19-directed therapy in general or due to the prolonged antigen exposure and immunologic pressure caused by incomplete CD19 clearance. In fact, Myers and colleagues[42] recommend that blinatumomab exposure or non-response should not be a contraindication to CAR T cell therapy as most patients will achieve CR with CAR T cell therapy despite this history.

Inotuzumab ozogamicin is an antibody-drug conjugate which targets CD22 and has demonstrated success in both pediatric and adult ALL, with further studies ongoing.[15,16,55] While Inotuzumab would not be expected to directly alter CD19 expression on leukemic blasts, it can induce widespread B cell aplasia (BCA) due to the expression of CD22 on endogenous, healthy B cells. This BCA decreases the overall CD19$^+$ antigen load within the body, which may be important for CD19-directed CAR T cell expansion and persistence.[42,56] Furthermore, inotuzumab significantly increases the risk of sinusoidal obstructive syndrome following stem cell transplant, and this may be a significant consideration for patients proceeding to HSCT following CAR T cell infusion.[55] Thus, the timing of inotuzumab prior to CAR T cell therapy should be carefully considered.

How CAR T cell response after infusion can inform the likelihood of future relapse

Thus far, following infusion of CAR T cells for B-ALL there are two primary post-infusion factors that can inform the likelihood of future relapse: (1) duration of B cell aplasia and (2) next-generation sequencing (NGS)-MRD status at 1- and 3-months following infusion. B cell aplasia is a well-accepted proxy for CAR T cell persistence given that CD19 is expressed by healthy B cells as well as B cell leukemia.[30,42,57] In general, early B cell recovery is associated with a high risk of CD19$^+$ relapse,[30,42,56,57] in contrast to CD19$^-$ relapse thought to be associated with leukemic factors that drive immune evasion. In adults, loss of B cell aplasia with loss of CAR T cell persistence was highly associated with CD19$^+$ leukemic relapse.[30] Furthermore, in pediatric and young adult patients, loss of B cell aplasia within 1 year of tisagenlecleucel infusion significantly increased the risk of relapse, with highest risk associated with loss within 6 months.[57] In a trial of a humanized CD19 CAR T cell therapy for pediatric and young adult B-ALL, recovery of B cells within 6 months shortened EFS and RFS.[48] However, whether B cell aplasia beyond the first year after infusion is associated with higher rates of relapse remains unclear. Secondly, NGS-MRD positivity is highly associated with relapse following tisagenlecleucel in pediatric and young adult patients, both at day 28 and 3 months following infusion.[57] Better understanding of the predictive value of both CAR T cell persistence and NGS-MRD positivity for future relapse and how that may inform post-CAR T cell therapy treatment decisions remains an important focus of current CAR T cell investigation.

The role for consolidative hematopoietic stem cell transplant following CAR T cell therapy for B-ALL

CAR T cell therapy for B-ALL has demonstrated remarkable results with most patients experiencing a complete remission following treatment, more than half remaining disease-free one year after infusion,[40,46] and nearly half of the patients that responded to tisagenlecleucel remaining relapse-free without further therapy at the 3-year mark.[33] However, treatment options for relapsed leukemia after CAR T cell therapy are incredibly limited, and in pediatric patients, relapse after tisagenlecleucel is associated with poor prognosis.[36] Thus, there is considerable debate in the field regarding which patients would benefit from consolidative allogeneic hematopoietic stem cell transplant (alloHSCT) following CAR T cell infusion in an attempt to decrease the risk of disease recurrence. Importantly, there have been no prospective clinical trials designed to directly evaluate the role of alloHSCT after CAR T cell therapy for adults or children.[3] Yet, several trials have provided some important information that may help guide decisions. In ZUMA-3 and ELIANA, only 17% and 14%, respectively, of the patients enrolled underwent post-infusion consolidative alloHSCT while in remission,[5,33,40,41] suggesting that many patients can sustain a durable remission without a consolidative transplant. Furthermore, neither trial demonstrated an obvious survival benefit to alloHSCT following CAR T cell therapy,[5,33,40,41] but neither trial was designed or large enough to directly ask this question. In general, CD28-based CAR T cells have decreased cell persistence compared to 4-1BB constructs, including tisagenlecleucel, and recent recommendations have supported alloHSCT following CD28-directed CAR T cell therapy in pediatric and young adult patients.[42,58] However, for older adults or patients with significant co-morbidities, the risk/benefit of alloHSCT is less clear given the increased risk of non-relapse death following transplants in these patient populations.[59] Thus, there remains no explicit guidance for who should and should not go to transplant following CAR T cell therapy for B-ALL, rather the decision should be made based on the CAR T cell construct received, age and co-morbidities of the patient, and disease assessments and bone marrow recovery post-infusion.[3,42]

Ongoing Clinical Trials and Future Directions

While CAR T cell therapy has drastically improved treatment options for patients with multiply relapsed or refractory B-ALL, up to 50% of patients who receive CAR T cells will ultimately relapse. Thus, optimization in manufacturing or engineering to improve persistence and efficacy as well as investigations into additional CAR T cell targets remain critical to further advance the field and improve patient outcomes.

Humanized CD19 CAR T cells for B-ALL

CD19+ relapses are associated with early B cell recovery, poor CAR T cell persistence, and account for the majority of post-CAR T cell relapses in B-ALL.[28,56,60] Thus, efforts are underway to address factors that may contribute to early CAR T cell clearance. Tisagenlecleucel, brexucabtagene autoleucel, and most CD19-directed CAR T cells, contain an scFv domain derived from mouse monoclonal antibodies, which may cause unwanted immunogenicity that promotes CAR T cell loss.[61] To mitigate this, several groups have developed humanized or fully human constructs. The University of Pennsylvania developed a CAR T cell containing a humanized anti-CD19 scFv domain with the 4-1BB costimulatory domain (huCART19).[48] In the phase I huCART19 trial at CHOP, 74 patients were infused, with day 28 CR rates of 98% and 64% for patients without and with prior CAR T cell exposure, respectively. Patients who had received no prior CD19-directed CAR T cell therapy had an 84% RFS at 12 months and 74% at 24 months, whereas patients who had received prior CAR T cell therapy had a 74% RFS at 12 months and 58% at 24 months, demonstrating that while outcomes were better for CAR T cell naïve patients, patients who had received prior CAR T cell therapy also could experience a durable remission after huCART19 treatment.[48] Furthermore, while B cell recovery at 6 months was higher in patients who had received prior CAR T cell therapy compared to those who had not

(58% vs 15%),[48] these initial results also demonstrate that huCART19 can induce BCA and can persist in patients with prior CAR T cell therapy. Further trials assessing huCART19 are underway.

CD22-directed CAR T cell therapy for B-ALL

CD19 antigen loss on relapsed leukemia following upfront therapy or after prior CD19 CAR T cell therapy is a challenging mechanism of resistance to CD19-targeted immunotherapy. However, several trials are investigating alternative B-ALL targets. CD22 is expressed on most B-ALL cases, even after CD19 loss[62–64] and its expression is restricted to the B cell lineage. Furthermore, the success of the antibody-drug conjugate inotuzumab ozogamicin, which targets CD22,[15,16] suggests that CD22 may be a potent target for CAR T cell therapies in B-ALL. In a phase I trial investigating a fully human CD22-directed CAR T cell, 73% of 15 patients experienced a CR,[62] and in an updated report of 58 patients from the same trial, 70% experienced a CR, but median RFS was short at 6 months.[17] Rates of HLH-like CRS were high (32%).[17] Yet, these studies demonstrate that CAR T cells targeting CD22 may induce remission and may be a useful tool in addressing CD19 antigen loss. Further trials developing anti-CD22 CAR T cells are underway at multiple institutions.

Another attractive method of targeting CD22 with CAR T cell therapy is to combine an anti-CD22 CAR with a CD19 CAR in order to prevent antigen escape from either CD19 or CD22 alone. Multiple trials have now reported variable success with combinatory CAR T therapy using the co-administration of CD19-and CD22-directed CAR T cells[18,19] or bispecific CD19/CD22 CAR T cells,[20–22] with poor persistence emerging as a limitation, and trials are ongoing at multiple institutions. Constructs targeting three targets, including CD19, CD22, and CD20, are all in pre-clinical development.[23,24]

Allogeneic CAR T cell therapy for B-ALL

The two FDA-approved CAR T cell constructs and most other CAR T cell products in development for B-ALL have all been autologous therapies; that is, the CAR T cells are manufactured from T cells leukapheresed directly from the recipient patient. This poses several challenges. First, not all patients are able to produce an adequate T cell collection due to prior treatment, ongoing cytopenias, high peripheral blast burden, or poor medical suitability for apheresis. Secondly, autologous CAR T cell manufacturing is time-consuming. Thus, there is significant interest in the development of an allogeneic CAR T cell product for B-ALL.[3] Multiple trials in children and adults have now reported preliminary findings suggesting that allogeneic donor-derived CAR T cell therapy may be possible[65,66]; however, limitations have been encountered, including rejection causing poor expansion or persistence. Further trials are ongoing to assess safety, efficacy, and scalability of a universal CAR T cell product.

SUMMARY

Over the past decade, CAR T cell therapy has transformed the treatment paradigm for relapsed or refractory B-ALL in both adults and children. With the FDA approval of two CD19-directed CAR T cells for B-ALL and with many other constructs in clinical trials, the landscape of available cell therapies for B-ALL has never been wider. Indeed, CAR T cell therapy has the power to induce remission in a large majority of B-ALL patients and can provide long-term durable remissions for many. However, significant challenges remain for patients who experience CAR T cell non-response or post-infusion relapse. How to mitigate these challenges is a highly important focus of CAR T cell research.

CLINICS CARE POINTS

- CAR T cell therapy induces durable, MRD-negative remissions for many patients with relapsed or refractory B-ALL.
- Tisagenlecleucel is currently approved for patients up to 25 years old with multiply relapsed or refractory B-ALL.
- Brexucabtagene autoleucel is currently approved for patients 18 years or older with relapsed or refractory B-ALL.
- Factors such as patient age, co-morbidities, post-infusion NGS-MRD, presence of BCA, and bone marrow recovery should all inform the decision on consolidative alloHSCT following CAR T cell therapy for B-ALL.
- Many patients remain eligible for a number of clinical trials investigating current or new CAR T cell strategies for B-ALL and these should be discussed on an individual basis.

DISCLOSURE

S.E. McClory has no financial disclosures to report. S.L. Maude reports clinical trial support: Novartis, Switzerland, Wugen; consulting, advisory boards, or study steering committee: Novartis; patent pending and licensed to Novartis Pharmaceuticals for PCT/US2017/044425: Combination Therapies of Car and PD-1 Inhibitors.

REFERENCES

1. Hunger SP, Mullighan CG. Acute lymphoblastic leukemia in children. N Engl J Med 2015;373(16):1541–52.
2. Lennmyr E, Karlsson K, Ahlberg L, et al. Survival in adult acute lymphoblastic leukaemia (ALL): A report from the Swedish ALL Registry. Eur J Haematol 2019;103(2):88–98.
3. Pasvolsky O, Kebriaei P, Shah BD, et al. Chimeric antigen receptor T therapy for adult B-cell acute lymphoblastic leukemia: state-of the-(C)ART and road ahead. Blood Adv 2023. https://doi.org/10.1182/bloodadvances.2022009462.
4. Maude SL, Frey N, Shaw PA, et al. Chimeric antigen receptor T cells for sustained remissions in leukemia. N Engl J Med 2014;371(16):1507–17.
5. Maude SL, Laetsch TW, Buechner J, et al. Tisagenlecleucel in children and young adults with B-Cell lymphoblastic leukemia. N Engl J Med 2018;378(5): 439–48.
6. Schultz L. Chimeric antigen receptor T cell therapy for pediatric B-ALL: narrowing the gap between early and long-term outcomes. Front Immunol 2020;11:1985.
7. Sadelain M, Brentjens R, Rivière I. The basic principles of chimeric antigen receptor design. Cancer Discov 2013;3(4):388–98.
8. Brentjens RJ, Santos E, Nikhamin Y, et al. Genetically targeted T cells eradicate systemic acute lymphoblastic leukemia xenografts. Clin Cancer Res 2007; 13(18 Pt 1):5426–35.
9. Imai C, Mihara K, Andreansky M, et al. Chimeric receptors with 4-1BB signaling capacity provoke potent cytotoxicity against acute lymphoblastic leukemia. Leukemia 2004;18(4):676–84.
10. Carpenito C, Milone MC, Hassan R, et al. Control of large, established tumor xenografts with genetically retargeted human T cells containing CD28 and CD137 domains. Proc Natl Acad Sci U S A 2009;106(9):3360–5.

11. Milone MC, Fish JD, Carpenito C, et al. Chimeric receptors containing CD137 signal transduction domains mediate enhanced survival of T cells and increased antileukemic efficacy in vivo. Mol Ther 2009;17(8):1453–64.

12. Kochenderfer JN, Wilson WH, Janik JE, et al. Eradication of B-lineage cells and regression of lymphoma in a patient treated with autologous T cells genetically engineered to recognize CD19. Blood 2010;116(20):4099–102.

13. Porter DL, Levine BL, Kalos M, et al. Chimeric antigen receptor-modified T cells in chronic lymphoid leukemia. N Engl J Med 2011;365(8):725–33.

14. Kalos M, Levine BL, Porter DL, et al. T cells with chimeric antigen receptors have potent antitumor effects and can establish memory in patients with advanced leukemia. Sci Transl Med 2011;3(95):95ra73.

15. Kantarjian H, Thomas D, Jorgensen J, et al. Results of inotuzumab ozogamicin, a CD22 monoclonal antibody, in refractory and relapsed acute lymphocytic leukemia. Cancer 2013;119(15):2728–36.

16. Kantarjian HM, DeAngelo DJ, Stelljes M, et al. Inotuzumab ozogamicin versus standard therapy for acute lymphoblastic leukemia. N Engl J Med 2016;375(8): 740–53.

17. Shah NN, Highfill SL, Shalabi H, et al. CD4/CD8 T-cell selection affects chimeric antigen receptor (CAR) T-cell potency and toxicity: updated results from a phase I anti-CD22 CAR T-cell trial. J Clin Oncol 2020;38(17):1938–50.

18. Wang N, Hu X, Cao W, et al. Efficacy and safety of CAR19/22 T-cell cocktail therapy in patients with refractory/relapsed B-cell malignancies. Blood 2020;135(1): 17–27.

19. Liu S, Deng B, Yin Z, et al. Combination of CD19 and CD22 CAR-T cell therapy in relapsed B-cell acute lymphoblastic leukemia after allogeneic transplantation. Am J Hematol 2021;96(6):671–9.

20. Dai H, Wu Z, Jia H, et al. Bispecific CAR-T cells targeting both CD19 and CD22 for therapy of adults with relapsed or refractory B cell acute lymphoblastic leukemia. J Hematol Oncol 2020;13(1):30.

21. Spiegel JY, Patel S, Muffly L, et al. CAR T cells with dual targeting of CD19 and CD22 in adult patients with recurrent or refractory B cell malignancies: a phase 1 trial. Nat Med 2021;27(8):1419–31.

22. Cordoba S, Onuoha S, Thomas S, et al. CAR T cells with dual targeting of CD19 and CD22 in pediatric and young adult patients with relapsed or refractory B cell acute lymphoblastic leukemia: a phase 1 trial. Nat Med 2021;27(10):1797–805.

23. Fousek K, Watanabe J, Joseph SK, et al. CAR T-cells that target acute B-lineage leukemia irrespective of CD19 expression. Leukemia 2021;35(1):75–89.

24. Schneider D, Xiong Y, Wu D, et al. Trispecific CD19-CD20-CD22-targeting duo-CAR-T cells eliminate antigen-heterogeneous B cell tumors in preclinical models. Sci Transl Med 2021;13(586). https://doi.org/10.1126/scitranslmed.abc6401.

25. Grupp SA, Kalos M, Barrett D, et al. Chimeric antigen receptor-modified T cells for acute lymphoid leukemia. N Engl J Med 2013;368(16):1509–18.

26. Lee DW, Kochenderfer JN, Stetler-Stevenson M, et al. T cells expressing CD19 chimeric antigen receptors for acute lymphoblastic leukaemia in children and young adults: a phase 1 dose-escalation trial. Lancet 2015;385(9967):517–28.

27. Brentjens RJ, Davila ML, Riviere I, et al. CD19-targeted T cells rapidly induce molecular remissions in adults with chemotherapy-refractory acute lymphoblastic leukemia. Sci Transl Med 2013;5(177):177ra38.

28. Park JH, Rivière I, Gonen M, et al. Long-term follow-up of CD19 CAR therapy in acute lymphoblastic leukemia. N Engl J Med 2018;378(5):449–59.

29. Davila ML, Riviere I, Wang X, et al. Efficacy and toxicity management of 19-28z CAR T cell therapy in B cell acute lymphoblastic leukemia. Sci Transl Med 2014;6(224):224ra25.

30. Hay KA, Gauthier J, Hirayama AV, et al. Factors associated with durable EFS in adult B-cell ALL patients achieving MRD-negative CR after CD19 CAR T-cell therapy. Blood 2019;133(15):1652–63.

31. O'Leary MC, Lu X, Huang Y, et al. FDA Approval Summary: Tisagenlecleucel for Treatment of Patients with Relapsed or Refractory B-cell Precursor Acute Lymphoblastic Leukemia. Clin Cancer Res 2019;25(4):1142–6.

32. Bouchkouj N, Lin X, Wang X, et al. FDA approval summary: brexucabtagene autoleucel for treatment of adults with relapsed or refractory B-cell precursor acute lymphoblastic leukemia. Oncol 2022;27(10):892–9.

33. Laetsch TW, Maude SL, Rives S, et al. Three-year update of tisagenlecleucel in pediatric and young adult patients with relapsed/refractory acute lymphoblastic leukemia in the ELIANA trial. J Clin Oncol 2023;41(9):1664–9.

34. Pasquini MC, Hu ZH, Curran K, et al. Real-world evidence of tisagenlecleucel for pediatric acute lymphoblastic leukemia and non-Hodgkin lymphoma. Blood Adv 2020;4(21):5414–24.

35. Schultz LM, Baggott C, Prabhu S, et al. Disease burden affects outcomes in pediatric and young adult B-Cell lymphoblastic leukemia after commercial tisagenlecleucel: a pediatric real-world chimeric antigen receptor consortium report. J Clin Oncol 2022;40(9):945–55.

36. Schultz LM, Eaton A, Baggott C, et al. Outcomes after nonresponse and relapse post-tisagenlecleucel in children, adolescents, and young adults with B-cell acute lymphoblastic leukemia. J Clin Oncol 2023;41(2):354–63.

37. Wang M, Munoz J, Goy A, et al. KTE-X19 CAR T-cell therapy in relapsed or refractory mantle-cell lymphoma. N Engl J Med 2020;382(14):1331–42.

38. Roberts ZJ, Better M, Bot A, et al. Axicabtagene ciloleucel, a first-in-class CAR T cell therapy for aggressive NHL. Leuk Lymphoma 2018;59(8):1785–96.

39. Shah BD, Bishop MR, Oluwole OO, et al. KTE-X19 anti-CD19 CAR T-cell therapy in adult relapsed/refractory acute lymphoblastic leukemia: ZUMA-3 phase 1 results. Blood 2021;138(1):11–22.

40. Shah BD, Ghobadi A, Oluwole OO, et al. KTE-X19 for relapsed or refractory adult B-cell acute lymphoblastic leukaemia: phase 2 results of the single-arm, open-label, multicentre ZUMA-3 study. Lancet 2021;398(10299):491–502.

41. Shah BD, Ghobadi A, Oluwole OO, et al. Two-year follow-up of KTE-X19 in patients with relapsed or refractory adult B-cell acute lymphoblastic leukemia in ZUMA-3 and its contextualization with SCHOLAR-3, an external historical control study. J Hematol Oncol 2022;15(1):170.

42. Myers RM, Shah NN, Pulsipher MA. How I use risk factors for success or failure of CD19 CAR T cells to guide management of children and AYA with B-cell ALL. Blood 2023;141(11):1251–64.

43. Park JH, Geyer MB, Brentjens RJ. CD19-targeted CAR T-cell therapeutics for hematologic malignancies: interpreting clinical outcomes to date. Blood 2016; 127(26):3312–20.

44. Jain MD, Smith M, Shah NN. How I treat refractory CRS and ICANS after CAR T-cell therapy. Blood 2023;141(20):2430–42.

45. Lee DW, Santomasso BD, Locke FL, et al. ASTCT consensus grading for cytokine release syndrome and neurologic toxicity associated with immune effector cells. Biol Blood Marrow Transplant 2019;25(4):625–38.

46. Maude SL. Tisagenlecleucel in pediatric patients with acute lymphoblastic leukemia. Clin Adv Hematol Oncol 2018;16(10):664–6.

47. Kadauke S, Myers RM, Li Y, et al. Risk-Adapted preemptive tocilizumab to prevent severe cytokine release syndrome after CTL019 for pediatric B-cell acute lymphoblastic leukemia: a prospective clinical trial. J Clin Oncol 2021;39(8): 920–30.

48. Myers RM, Li Y, Barz Leahy A, et al. Humanized CD19-targeted chimeric antigen receptor (CAR) T cells in CAR-naive and CAR-exposed children and young adults with relapsed or refractory acute lymphoblastic leukemia. J Clin Oncol 2021; 39(27):3044–55.

49. Myers RM, Taraseviciute A, Steinberg SM, et al. Blinatumomab nonresponse and high-disease burden are associated with inferior outcomes after CD19-CAR for B-ALL. J Clin Oncol 2022;40(9):932–44.

50. Lamble AJ, Myers RM, Taraseviciute A, et al. Preinfusion factors impacting relapse immunophenotype following CD19 CAR T cells. Blood Adv 2023;7(4): 575–85.

51. Ravich JW, Huang S, Zhou Y, et al. Impact of high disease burden on survival in pediatric patients with B-ALL treated with Tisagenlecleucel. Transplant Cell Ther 2022;28(2):73.e1–9.

52. Fabrizio VA, Phillips CL, Lane A, et al. Tisagenlecleucel outcomes in relapsed/refractory extramedullary ALL: a pediatric real world CAR consortium report. Blood Adv 2022;6(2):600–10.

53. Mejstríková E, Hrusak O, Borowitz MJ, et al. CD19-negative relapse of pediatric B-cell precursor acute lymphoblastic leukemia following blinatumomab treatment. Blood Cancer J 2017;7(12):659.

54. Pillai V, Muralidharan K, Meng W, et al. CAR T-cell therapy is effective for CD19-dim B-lymphoblastic leukemia but is impacted by prior blinatumomab therapy. Blood Adv 2019;3(22):3539–49.

55. O'Brien MM, Ji L, Shah NN, et al. Phase II trial of inotuzumab ozogamicin in children and adolescents with relapsed or refractory B-cell acute lymphoblastic leukemia: children's oncology group protocol AALL1621. J Clin Oncol 2022;40(9): 956–67.

56. Gardner RA, Finney O, Annesley C, et al. Intent-to-treat leukemia remission by CD19 CAR T cells of defined formulation and dose in children and young adults. Blood 2017;129(25):3322–31.

57. Pulsipher MA, Han X, Maude SL, et al. Next-generation sequencing of minimal residual disease for predicting relapse after tisagenlecleucel in children and young adults with acute lymphoblastic leukemia. Blood Cancer Discov 2022; 3(1):66–81.

58. Shah NN, Lee DW, Yates B, et al. Long-term follow-up of CD19-CAR T-cell therapy in children and young adults with B-ALL. J Clin Oncol 2021;39(15):1650–9.

59. Sorror ML, Maris MB, Storb R, et al. Hematopoietic cell transplantation (HCT)-specific comorbidity index: a new tool for risk assessment before allogeneic HCT. Blood 2005;106(8):2912–9.

60. Xu X, Sun Q, Liang X, et al. Mechanisms of relapse after cd19 car t-cell therapy for acute lymphoblastic leukemia and its prevention and treatment strategies. Front Immunol 2019;10:2664.

61. Turtle CJ, Hanafi LA, Berger C, et al. CD19 CAR-T cells of defined CD4+:CD8+ composition in adult B cell ALL patients. J Clin Invest 2016;126(6):2123–38.

62. Fry TJ, Shah NN, Orentas RJ, et al. CD22-targeted CAR T cells induce remission in B-ALL that is naive or resistant to CD19-targeted CAR immunotherapy. Nat Med 2018;24(1):20–8.

63. Shah NN, Stevenson MS, Yuan CM, et al. Characterization of CD22 expression in acute lymphoblastic leukemia. Pediatr Blood Cancer 2015;62(6):964–9.

64. Raponi S, De Propris MS, Intoppa S, et al. Flow cytometric study of potential target antigens (CD19, CD20, CD22, CD33) for antibody-based immunotherapy in acute lymphoblastic leukemia: analysis of 552 cases. Leuk Lymphoma 2011; 52(6):1098–107.

65. Benjamin R, Graham C, Yallop D, et al. Genome-edited, donor-derived allogeneic anti-CD19 chimeric antigen receptor T cells in paediatric and adult B-cell acute lymphoblastic leukaemia: results of two phase 1 studies. Lancet 2020;396(10266): 1885–94.

66. Benjamin R, Jain N, Maus MV, et al. UCART19, a first-in-class allogeneic anti-CD19 chimeric antigen receptor T-cell therapy for adults with relapsed or refractory B-cell acute lymphoblastic leukaemia (CALM): a phase 1, dose-escalation trial. Lancet Haematol 2022;9(11):e833–43.

Chimeric Antigen Receptor T-Cell Therapy in Aggressive B-Cell Lymphoma

Mark P. Hamilton, MD, PhD[a,b,c,*], David B. Miklos, MD, PhD[a,b]

KEYWORDS

- CAR T-cell • Large B-cell lymphoma • Aggressive lymphoma • CAR T-cell toxicity
- CAR T-cell resistance • Review • CD19

KEY POINTS

- Chimeric antigen receptor (CAR) T-cell therapy with axi-cel and liso-cel is approved for second-line treatment of large B-cell lymphoma (LBCL).
- CAR T-cell therapy with axi-cel, liso-cel, and tisa-cel is approved for the third-line treatment LBCL.
- Early CAR T-cell toxicity of cytokine release syndrome and immune effector cell associated neurotoxicity syndrome should be treated promptly with steroids and tocilizumab.
- Prolonged CAR T-cell toxicity includes persistent cytopenia and infection that can last more than a year postinfusion.

INTRODUCTION

Chimeric antigen receptor (CAR) T-cell therapy is a cellular therapy that uses an engineered T-cell receptor on the surface of donor T cells to kill cancer. The most common antigen targeted clinically in this context is CD19 which was chosen because of broad and high expression in leukemia and lymphomas.[1]

CAR T-cell therapy is increasingly an integral tool in the treatment of non-Hodgkin lymphomas (NHL). Though many initial clinical CAR T-cell studies debuted in leukemia,[2–5] the use of CAR has expanded dramatically in NHL in recent years where it is now approved as an early line of therapy in multiple lymphoma types. This review focuses on the clinical role of CAR-T cells in aggressive B-cell lymphoma including indications, determinants of outcomes, toxicities, and future areas of study.

[a] Center for Cancer Cell Therapy, Stanford Cancer Institute, Stanford University School of Medicine, Stanford, CA 94305, USA; [b] Division of Blood and Marrow Transplantation and Cellular Therapy, Department of Medicine, Stanford University School of Medicine, Stanford, CA 94305, USA; [c] Division of Hematology, Department of Medicine, Stanford University School of Medicine, Stanford, CA 94305, USA
* Corresponding author.
E-mail address: mphamilt@stanford.edu

Hematol Oncol Clin N Am 37 (2023) 1053–1075
https://doi.org/10.1016/j.hoc.2023.05.007
0889-8588/23/© 2023 Elsevier Inc. All rights reserved.

Section I–Indications for Chimeric Antigen Receptor T-Cell Therapy in Aggressive Lymphoma

Large B-cell lymphoma (LBCL) is the most common lymphoid malignancy. Though 5-year survival rates after first-line chemotherapy are 60%–70%, up to 50% of patients develop relapsed or refractory disease.[6,7] CAR T-cell therapy has revolutionized treatment of LBCL by using CD19 targeting chimeric antigen receptors expressed on the surface of genetically manipulated T cells to drive durable complete responses (CRs) in previously relapsed and refractory tumors.[1,8]

Currently, 3 CAR T-cell constructs are approved for the treatment of relapsed and refractory LBCL (**Table 1**): axicabtagene ciloleucel (axi-cel, brand name Yescarta),[8,9] lisocabtagene ciloleucel (liso-cel, brand name Breyanzi),[10,11] and tisagenlecleucel (tisa-cel, brand name Kymriah).[12,13] All 3 constructs involve use of autologous CAR-T cells to target the CD19 antigen with the single-chain monoclonal antibody FMC63[14,15] in a second generation[16] CAR T-cell construct. Axi-cel is engineered from a retroviral construct and uses a CD28 hinge, transmembrane, and activation domain. Liso-cel is a lentiviral construct engineered with a IgG4 hinge region, a CD28 transmembrane domain, and a 41BB transactivation domain. Tisa-cel is also a lentiviral construct engineered with a CD8 hinge and transmembrane domain with a 41BB transactivation domain (**Fig. 1**).

The axi-cel product is not balanced for CD4+:CD8+ T-cell ratio and is given at a standard dose of 2×10^6 CAR-positive viable T cells per kilogram. Liso-cel is given at a dose of $90 - 110 \times 10^6$ CAR-positive viable T cells. The liso-cel apheresis product is sorted into CD4+ and CD8+ populations prior to transduction and the final CAR T-cell product is then infused as separate CD4+ and CD8+ CAR-T cells in a 1:1 ratio. Tisa-cel is also unsorted and given at a dose of $0.6 - 6 \times 10^8$ CAR-positive vaiable T cells. Patients are typically treated with fludarabine and cyclophosphamide lympho-depleting chemotherapy generally starting on day minus 5 prior to cellular infusion. Recently, single-agent bendamustine has been successfully used as lymphodepleting chemotherapy in patients treated with tisa-cel,[17] and this may offer a less immune suppressive therapeutic option for other CAR T-cell vectors in the future.

All 3 constructs were initially approved for third-line treatment of relapsed and refractory LBCL. Axi-cel and liso-cel received additional approval for second-line treatment of patients with refractory disease or disease that relapsed less than 12 months from initial therapy after 1:1 randomization versus standard of care (SOC) autologous hematopoietic cellular transplant (HCT).

Axi-cel

Axi-cel was initially approved by the Food and Drug Administration in the United States on October 18, 2017. This approval followed the success of the pivotal phase 2 ZUMA-1 study[8,18,19] which targeted LBCL (including high grade B-cell lymphoma with MYC and BCL-2 or BCL-6 translocation, transformed follicular lymphoma, and primary mediastinal B-cell lymphoma) in the third line or later setting. This trial demonstrated an 82% objective response rate (ORR) with a 54% CR rate.[8] The median duration of response was 11.1 months, and the median overall survival (OS) was not reached after 27.1 months of follow-up.[19] Similar results were noted in consortium studies of patients treated in the SOC setting.[20]

Following the success of ZUMA-1, axi-cel was tested versus SOC HCT in the second-line setting in the ZUMA-7 trial.[9] In this trial, 180 patients were randomized to second-line CAR T-cell therapy versus 179 patients randomized to HCT. At a median of 24.9 months, the event free survival (EFS) was 8.3 months in the axi-cel arm and only 2 months in the SOC arm. Subsequent follow up also demonstrated an OS

Table 1
Overview of pivotal chimeric antigen receptor T-cell trials in large B-cell lymphoma

Product	Trial	Disease	Randomization	Bridging Therapy Allowed	Primary Endpoint	Objective Response Rate	Complete Response Rate
Axi-cel	ZUMA-1	3rd line LBCL	Single arm	No	Response rate	82%	54%
Liso-cel	TRANSCEND	3rd line LBCL	Single arm	Yes	Response rate	73%	53%
Tisa-cel	JULIET	3rd line LBCL	Single arm	Yes	Response rate	52%	40%
Axi-cel	ZUMA-7	2nd line LBCL vs SOC	1:1, open label	No	Event free survival (met)	83%	65%
Liso-cel	TRANSFORM	2nd line LBCL vs SOC	1:1, open label	Yes	Event free survival (met)	86%	66%
Tisa-cel	BELINDA	2nd line LBCL vs SOC	1:1, open label	Yes	Event free survival (not met)	46%	28%
Axi-cel	ZUMA-12	1st line high risk LBCL	Single arm vs historic control	Yes	Efficacy	89%	78%

CAR T-cell therapy has high response rates in relapsed and refractory LBCL.

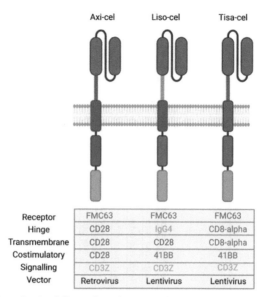

Fig. 1. Vector design of axi-cel, liso-cel, and tisa-cel, the 3 primary vectors used in LBCL. Axi-cel is a retroviral-based vector that relies on CD28 costimulation which liso-cel and tisa-cel utilize lentiviral vectors with 41BB costimulation.

difference favoring axi-cel (OS not reached in axi-cel vs 31.1 months in SOC).[21] Based on the success of the ZUMA-7 trial, axi-cel was approved on April 1, 2022 for second-line treatment of LCBL in patients who are refractory to first line treatment or who relapse before 12 months.

Finally, in the recent ZUMA-12 trial axi-cel was tested as a first-line treatment[22] for high-risk LBCL. In this phase 2, single-arm study patients with high-risk LBCL defined as high grade B-cell lymphoma (HGBCL) or LBCL with international prognostic index (IPI) score $\geq$ 3, were treated with axi-cel as part of risk adapted therapy in the first line. Patients with Deauville positive (Deauville 4–5) after 2 cycles of chemoimmunotherapy with anti-CD20 antibody and an anthracycline were recruited and the primary endpoint was CR rate (as determined by study investigators). The goal CR rate was 60% based on historic data from the Groupe d'Etude des Lymphomes de l'Adulte (GELA) study[23] and CALGB50303.[24] The result of the study was an impressive 78% CR rate which was substantially improved over historic controls. Though this study offers an excellent framework for considering CAR T-cell therapy in the first line, there is currently not approval for CAR-T cells in first-line LBCL.

Liso-cel

Liso-cel was initially approved for third line and beyond relapsed refractory LBCL on February 5, 2021 following results of the phase 2 TRANSCEND study.[10] This study demonstrated similar results to the ZUMA-1 study with an ORR of 73% and a CR rate of 53% in 256 patients evaluable in the efficacy set. The TRANSCEND study was followed by the phase 3 TRANSFORM study which, similar to ZUMA-7, randomized patients to receive either the CAR T-cell therapy or HCT in the second-line setting.[11] When comparing 92 patients treated with liso-cel with 92 patients receiving SOC, the EFS was significantly improved in the liso-cel group at 10.1 months versus 2.3 months in the HCT arm. There was no OS benefit in the CAR arm of the study despite an excellent EFS benefit. In this case, the cross-over designed within the study may have confounded OS results. Based on results from the TRANSFORM study, liso-cel was approved by the FDA for second-line treatment of relapsed and refractory LBCL on June 24, 2022.

Tisa-cel

Tisa-cel was similarly approved on May 1, 2018 for the treatment of third line and beyond relapsed and refractory LBCL after the phase 2 JULIET study.[12] In this study, 93 patients were evaluated and 52% had ORR with 40% obtaining a CR. The 12-month relapse free survival was 65%. Similar to axi-cel and liso-cel, tisa-cel was also then compared to SOC HCT in the second line 1:1 randomized phase 3 BELINDA study.[13] In this study, 162 patients were randomized to the CAR group and 160 patients were randomized to the SOC group. There were no differences in median EFS which was 3 months in both groups.

The cause of the failure of the BELINDA study is unclear. Multiple factors likely played a role including (1) imbalance between groups as the CAR arm of the BELINDA had significantly more patients with HGBCL and higher IPI scores, (2) delays in care with a median of 52 days from apheresis to infusion compared to a median of 13 days in ZUMA-7 and 26 days in TRANSFORM, and (3) possibly the construct itself that may have less transactivation than other constructs.

The final possible cause of a weaker overall construct was recently supported in propensity matched study of 809 patients treated in the third line with SOC comparing tisa-cel with axi-cel.[25] In this study, patients were 1:1 matched and the axi-cel group demonstrated a best ORR/CR rate of 80% and 60% versus 66% and 42% in the tisa-cel group with 1-year progression free survival (PFS) and OS of 46.6% and 63.5% in the axi-cel group versus 33.2% and 48.8% in the tisa-cel group. All these differences were significant in the study potentially indicating improved outcomes in the axi-cel group when comparing constructs.

Whatever the cause of failure to meet the BELINDA trial endpoints, tisa-cel was not approved in the second line for LBCL which limits its clinical utility in aggressive lymphoma relative to axi-cel and liso-cel. The same SOC study[25] comparing axi-cel versus tisa-cel did demonstrate greater cytokine release syndrome (CRS) and immune effector cell associated neurotoxicity syndrome (ICANS), including high grade (grade $\geq$ 3) ICANS in the axi-cel group which possibly leaves open a role for tisa-cel in the third line for frail patients.

Bridging therapy

There is no clear consensus on the impact of bridging therapy or the best choice of bridging therapy prior to CAR T-cell therapy. In the original ZUMA trials patients requiring bridging therapy were excluded (see **Table 1**). The main goal of bridging is to temporally control tumor progression and preferably reduce tumor burden prior to CAR T-cell therapy. Such bridging could also provide additional time for CAR T-cell manufacturing, improve CAR-mediated responses, or provide for CAR T-cell eligibility by improving performance status.

Common forms of bridging therapy include chemotherapy, corticosteroids, targeted therapy such as ibrutinib or lenalidomide, and radiation.[20,26] More than 50% of patients reported in both trials and SOC studies received bridging therapy.[10,20,26,27] In general patients receiving bridging therapy have inferior outcomes[20,26,28] but this may vary by bridging therapy type with patients receiving systemic therapy bridging potentially having worse outcome, whereas those receiving radiation therapy bridging having similar or improved outcomes.[26] Given that patients requiring bridging therapy are likely to have a higher overall disease burden prior to CAR, any notable adverse outcomes could be attributable to the difference in patient population rather than the bridging therapy itself. Because of these limitations in the retrospective setting, it is currently difficult to clearly establish any positive or negative overall impact of bridging therapy. Certainly, if a patient requires bridging therapy to maintain disease control while awaiting product, then it is appropriate to treat. Rapid referral to CAR T-cell centers may help abrogate the need for bridging therapy.

There is no standard bridging therapy regimen. Bendamustine likely should not be provided to patients prior to apheresis due to potential toxicity to the T-cell repertoire[29,30] which has led to our avoidance as a bridging therapy. Radiation therapy does offer good disease control with reduced systemic toxicity[31] but is only appropriate for localized disease. Steroid only bridging is frequently reported[20,26,27] but may not sufficient for patients with more rapidly progressive disease. Steroid-only bridging provides a reasonable short-term option that is unlikely to cause severe toxicity.

CD19 antibody–drug conjugate therapy such as loncastuximab and tafasitamab has not demonstrated subsequent loss of CD19 surface antigen or reduced response to subsequent CAR T-cell therapy in limited studies.[32,33] This is presumably due to the well described "bystander effect" associated with antibody–drug conjugates.[34] Despite this preliminary data, the number of patients in these reports is small and we do typically avoid these agents as a bridge to CAR due to CD19 co-targeting. The use of CD20 targeting bispecific antibodies[35–40] as a bridge to CAR is a novel possibility. However, these agents may represent a separate mechanism for long-term disease control making their sequencing in regard to CAR T-cell therapy unclear. Further, these therapies enjoy a rather long half-life similar to native antibodies and the impact of residual bispecific antibody on CAR function after infusion is unknown.

Ultimately if more aggressive systemic therapy is necessary, our practice is typically to use polatuzumab vedotin and rituximab (R-pola) which provides high ORRs with minimal toxicity.[41] We try to provide bridging after apheresis to minimize potential impact on T-cell fitness. Other standard salvage regimens such as rituximab with gemcitabine and oxaliplatin (R-GemOx) or rituximab with ifosfamide, carboplatin, and etoposide (R-ICE) are also options. Importantly, one goal of bridging therapy is to minimize systemic toxicity from the treatment itself so that the patient has sufficient performance status for CAR T-cell infusion. The clinical impact of bridging therapy is an area in clear need of additional research to improve outcomes and standardize care.

Section II–Factors Impacting Chimeric Antigen Receptor T-Cell Efficacy in Large B-cell Lymphoma

There is limited data suggesting which factors limit efficacy after CAR T-cell treatment in aggressive lymphoma. Risk factors can be differentiated into patient-specific factors, tumor-specific factors, and CAR-specific factors (**Fig. 2**).

Chimeric antigen receptor specific determinants of efficacy

The major CAR specific determinant of function is the CAR T-cell vector itself which is described in detail above. Study of the CAR-T cell is a complex process that requires correlative analysis between the CAR-T cell and requisite patient data. Single-cell RNA (scRNA) study of CAR T-cell product has indicated that presence of CD8 T cells expressing memory signatures had improved outcomes, whereas T-cell senescence signals in the product were associated with inferior outcomes.[42] In a recently published companion study, the presence of post-infusion CAR T-regulatory cells was

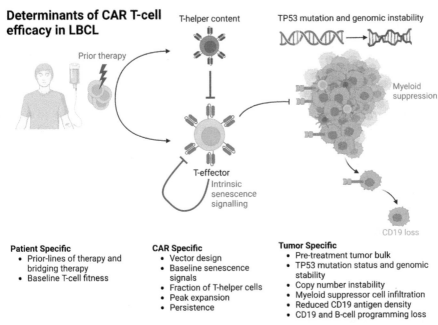

Fig. 2. Patient-specific, CAR-specific, and tumor-specific determinants of CAR T-cell efficacy described in LBCL. CAR T-cells are safe in many patient populations and there are few patient-specific determinants that are detrimental to CAR treatment. CAR-specific determinants have centered on the vector design itself and the ability of the CAR to expand and persist in some studies. Tumor-specific determinants of CAR T-cell efficacy are largely tumor bulk and the ability of the tumor to lose CD19 expression. Tumors with TP53 mutation and unstable genomes may also have worse outcomes. Traditional factors associated with poor outcomes such as HGBCL have not demonstrated worse outcomes in CAR T-cell therapy.

associated with worse outcomes possibly due to suppression of effector CAR T-cell populations.[43,44] Currently, there is no clearly dominant CAR T-cell population but identification of an "ideal" CAR-T cell may improve product development in the future.

One major focus of study within each vector is expansion of the CAR-T cell as an indirect measure of CAR T-cell fitness. CAR T-cell expansion occurs logarithmically after infusion and typically peaks between D7 and D14. CAR19 constructs with 41BB costimulatory molecules expand more slowly than those with CD28. So far there has not been clearly discerned differences in CAR T-cell expansion between tumor types, though additional persistence at later timepoints is notable in brexu-cel treatment of MCL in the ZUMA-2 trial,[45] and there appeared to be slightly higher peak expansion in marginal zone lymphoma relative to follicular lymphoma in the ZUMA-5 trial.[46]

CAR19 expansion is associated with limited impact on efficacy. There were greater CAR-positive cells noted by qPCR in patients with an objective response in the third-line ZUMA-1 study[8] though significant association between expansion and response was not reported in the ZUMA-7 study[9] or the ZUMA-12 study.[22] In independent analysis of third-line CAR T-cell treatment, there was an association between D7 axi-cel cell free DNA and EFS[47] as well as peak expansion and response by qPCR.[48] Similarly, there was increased liso-cel expansion noted in responders in the third-line TRANSCEND study but no relationship between liso-cel expansion and outcomes was noted in the second-line TRANSFORM study.[10,11] In the third-line JULIET study, tisa-cel had increased persistence in patients with a response, but there was no difference in expansion in the first 28 days between responders and nonresponders.[12] Ultimately, the importance of CAR T-cell expansion and persistence remains indeterminate and may be variable based on line of therapy, method of CAR T-cell measurement, CAR vector, and pre-treatment tumor burden.

Patient-specific determinants of efficacy

In terms of patient-specific factors, CAR T-cell therapy has proven equally effective in patients who would typically have trouble tolerating high-risk therapy. In the ZUMA-1 study elderly (age >65 years) patients treated with CAR T-cell therapy had no difference in CAR T-cell expansion or difference in PFS relative to younger patients with similar toxicity.[49] This finding has been reproduced in single-center studies that also fail to find differences in efficacy in older patient populations.[50]

Another major pretreatment determinant of efficacy is prior therapies. Patients who have rapid tumor progression often require bridging therapy which is associated with worse outcomes and prolonged toxicity.[51] Patients who have lower peripheral T-cell counts at leukapheresis may also have inferior outcomes.[52] In particular, recent use of bendamustine prior to apheresis is associated with inferior outcomes.[29,30]

Finally, there is initial data suggesting that the fecal microbiota may impact CAR efficacy.[53] In this study, pretreatment exposure to antibiotics was associated with worse survival rates and increased toxicity. Subsequent analysis showed that specific gut microbiota composition is associated with improved responses, specifically the clostridial species *Ruminococcus* and *Bacteroides*.

The sum of this data suggests that though CAR T-cell therapy is safe and effective in frail patients, pretreatment T-cell fitness and other pretreatment parameters do play a role in outcomes. Additional study is necessary to understand which patients are at risk for CAR T-cell kinetic failure due to T-cell fitness at apheresis, or which patients who are at lower risk for kinetic failure could benefit from the use of less aggressive T-cell constructs or lymphodepletion regimens.

Tumor-specific determinants of efficacy

Tumor-associated factors are likely the major driver of treatment failure. The most commonly described mechanism of resistance to CD19-directed CAR T-cell therapy is loss of the CD19 cell surface antigen (**Figs 3**).[54–57] Mechanisms of antigen loss include downregulation of the CD19 antigen at the mRNA level and through alternate splicing[58] as well as mutation and copy number alteration at the DNA level.[47] Still loss of CD19 antigen has only been observe in 1/12 to 1/3 of cases in prior studies.[55,56,59] Other potential intratumoral mechanisms of resistance in LCBL include tumor microenvironmental characteristics such as tumor interferon response[60] and direct mutation of genes involved in B-cell identity such as PAX5 and genes involved in immune microenvironment modulation such as TMEM30A. Pretreatment tumor microenvironment enriched for cytokines that foster T-cell development is also associated with higher CR rates.[61]

One of the most frequently cited risk factors for poor outcomes is elevated lactate dehydrogenase (LDH)[20,43,47,62,63] which clearly carries a worse overall prognosis. LDH correlates with tumor burden and in keeping with this observation higher pretreatment ctDNA levels and increased metabolic tumor volume are noted in multiple studies to be major determinants of treatment failure.[47,64,65] High LDH may also have association with interferon signaling and myeloid suppressor cells in the tumor.[60]

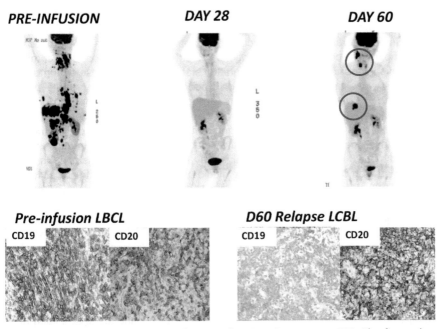

Fig. 3. Loss of CD19 is a common mechanism of LBCL resistance post CAR. The figure demonstrates loss of CD19 in a patient relapsing on D60 post-infusion with CD19 negative disease.

Molecular determinants of poor prognosis include TP53 genomic alterations[66] which may be associated with dysregulation of CAR T-cell-mediated cytotoxicity pathways. Notably, in this study patients who received CAR T-cell therapy with a CD28 costimulatory domain has improved survival relative to those that did not

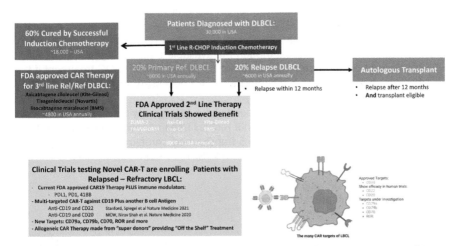

Fig. 4. Flow chart of CAR T-cell therapy in the new era. CAR T-cell therapy is approved in second line treatment of LBCL in patients with refractory disease or relapse before 12 months from the end of therapy. CD19-directed CAR T-cell therapy is the first of many potential cellular targets in LCBL indicating multiple new lines of therapy will become available in the future.

providing weak evidence that therapy could be risk stratified based on TP53 status. Additionally, using low pass whole-genome sequencing the presence of pretreatment copy number alterations were associated with inferior outcomes[67] though it remains unclear how these copy number alterations interact with tumor bulk and other markers of genomic instability such as TP53 mutation status. In a separate study tumor chromothripsis was associated with inferior outcomes as defined by whole genome sequencing.[68] Overall, these studies are strong evidence that genomic complexity is a mechanism of aggressive lymphoma resistance to CAR T-cell therapy.

Finally, there is limited data that antigen density of CD19 on the cell surface may impact CAR efficacy.[56,69] Increased activity along the more efficient immune synapse formed by CD28 co-stimulatory domains may help overcome resistance in tumors with low antigen density.[70] Prospective elucidation of higher risk molecular features such as TP53 mutation and low antigen density could lead to tailored CAR T-cell therapies directed against higher and lower risk to balance efficacy and toxicity.

Traditional factors associated with worse outcomes in LBCL include HGBCL which typically requires a MYC and BCL2 or BCL6 translocation (based on the WHO 2016 classification). More recently, more lymphomas with MYC and BLC6 translocations are not included as higher grade. CAR T-cell therapy has not demonstrated worse outcomes for HGBCL patients (reviewed in Ali and colleagues[71]). These findings are partially skewed by the fact that the comparator LBCL groups are so far by definition higher risk relapsed and refractory disease. Still the remarkable efficacy of CAR T-cell therapy on this traditionally difficult to treat histology may suggest that unique tumor resistance mechanisms underly resistance to CAR T-cell activity versus traditional chemoimmunotherapy.

Another common LBCL pathology that is traditionally difficult to treat is in primary and secondary central nervous system (CNS) lymphoma. Patients with CNS lymphoma so far have been excluded from major CAR T-cell trials. However, CAR-T cells do traffic to the brain and are easily discernable in the cerebral spinal fluid. Recently, a phase 1/2 trial of tisa-cel in primary CNS lymphoma demonstrated CR in 6/12 (50%) of patients with highly refractory primary CNS lymphoma. Of these, 3 had ongoing response at the time of data cutoff. CAR T-cell therapy is also effective in secondary CNS lymphoma with an 85.7% day 28 CR rate noted in one retrospective analysis.[72] Despite these promising results, there remains limited data on the efficacy of CAR T-cell therapy in CNS lymphoma though the available data do suggest that patients with a history of CNS lymphoma should not be excluded from SOC treatment if they also have systemic disease. Dedicated trials are necessary to further elucidate the impact of CNS involvement on efficacy.

Finally, Richter transformation is an additional tumor type with limited treatment options and a poor prognosis. Patients with Richter transformation were excluded from most early CAR T-cell trials excepting 5 transformed chronic lymphocytic leukemia/lymphoma (CLL) patients enrolled in the TRANSCEND study. Response assessment of Richter patients treated with CAR T-cell therapy are nearly absent from the literature. The minimal information available does indicate these tumors can response to CAR19 treatment[73–75] and should not be excluded from receiving CAR T-cell therapy if relapsed or refractory from standard therapy.[76] For Richter patients, we typically use liso-cel because (1) liso-cel is approved for LBCL in the second and third line, (2) transformed CLL was minimally included in the TRANSCEND study, (3) liso-cel has evidence in CLL alone,[77] and (4) the FDA label for liso-cel nonspecifically approves for transformed indolent lymphoma.

In sum, the overall tumor burden, pretreatment tumor characteristics such as TP53 mutation status, and tumor escape mechanisms such as CD19 loss work together to drive relapse. Preinfusion patient characteristics limiting T-cell fitness may also contribute to kinetic failure of the CAR-T cell. Additional work in modeling which tumors are at highest risk may inform future trials such as use of less toxic CAR19 therapy for lower risk patients or using multiple infusions or CAR T-cell products directed against multiple antigens for higher risk patients. Additional molecular assessments of tumor burden such as ctDNA may help direct risk-adapted infusion strategies.

Section III–Chimeric Antigen Receptor T-Cell Toxicity

The success of CAR-T therapy makes thorough understanding of how the CAR-T cells work within the clinical setting of paramount importance. Despite their promise in treating patients with previously limited therapeutic options, CAR T-cell therapy suffers from novel toxicities such as CRS, ICANS, B-cell aplasia, prolonged cytopenia, and infection risk. This section will focus on known CAR T-cell toxicities.

Cytokine release syndrome and immune effector cell associated neurotoxicity syndrome

CRS and ICANS are the 2 hallmark toxicities of CAR T-cell therapy (**Table 2**). CRS is defined by the presence of fever with or without hypotension or increased oxygen requirement. CRS is typically the first CAR T-cell toxicity that occurs clinically with a median of onset of approximately 3 to 5 days. Initial studies focused on neurologic toxicity rather than the now more commonly used ICANS to define general neurologic impacts caused by CAR-T cells. ICANS itself is intimately associated with increased absolute CAR T-cell expansion in CD19 CAR T-cell vectors.[8,10,43,45] ICANS typically follows development of CRS but is much less common than CRS. The median onset of ICANS is approximately 6 days.

It is difficult to compare rates of CRS and ICANS across CAR T-cell vectors because of lack of head-to-head studies. That said the average rate of CRS in axi-cel constructs is 92% (ZUMA-1, ZUMA-7, ZUMA-12, ZUMA-5[46]) with an average of CRS greater than or equal to grade 3 of 9%. Average neurologic toxicity in the same group is 64% with 23% grade greater than or equal to 3. In the TRANSFORM and TRANSCEND trials an average of 42% of patients treated with liso-cel developed CRS with 2% having grade greater than or equal to 3 CRS; 21% developed neurologic toxicity with 7% developing grade greater than or equal to 3 neurotoxicity. Finally, the

Table 2
Overview of chimeric antigen receptor (CAR) T-cell mediated toxicities in CAR T-cell trials

CAR	Study	Pathology	CRS	CRS ≥3	Neurological	Neurological ≥3	N
Axi-cel	ZUMA-1	LBCL	93%	13%	64%	28%	101
Axi-cel	ZUMA-7	LCBL	92%	6%	60%	21%	170
Axi-cel	ZUMA-12	LBCL	100%	8%	73%	23%	40
Axi-cel	ZUMA-5	FL, MZL	82%	7%	59%	19%	148
Brexu-cel	ZUMA-2	MCL	91%	15%	63%	31%	68
Brexu-cel	ZUMA-3	ALL	89%	24%	60%	25%	55
Liso-cel	TRANSCEND	LBCL	42%	2%	30%	10%	269
Liso-cel	TRANSFORM	LBCL	49%	1%	12%	4%	92
Tisa-cel	JULIET	LBCL	58%	22%	21%	12%	111
Tisa-cel	BELINDA	LBCL	61%	5%	10%	2%	155

The axi-cel vector may have greater toxicity than the liso-cel and tisa-cel vectors based on limited cross-trial comparisons.

average rate of CRS in the JULIET and BELINDA trials was 60% with 14% grade greater than or equal to 3 and the rate of neurologic toxicity was 16% with 7% grade greater than or equal to 3.

Because of these numeric differences in the rate of CAR T-cell toxicity axi-cel is generally considered to have greater rates of severe ICANS which is also backed by propensity matched comparisons.[25] These differences are supported by initial observations suggesting increased toxicity in CD28 constructs,[78] increased cytokine signalling associated with CD28 transactivation in preclinical models,[79] and observed rapid increases in CAR T-cell expansion in CD28 constructs versus 41BB.[80] Consistent with these findings, high blood expansion of CAR T-cells is clearly associated with development of ICANS.[8,10,43]

Cytopenia

Currently, cytopenia after CAR has been defined relative to infusion as early (<30 days after infusion), prolonged (30–90 days after infusion), and late (>90 days after infusion).[81] Lymphodepleting chemotherapy is frequently associated with the development of early grade 3 cytopenias. In the ZUMA-1 trial, neutropenia occurred in 84% of patients with 78% grade greater than or equal to 3, thrombocytopenia occurred in 58% with 38% grade greater than or equal to 3, and anemia occurred in 66% with 43% grade greater than or equal to 3.[82] The TRANSCEND study had similar results of neutropenia in 63% of patients and 60% grade greater than or equal to 3, 31% had thrombocytopenia with 27% grade greater than or equal to 3, and 48% of patients had anemia with 37% grade greater than or equal to 3.[10] Results were similar in the ZUMA-7, ZUMA-12, and TRANSFORM studies. Close monitoring is required in the immediate postinfusion period while lymphodepleting chemotherapy takes effect and until counts have an opportunity to recover.

An unexpected but significant toxicity after CAR T-cell therapy in aggressive lymphoma is persistent cytopenia.[83] Early studies indicate that cytopenias can frequently persist for 1 year or longer postinfusion.[84,85] In the ZUMA-1 extended cohort 17% of patients maintained grade 3 or worse cytopenia 3 months after infusion.[82] Though neutrophils typically recover to normal levels, B-cell aplasia post-CAR, presumably due to on-target but off-tumor activity of the CAR T-cell itself, can persistent for longer periods of time. In CLL CAR T-cell persistence with associated B-cell aplasia has followed for over 10 years.[86] In axi-cel treated patients, CAR-T cells and B-cell aplasia frequently persist for multiple years post-infusion as well.[9,82] The relationship between CAR persistence and persistent cytopenias is unclear, though persistent CAR is likely associated at least with persistent B-cell aplasia. Consequent with these cytopenias, patents are at a high risk for infection after CAR T-cell therapy.[83,85,87–90]

Predictive scoring mechanisms for prolonged cytopenia in LBCL post-CAR are developed,[91] and pre-infusion predictive factors increasing the risk of developing post-CAR prolonged cytopenia include low platelet count, low absolute neutrophil count, low hemoglobin, high C-reactive protein, and high ferritin. These studies suggest patients with increased inflammatory markers and pretreatment cytopenias are at greater risk for additional cytopenia. It is difficult to use this data clinically as CAR T-cells are often the only reasonable line of treatment for patients no matter the ultimate toxicity, but with increased research and new anti-cancer agents these scoring systems may improve toxicity response or therapeutic choice.

In sum, post-CAR cytopenias are a durable consequence of CAR T-cell infusion and are likely multifactorial related to prior treatments, lymphodepleting chemotherapy, and the CAR T-cell itself including the inflammatory impact of initial CAR T-cell expansion and the on-target but off-tumor effect of persistent CAR T-cell targeting of CD19.

These toxicities are difficult to avoid and providers should be considered infectious prophylaxis and close immune surveillance. There are not clear differences in the rates of cytopenias between vectors. A separate article of this review covers post-CAR toxicity management in detail. Treatment of CAR T-cell-related toxicity and toxicity mechanisms is reviewed in detail by Neelapu and colleagues[92] and Siegler and colleagues.[93] Management of post-CAR cytopenias is discussed in Hill and colleagues[94] and Jain and colleagues.[81]

Secondary malignancy

Several recent studies suggest there is increased potential for development therapy related myeloid neoplasms (t-MN) after CAR T-cell therapy.[95,96] The most comprehensive of these studies indicates reduced latency between CAR T-cell treatment and development of t-MN post CAR. An additional study demonstrated that clonal hematopoiesis of indeterminate potential (CHIP) was present in 34% to 48% of patients prior to CAR T-cell therapy.[97,98] A separate study did associate the presence of CHIP mutations prior to infusion with increased severity of ICANS.[99] The presence of CHIP in this context was associated with increased response rates in one study, but none of these studies described differences in long-term outcomes in patients with CHIP mutations prior to infusion. The known prolonged cytopenias associated with CAR T-cell therapy which often recover over time combined with the often-substantial pretreatment chemotherapy received by patients prior to CAR infusion make the causative factor in the development of myeloid malignancies after CAR difficult. Further study into secondary malignancy after CAR T-cell therapy is warranted, but must be balanced by careful discrimination versus other causes of cytopenia in the setting of a patient population that is known to have a high prevalence of CHIP mutations and prolonged cytopenias that are likely not attributable to myeloid neoplasms.

Section IV–Novel Chimeric Antigen Receptor T-Cell Constructs and Bispecific T-Cell Engagers

Novel chimeric antigen receptor T-cell constructs

Despite the remarkable success of autologous CD19-directed therapies in LBCL, the high relapse rate after CD19-directed therapy necessitates additional tumor-directed therapies in up to half of treated patients. Multiple new CAR T-cell constructs are currently in clinical trials. Recently, the first CD19-22-directed bispecific CAR-T cell was published though this therapy unfortunately was met with high rates of CD19 antigen loss and relapse, possibly without substantial CD22-directed activity.[56] Similarly a CD19-20 bispecific CAR demonstrates anti-tumor activity in humans without antigen escape.[100] Promising single targets against CD22 are also in production and have recently been granted accelerated approval based on successful phase 1 trial results.[101] Notably, the development of multiple single target CAR-T cells raises the possibility of tandem[102] or cocktail[103,104] infusions in the future that may abrogate tumor-mediated antigen escape. In initial trials, these therapies have demonstrated response rates up to 90% highlighting the promise of multi-antigen targeting. Despite this promise, larger trials are necessary to more clearly define the safety and efficacy of combining constructs. Finally, multiple additional autologous targets are under investigation. These include CD79ab,[105,106] CD70,[107] and ROR1.[108]

Another important development in the CAR T-cell field is generation of allogeneic CAR T-cell therapy.[109,110] Autologous CAR-T cells are limited by the need for patients to undergo apheresis, have CAR T-cells generated and subsequently shipped, and then undergo infusion. This prevents dissemination of CAR T-cell treatments outside of academic centers with the logistic capacity to handle these complex pathways. The promise of allogeneic CAR T-cell therapy is effective off-the-shelf agents without the need for patient-specific products. These products promise activity in any patient including those with T cells that may have reduced function after multiple lines of chemotherapy. Despite this promise these agents are limited by host versus graft responses that requires sometimes more intensive immune suppression to overcome as well as multiple infusions.

Bispecific T-cell antibodies

Bispecific T-cell antibodies, though not CAR T-cell therapies, represent a similar mechanism of engaging T cells against B-cell-specific surface antigens. Multiple CD3–CD20 bispecific antibodies have been tested with some success in LBCL.[35–40] The most clinically advanced of these agents in LBCL is glofitamab and epcoritamab which have completed phase 2 trials. In a recent phase 2 study, glofitamab had a 39% CR rate at a 12.6 month follow-up in 154 treated patients with at least 2 prior lines of therapy as a single agent.[36] These results were consistent in 52 patients who had received prior CAR T-cell therapy. Epcoritamab similarly had a high response rate of 63.1% with a 38.9% CR rate in 157 patients with pretreated LBCL.[40] Results again were not different in the 61 study patients who had prior CAR T-cell therapy. The success of bispecific antibodies in the setting of LBCL as well as other NHLs[111] represents a potential challenge to the dominance of CAR T-cell therapy as the preferred T-cell agent directed against cell-surface antigens. Reflecting the rapid pace of these agents entering clinical practice, epcoritamab was granted accelerated FDA approval on May 19, 2023 for relapsed and refractory LBCL after two or more lines of systemic therapy.

Benefits of bispecific antibodies include ease of construction and treatment relative to CAR-T cells. These therapies are off-the-shelf meaning that they have less requirement for treatment in large academic cell therapy centers. Bispecific therapy with glofitamab does require pretreatment depletion of CD19 with obinutuzumab, but bispecific antibody treatments do not require lymphodepletion leading to substantially lower rates of high grade cytopenia. Glofitamab and epcoritamab require hospitalization for the first cycle, but do not require hospitalization for subsequent infusions. CRS and ICANS are major adverse effects of bispecific antibodies similar to CAR19 therapy, but occur with less frequency and intensity.

Another potential benefit of bispecific therapy is certain breakdown of the monoclonal antibody over time. The typical half-life of a bispecific antibody containing an Fc domain is similar to that of other monoclonal antibody treatments (typically 6–11 days)[112] which would potentially counteract some of the longer term impacts of persistent CAR. This benefit is likely confounded by the possibility of persistent CAR-T cells to act in longer term tumor surveillance, though the importance of this potential feature and the necessary duration of effect remains unclear. Finally, bispecific antibody treatments require multiple infusions over time rather than a single infusion meaning the duration of therapy as well as frequency of clinic visits is substantially increased relative to a single CAR19 infusion. Both therapies are likely to suffer from geographic and racial disparities in access[113] which is an issue of major concern moving forward.

Sequencing of bispecific versus CAR T-cell therapy is undetermined. Theoretically similar mechanisms of anti-tumor function such as epitope spreading[114] should be shared, and thus mechanisms of resistance could overlap. Despite this theoretical limitation so far patients pre-treated with CAR T-cell therapies have not had reduced efficacy when subsequently treated with bispecific antibodies[36,40,111] though the total number of such treated patients is low.

Similar theoretical limitations in potential cross resistance apply when considering bispecific antibodies prior to CAR. An additional concern with CAR sequenced after bispecific antibodies is the potential of exhausting the T-cell population prior to creating the CAR T-cell product. Despite this potential limitation, data on the efficacy of CAR T-cell therapy after a bispecific antibody in LBCL in a preliminary registry study suggest the CAR may remain effective when sequenced after bispecific antibodies.[115] Additionally in B-ALL CD19-directed CAR T-cell therapy did remain effective after pretreatment with the CD19 bispecific T-cell engager (BITE) blinatumomab in patients who initially responded to the BITE.[116] Future research is necessary to assess for these potential interactions. Ultimately, the long-term outcome data will determine the relative place of each therapy in the sequencing of LBCL treatment and both types of therapies will have increasing use in the treatment of lymphoma for the foreseeable future.

Section V–Summary

CAR T-cell therapy targeting CD19 has revolutionized the treatment aggressive lymphomas. This treatment has provided durable responses and likely cures in over 40% of patients. In addition, CAR T-cell therapy use is now extended to adult ALL,[117] multiple myeloma,[119–122] mantle cell lymphoma,[45] follicular lymphoma,[46,118] and marginal zone lymphoma[46] providing broad utility across most B-cell malignancies. Use of axi-cel and liso-cel in the second-line treatment of LBCL is approved following the ZUMA-7 and TRANSFORM studies (**Fig. 4**). CAR-T cells are now actively studied in first-line clinical trials and may soon become front-line therapy in LBCL.

Despite immense clinical promise in treating relapsed and refractory aggressive lymphomas, CAR T-cell therapies have a number of well-documented toxicities. Early toxicities of CRS and ICANS are so-far manageable with algorithmic approaches that involve multi-modal immune suppression. As CAR T-cell therapy is a living therapy there is also a concern for persistent CAR T-cell toxicity resulting in long-term cytopenia and infection. These persistent toxicities will require close monitoring and follow-up of CAR T-cell patients and perhaps novel interventions yet to be determined.

Even with the success of CD19-directed CAR T-cell therapy in LBCL more than half of patients relapse and the complexity and logistics of autologous CAR T-cell therapy is largely restricted to major academic centers. New CAR T-cell therapies with strong efficacy profiles are in development to ensure multiple additional lines of curative therapy are available to patients well after initial CAR T-cell treatment. Continuous development of new constructs, off-the-shelf allogeneic products, and related bispecific immune therapies will extend the curative benefits of cell therapy to most patients with aggressive lymphoma.

CLINICS CARE POINTS

- CAR T-cell therapy with axi-cel and liso-cel is approved for second-line treatment of LBCL in patients who are refractory to front-line chemotherapy, and patients who relapse within 12 months of completing first-line therapy.
- CAR T-cell therapy with axi-cel, liso-cel, and tisa-cel is approved for the third-line treatment LBCL.
- Early CAR T-cell toxicity of CRS and ICANS should be treated promptly with steroids and tocilizumab.

> • Prolonged CAR T-cell toxicity includes persistent cytopenia and infection that can last more than a year post-infusion. Long-term monitoring of CAR treated patients is warranted.

DISCLOSURE

M.P. Hamilton receives consulting fees as an advisor from Kite Pharma. D.B. Miklos holds a patent with Pharmacyclics supporting ibrutinib for chronic graft-versus-host disease and receives consulting or research fees or serves as an advisor for Pharmacyclics, Kite Pharma, Adaptive Biotechnologies, Novartis, Juno Therapeutics, Celgene, Janssen Pharmaceuticals, Roche, Genentech, Precision Bioscience, Allogene and Miltenyi Biotec.

FUNDING

M.P. Hamilton is funded by the Leukemia and Lymphoma Society Fellow Award. D. B. Miklos is funded by NCI PO1 CA049605, CIRM CLIN2-10846, Kite Scientific research agreement and multiple clinical trials with sponsors including: Kite-Gilead, BMS, Novartis, Miltenyi, Allogene, 2Seventy, Adicet, and Fate Therapeutics.

REFERENCES

1. June CH, Sadelain M. Chimeric antigen receptor therapy. N Engl J Med 2018; 379(1):64–73.
2. Porter DL, Levine BL, Kalos M, et al. Chimeric antigen receptor–modified t cells in chronic lymphoid leukemia. N Engl J Med 2011;365(8):725–33.
3. Davila ML, Riviere I, Wang X, et al. Efficacy and toxicity management of 19-28z CAR T cell therapy in B cell acute lymphoblastic leukemia. Sci Transl Med 2014; 6(224):224ra25.
4. Grupp SA, Kalos M, Barrett D, et al. Chimeric antigen receptor-modified T cells for acute lymphoid leukemia. N Engl J Med 2013;368(16):1509–18.
5. Kalos M, Levine BL, Porter DL, et al. T cells with chimeric antigen receptors have potent antitumor effects and can establish memory in patients with advanced leukemia. Sci Transl Med 2011;3(95):95ra73.
6. Crump M, Neelapu SS, Farooq U, et al. Outcomes in refractory diffuse large B-cell lymphoma: results from the international SCHOLAR-1 study. Blood 2017;130(16):1800–8.
7. Gisselbrecht C, Glass B, Mounier N, et al. Salvage regimens with autologous transplantation for relapsed large B-cell lymphoma in the rituximab era. J Clin Oncol 2010;28(27):4184–90.
8. Neelapu SS, Locke FL, Bartlett NL, et al. Axicabtagene ciloleucel CAR T-cell therapy in refractory large B-cell lymphoma. N Engl J Med 2017;377(26): 2531–44.
9. Locke FL, Miklos DB, Jacobson CA, et al. Axicabtagene ciloleucel as second-line therapy for large B-cell lymphoma. N Engl J Med 2022;386(7):640–54.
10. Abramson JS, Palomba ML, Gordon LI, et al. Lisocabtagene maraleucel for patients with relapsed or refractory large B-cell lymphomas (TRANSCEND NHL 001): a multicentre seamless design study. Lancet 2020;396(10254):839–52.
11. Kamdar M, Solomon SR, Arnason J, et al. Lisocabtagene maraleucel versus standard of care with salvage chemotherapy followed by autologous stem cell transplantation as second-line treatment in patients with relapsed or refractory

large B-cell lymphoma (TRANSFORM): results from an interim analysis of an open-label, randomised, phase 3 trial. Lancet 2022;399(10343):2294–308.

12. Schuster SJ, Bishop MR, Tam CS, et al. Tisagenlecleucel in adult relapsed or refractory diffuse large B-cell lymphoma. N Engl J Med 2019;380(1):45–56.

13. Bishop MR, Dickinson M, Purtill D, et al. Second-line tisagenlecleucel or standard care in aggressive B-cell lymphoma. N Engl J Med 2022;386(7):629–39.

14. Zola H, Macardle PJ, Bradford T, et al. Preparation and characterization of a chimeric CD 19 monoclonal antibody. Immunol Cell Biol 1991;69(6):411–22.

15. Nicholson IC, Lenton KA, Little DJ, et al. Construction and characterisation of a functional CD19 specific single chain Fv fragment for immunotherapy of B lineage leukaemia and lymphoma. Mol Immunol 1997;34(16):1157–65.

16. Meng J, Wu X, Sun Z, et al. Efficacy and safety of CAR-T cell products axicabtagene ciloleucel, tisagenlecleucel, and lisocabtagene maraleucel for the treatment of hematologic malignancies: a systematic review and meta-analysis. systematic review. Front Oncol 2021;11. https://doi.org/10.3389/fonc.2021.698607.

17. Ghilardi G, Chong EA, Svoboda J, et al. Bendamustine is safe and effective for lymphodepletion before tisagenlecleucel in patients with refractory or relapsed large B-cell lymphomas. Ann Oncol 2022;33(9):916–28.

18. Locke FL, Neelapu SS, Bartlett NL, et al. Phase 1 Results of ZUMA-1: a multicenter study of KTE-C19 Anti-CD19 CAR T cell therapy in refractory aggressive lymphoma. Mol Ther 2017;25(1):285–95.

19. Jacobson C, Locke FL, Ghobadi A, et al. Long-term survival and gradual recovery of B cells in patients with refractory large b cell lymphoma treated with axicabtagene ciloleucel (Axi-Cel). Blood 2020;136(Supplement 1):40–2.

20. Nastoupil LJ, Jain MD, Feng L, et al. Standard-of-care axicabtagene ciloleucel for relapsed or refractory large b-cell lymphoma: results from the US lymphoma CAR T consortium. J Clin Oncol 2020;38(27):3119–28.

21. Westin JR, Oluwole OO, Kersten MJ, et al. Survival with Axicabtagene Ciloleucel in Large B-Cell Lymphoma. N Engl J Med 2023. https://doi.org/10.1056/NEJMoa2301665.

22. Neelapu SS, Dickinson M, Munoz J, et al. Axicabtagene ciloleucel as first-line therapy in high-risk large B-cell lymphoma: the phase 2 ZUMA-12 trial. Nat Med 2022;28(4):735–42.

23. Coiffier B, Thieblemont C, Van Den Neste E, et al. Long-term outcome of patients in the LNH-98.5 trial, the first randomized study comparing rituximab-CHOP to standard CHOP chemotherapy in DLBCL patients: a study by the Groupe d'Etudes des Lymphomes de l'Adulte. Blood 2010;116(12):2040–5.

24. Bartlett NL, Wilson WH, Jung SH, et al. Dose-Adjusted EPOCH-R compared with R-CHOP as frontline therapy for diffuse large B-cell lymphoma: clinical outcomes of the phase III intergroup trial alliance/CALGB 50303. J Clin Oncol 2019;37(21):1790–9.

25. Bachy E, Le Gouill S, Di Blasi R, et al. A real-world comparison of tisagenlecleucel and axicabtagene ciloleucel CAR T cells in relapsed or refractory diffuse large B cell lymphoma. Nat Med 2022;28(10):2145–54.

26. Pinnix CC, Gunther JR, Dabaja BS, et al. Bridging therapy prior to axicabtagene ciloleucel for relapsed/refractory large B-cell lymphoma. Blood Advances 2020;4(13):2871–83.

27. Oluwole OO, Bouabdallah K, Muñoz J, et al. Prophylactic corticosteroid use in patients receiving axicabtagene ciloleucel for large B-cell lymphoma. Br J Haematol 2021;194(4):690–700.

28. Spiegel JY, Dahiya S, Jain MD, et al. Outcomes of patients with large B-cell lymphoma progressing after axicabtagene ciloleucel therapy. Blood 2021;137(13): 1832–5.

29. Iacoboni G, Martin Lopez AA, Jalowiec KA, et al. Recent Bendamustine Treatment before Apheresis Has a Negative Impact on Outcomes in Patients with Large B-Cell Lymphoma Receiving Chimeric Antigen Receptor T-Cell Therapy. Blood 2022;140(Supplement 1):1592–4.

30. Wang Y, Jain P, Locke FL, et al. Brexucabtagene Autoleucel for Relapsed or Refractory Mantle Cell Lymphoma in Standard-of-Care Practice: Results From the US Lymphoma CAR T Consortium. J Clin Oncol 2023. https://doi.org/10.1200/JCO.22.01797. :JCO.22.01797.

31. Saifi O, Breen WG, Lester SC, et al. Does bridging radiation therapy affect the pattern of failure after CAR T-cell therapy in non-Hodgkin lymphoma? Radiother Oncol 2022;166:171–9.

32. Thapa B, Caimi PF, Ardeshna KM, et al. CD19 antibody-drug conjugate therapy in DLBCL does not preclude subsequent responses to CD19-directed CAR T-cell therapy. Blood Advances 2020;4(16):3850–2.

33. Horvei P, Sakemura R, Cox MJ, et al. Targeting of CD19 by tafasitamab does not impair CD19 directed chimeric antigen receptor T cell activity in vitro. Blood 2019;134(Supplement_1):2859.

34. Calabretta E, Hamadani M, Zinzani PL, et al. The antibody-drug conjugate loncastuximab tesirine for the treatment of diffuse large B-cell lymphoma. Blood 2022;140(4):303–8.

35. Hutchings M, Morschhauser F, Iacoboni G, et al. Glofitamab, a novel, bivalent CD20-targeting T-Cell–engaging bispecific antibody, induces durable complete remissions in relapsed or refractory B-cell lymphoma: a phase I trial. J Clin Oncol 2021;39(18):1959–70.

36. Dickinson MJ, Carlo-Stella C, Morschhauser F, et al. Glofitamab for relapsed or refractory diffuse large B-cell lymphoma. N Engl J Med 2022;387(24):2220–31.

37. Hutchings M, Mous R, Clausen MR, et al. Dose escalation of subcutaneous epcoritamab in patients with relapsed or refractory B-cell non-Hodgkin lymphoma: an open-label, phase 1/2 study. Lancet 2021;398(10306):1157–69.

38. Bannerji R, Arnason JE, Advani RH, et al. Odronextamab, a human CD20xCD3 bispecific antibody in patients with CD20-positive B-cell malignancies (ELM-1): results from the relapsed or refractory non-Hodgkin lymphoma cohort in a single-arm, multicentre, phase 1 trial. Lancet Haematol 2022;9(5):e327–39.

39. Budde LE, Assouline S, Sehn LH, et al. Single-agent mosunetuzumab shows durable complete responses in patients with relapsed or refractory B-Cell lymphomas: phase I dose-escalation study. J Clin Oncol 2022;40(5):481–91.

40. Thieblemont C, Phillips T, Ghesquieres H, et al. Epcoritamab, a novel, subcutaneous CD3xCD20 bispecific T-cell–engaging antibody, in relapsed or refractory large B-cell lymphoma: dose expansion in a phase I/II trial. J Clin Oncol 2022;0(0). JCO.22.01725.

41. Morschhauser F, Flinn IW, Advani R, et al. Polatuzumab vedotin or pinatuzumab vedotin plus rituximab in patients with relapsed or refractory non-Hodgkin lymphoma: final results from a phase 2 randomised study (ROMULUS). Lancet Haematol 2019;6(5):e254–65.

42. Deng Q, Han G, Puebla-Osorio N, et al. Characteristics of anti-CD19 CAR T cell infusion products associated with efficacy and toxicity in patients with large B cell lymphomas. Nat Med 2020;26(12):1878–87.

43. Good Z, Spiegel JY, Sahaf B, et al. Post-infusion CAR TReg cells identify patients resistant to CD19-CAR therapy. Nat Med 2022;28(9):1860–71.

44. Haradhvala NJ, Leick MB, Maurer K, et al. Distinct cellular dynamics associated with response to CAR-T therapy for refractory B cell lymphoma. Nat Med 2022; 28(9):1848–59.

45. Wang M, Munoz J, Goy A, et al. KTE-X19 CAR T-cell therapy in relapsed or refractory mantle-cell lymphoma. N Engl J Med 2020;382(14):1331–42.

46. Jacobson CA, Chavez JC, Sehgal AR, et al. Axicabtagene ciloleucel in relapsed or refractory indolent non-Hodgkin lymphoma (ZUMA-5): a single-arm, multicentre, phase 2 trial. Lancet Oncol 2022;23(1):91–103.

47. Sworder BJ, Kurtz DM, Alig SK, et al. Determinants of resistance to engineered T cell therapies targeting CD19 in large B cell lymphomas. Cancer Cell 2022. https://doi.org/10.1016/j.ccell.2022.12.005.

48. Locke FL, Rossi JM, Neelapu SS, et al. Tumor burden, inflammation, and product attributes determine outcomes of axicabtagene ciloleucel in large B-cell lymphoma. Blood Adv 2020;4(19):4898–911.

49. Neelapu SS, Jacobson CA, Oluwole OO, et al. Outcomes of older patients in ZUMA-1, a pivotal study of axicabtagene ciloleucel in refractory large B-cell lymphoma. Blood 2020;135(23):2106–9.

50. Lin RJ, Lobaugh SM, Pennisi M, et al. Impact and safety of chimeric antigen receptor T-cell therapy in older, vulnerable patients with relapsed/refractory large B-cell lymphoma. Haematologica 2020;106(1):255–8.

51. Lutfi F, Holtzman NG, Kansagra AJ, et al. The impact of bridging therapy prior to CD19-directed chimeric antigen receptor T-cell therapy in patients with large B-cell lymphoma. Br J Haematol 2021;195(3):405–12.

52. Wada F, Jo T, Arai Y, et al. T-cell counts in peripheral blood at leukapheresis predict responses to subsequent CAR-T cell therapy. Sci Rep 2022;12(1):18696.

53. Smith M, Dai A, Ghilardi G, et al. Gut microbiome correlates of response and toxicity following anti-CD19 CAR T cell therapy. Nat Med 2022;28(4):713–23.

54. Sterner RC, Sterner RM. CAR-T cell therapy: current limitations and potential strategies. Blood Cancer J 2021;11(4):69.

55. Chong EA, Ruella M, Schuster SJ. Five-year outcomes for refractory B-cell lymphomas with CAR T-cell therapy. N Engl J Med 2021;384(7):673–4.

56. Spiegel JY, Patel S, Muffly L, et al. CAR T cells with dual targeting of CD19 and CD22 in adult patients with recurrent or refractory B cell malignancies: a phase 1 trial. Nat Med 2021. https://doi.org/10.1038/s41591-021-01436-0.

57. Plaks V, Rossi JM, Chou J, et al. CD19 target evasion as a mechanism of relapse in large B-cell lymphoma treated with axicabtagene ciloleucel. Blood 2021; 138(12):1081–5.

58. Shah NN, Fry TJ. Mechanisms of resistance to CAR T cell therapy. Nat Rev Clin Oncol 2019;16(6):372–85.

59. Neelapu SS, Rossi JM, Jacobson CA, et al. CD19-loss with preservation of other B cell lineage features in patients with large b cell lymphoma who relapsed post-axi-cel. Blood 2019;134(Supplement_1):203.

60. Jain MD, Zhao H, Wang X, et al. Tumor interferon signaling and suppressive myeloid cells are associated with CAR T-cell failure in large B-cell lymphoma. Blood 2021;137(19):2621–33.

61. Scholler N, Perbost R, Locke FL, et al. Tumor immune contexture is a determinant of anti-CD19 CAR T cell efficacy in large B cell lymphoma. Nat Med 2022;28(9):1872–82.

62. Vercellino L, Di Blasi R, Kanoun S, et al. Predictive factors of early progression after CAR T-cell therapy in relapsed/refractory diffuse large B-cell lymphoma. Blood Adv 2020;4(22):5607–15.

63. Rabinovich E, Pradhan K, Sica RA, et al. Elevated LDH greater than 400 U/L portends poorer overall survival in diffuse large B-cell lymphoma patients treated with CD19 CAR-T cell therapy in a real world multi-ethnic cohort. Exp Hematol Oncol 2021;10(1):55.

64. Frank MJ, Hossain NM, Bukhari A, et al. Monitoring of circulating tumor DNA improves early relapse detection after axicabtagene ciloleucel infusion in large B-cell lymphoma: results of a prospective multi-institutional trial. J Clin Oncol 2021;39(27):3034–43.

65. Dean EA, Mhaskar RS, Lu H, et al. High metabolic tumor volume is associated with decreased efficacy of axicabtagene ciloleucel in large B-cell lymphoma. Blood Advances 2020;4(14):3268–76.

66. Shouval R, Alarcon Tomas A, Fein JA, et al. Impact of TP53 genomic alterations in large B-cell lymphoma treated with CD19-chimeric antigen receptor T-Cell therapy. J Clin Oncol 2022;40(4):369–81.

67. Cherng H-JJ, Sun R, Sugg B, et al. Risk assessment with low-pass whole-genome sequencing of cell-free DNA before CD19 CAR T-cell therapy for large B-cell lymphoma. Blood 2022;140(5):504–15.

68. Jain MD, Ziccheddu B, Coughlin CA, et al. Whole-genome sequencing reveals complex genomic features underlying anti-CD19 CAR T-cell treatment failures in lymphoma. Blood 2022;140(5):491–503.

69. Majzner RG, Mackall CL. Tumor antigen escape from CAR T-cell therapy. Cancer Discov 2018;8(10):1219–26.

70. Majzner RG, Rietberg SP, Sotillo E, et al. Tuning the antigen density requirement for CAR T-cell activity. Cancer Discov 2020;10(5):702–23.

71. Ali A, Goy A, Dunleavy K. CAR T-cell therapy in highly aggressive B-cell lymphoma: emerging biological and clinical insights. Blood 2022;140(13):1461–9.

72. Ahmed G, Hamadani M, Shah NN. CAR T-cell therapy for secondary CNS DLBCL. Blood Advances 2021;5(24):5626–30.

73. Benjamini O, Shimoni A, Besser M, et al. Safety and Efficacy of CD19-CAR T cells in richter's transformation after targeted therapy for chronic lymphocytic leukemia. Blood 2020;136(Supplement 1):40.

74. Kittai AS, Bond DA, William B, et al. Clinical activity of axicabtagene ciloleucel in adult patients with Richter syndrome. Blood Advances 2020;4(19):4648–52.

75. Turtle CJ, Hay KA, Hanafi LA, et al. Durable molecular remissions in chronic lymphocytic leukemia treated with CD19-specific chimeric antigen receptor-modified T cells after failure of ibrutinib. J Clin Oncol 2017;35(26):3010–20.

76. Smyth E, Eyre TA, Cheah CY. Emerging therapies for the management of richter transformation. J Clin Oncol 2023;41(2):395–409.

77. Siddiqi T, Soumerai JD, Dorritie KA, et al. Phase 1 TRANSCEND CLL 004 study of lisocabtagene maraleucel in patients with relapsed/refractory CLL or SLL. Blood 2022;139(12):1794–806.

78. Ying Z, He T, Wang X, et al. Parallel comparison of 4-1BB or CD28 co-stimulated CD19-targeted CAR-T cells for b cell non-hodgkin's lymphoma. Mol Ther Oncolytics 2019;15:60–8.

79. Cappell KM, Kochenderfer JN. A comparison of chimeric antigen receptors containing CD28 versus 4-1BB costimulatory domains. Nat Rev Clin Oncol 2021;18(11):715–27.

80. Cheng Z, Wei R, Ma Q, et al. In vivo expansion and antitumor activity of coinfused CD28- and 4-1BB-engineered CAR-T cells in patients with B cell leukemia. Mol Ther 2018;26(4):976–85.
81. Jain T, Olson TS, Locke FL. How I treat cytopenias after CAR T-cell therapy. Blood 2023. https://doi.org/10.1182/blood.2022017415.
82. Locke FL, Ghobadi A, Jacobson CA, et al. Long-term safety and activity of axicabtagene ciloleucel in refractory large B-cell lymphoma (ZUMA-1): a single-arm, multicentre, phase 1–2 trial. Lancet Oncol 2019;20(1):31–42.
83. Wudhikarn K, Perales M-A. Infectious complications, immune reconstitution, and infection prophylaxis after CD19 chimeric antigen receptor T-cell therapy. Bone Marrow Transplant 2022;57(10):1477–88.
84. Jain T, Knezevic A, Pennisi M, et al. Hematopoietic recovery in patients receiving chimeric antigen receptor T-cell therapy for hematologic malignancies. Blood Adv 2020;4(15):3776–87.
85. Baird JH, Epstein DJ, Tamaresis JS, et al. Immune reconstitution and infectious complications following axicabtagene ciloleucel therapy for large B-cell lymphoma. Blood Adv 2021;5(1):143–55.
86. Melenhorst JJ, Chen GM, Wang M, et al. Decade-long leukaemia remissions with persistence of CD4(+) CAR T cells. Nature 2022;602(7897):503–9.
87. Spanjaart AM, Ljungman P, de La Camara R, et al. Poor outcome of patients with COVID-19 after CAR T-cell therapy for B-cell malignancies: results of a multicenter study on behalf of the European Society for Blood and Marrow Transplantation (EBMT) Infectious Diseases Working Party and the European Hematology Association (EHA) Lymphoma Group. Leukemia 2021;35(12):3585–8.
88. Busca A, Salmanton-García J, Corradini P, et al. COVID-19 and CAR T cells: a report on current challenges and future directions from the EPICOVIDEHA survey by EHA-IDWP. Blood Adv 2022;6(7):2427–33.
89. Aydillo T, Gonzalez-Reiche AS, Aslam S, et al. Shedding of viable SARS-CoV-2 after immunosuppressive therapy for cancer. N Engl J Med 2020;383(26):2586–8.
90. Hamilton MP, Liu-Fei FC, Alig SK, et al. Higher rates of severe infection and persistent cytopenias in long-term CAR19 responders than after autologous HCT: a single institution study of 139 subjects. Blood 2022;140(Supplement 1):7545–7.
91. Rejeski K, Perez A, Sesques P, et al. CAR-HEMATOTOX: a model for CAR T-cell–related hematologic toxicity in relapsed/refractory large B-cell lymphoma. Blood 2021;138(24):2499–513.
92. Neelapu SS, Tummala S, Kebriaei P, et al. Chimeric antigen receptor T-cell therapy — assessment and management of toxicities. Nat Rev Clin Oncol 2018;15(1):47–62.
93. Siegler EL, Kenderian SS. Neurotoxicity and cytokine release syndrome after chimeric antigen receptor T cell therapy: insights into mechanisms and novel therapies. Front Immunol 2020;11:1973.
94. Hill JA, Seo SK. How I prevent infections in patients receiving CD19-targeted chimeric antigen receptor T cells for B-cell malignancies. Blood 2020;136(8):925–35.
95. Alkhateeb HB, Mohty R, Greipp P, et al. Therapy-related myeloid neoplasms following chimeric antigen receptor T-cell therapy for Non-Hodgkin Lymphoma. Blood Cancer J 2022;12(7):113.
96. Andersen MJ Jr, Bindal P, Michaels P, et al. Clonal myeloid disorders following CAR T-cell therapy. Blood 2022;140(Supplement 1):10985–6.

97. Miller PG, Sperling AS, Brea EJ, et al. Clonal hematopoiesis in patients receiving chimeric antigen receptor T-cell therapy. Blood Adv 2021;5(15):2982–6.

98. Teipel R, Kroschinsky F, Kramer M, et al. Prevalence and variation of CHIP in patients with aggressive lymphomas undergoing CD19-directed CAR T-cell treatment. Blood Advances 2022;6(6):1941–6.

99. Saini NY, Swoboda DM, Greenbaum U, et al. Clonal hematopoiesis is associated with increased risk of severe neurotoxicity in axicabtagene ciloleucel therapy of large B-cell lymphoma. Blood Cancer Discov 2022;3(5):385–93.

100. Shah NN, Johnson BD, Schneider D, et al. Bispecific anti-CD20, anti-CD19 CAR T cells for relapsed B cell malignancies: a phase 1 dose escalation and expansion trial. Nat Med 2020;26(10):1569–75.

101. Baird JH, Frank MJ, Craig J, et al. CD22-directed CAR T-cell therapy induces complete remissions in CD19-directed CAR–refractory large B-cell lymphoma. Blood 2021;137(17):2321–5.

102. Wu J, Meng F, Cao Y, et al. Sequential CD19/22 CAR T-cell immunotherapy following autologous stem cell transplantation for central nervous system lymphoma. Blood Cancer J 2021;11(7):131.

103. Wang N, Hu X, Cao W, et al. Efficacy and safety of CAR19/22 T-cell cocktail therapy in patients with refractory/relapsed B-cell malignancies. Blood 2020;135(1): 17–27.

104. Cao Y, Xiao Y, Wang N, et al. CD19/CD22 chimeric antigen receptor t cell cocktail therapy following autologous transplantation in patients with relapsed/refractory aggressive B cell lymphomas. Transplantation and Cellular Therapy 2021; 27(11):910.e1–11.

105. Ormhøj M, Scarfò I, Cabral ML, et al. Chimeric antigen receptor T cells targeting CD79b show efficacy in lymphoma with or without cotargeting CD19. Clin Cancer Res 2019;25(23):7046–57.

106. Locke FL, Miklos DB, Tees M, et al. CRC-403: a phase 1/2 study of bbT369, a Dual CD79a and CD20 Targeting CAR T cell drug product with a gene edit, in relapsed and/or refractory B cell non-hodgkin's lymphoma (NHL). Blood 2022; 140(Supplement 1):12716–7.

107. Shaffer DR, Savoldo B, Yi Z, et al. T cells redirected against CD70 for the immunotherapy of CD70-positive malignancies. Blood 2011;117(16):4304–14.

108. Peng H, Nerreter T, Mestermann K, et al. ROR1-targeting switchable CAR-T cells for cancer therapy. Oncogene 2022;41(34):4104–14.

109. Depil S, Duchateau P, Grupp SA, et al. 'Off-the-shelf' allogeneic CAR T cells: development and challenges. Nat Rev Drug Discov 2020;19(3):185–99.

110. Sidaway P. Allogeneic CAR T cells show promise. Nat Rev Clin Oncol 2022; 19(12):748.

111. Budde LE, Sehn LH, Matasar M, et al. Safety and efficacy of mosunetuzumab, a bispecific antibody, in patients with relapsed or refractory follicular lymphoma: a single-arm, multicentre, phase 2 study. Lancet Oncol 2022;23(8):1055–65.

112. Falchi L, Vardhana SA, Salles GA. Bispecific antibodies for the treatment of B-cell lymphoma: promises, unknowns, and opportunities. Blood 2023;141(5): 467–80.

113. Alqazaqi R, Schinke C, Thanendrarajan S, et al. Geographic and racial disparities in access to chimeric antigen receptor–T Cells and Bispecific Antibodies Trials for Multiple Myeloma. JAMA Netw Open 2022;5(8):e2228877.

114. Brossart P. The role of antigen spreading in the efficacy of immunotherapies. Clin Cancer Res 2020;26(17):4442–7.

115. Crochet G, Audrey C, Bachy E, et al. CAR T-cell therapy remain effective in patients with relapse/refractory B-cell non-hodgkin lymphoma after bispecific antibodies exposure: results of a lysa study based on the descar-T registry. Blood 2022;140(Supplement 1):4639–41.

116. Myers RM, Taraseviciute A, Steinberg SM, et al. Blinatumomab nonresponse and high-disease burden are associated with inferior outcomes after CD19-CAR for B-ALL. J Clin Oncol 2022;40(9):932–44.

117. Shah BD, Ghobadi A, Oluwole OO, et al. KTE-X19 for relapsed or refractory adult B-cell acute lymphoblastic leukaemia: phase 2 results of the single-arm, open-label, multicentre ZUMA-3 study. Lancet 2021;398(10299):491–502.

118. Fowler NH, Dickinson M, Dreyling M, et al. Tisagenlecleucel in adult relapsed or refractory follicular lymphoma: the phase 2 ELARA trial. Nat Med 2022;28(2):325–32.

119. Berdeja JG, Madduri D, Usmani SZ, et al. Ciltacabtagene autoleucel, a B-cell maturation antigen-directed chimeric antigen receptor T-cell therapy in patients with relapsed or refractory multiple myeloma (CARTITUDE-1): a phase 1b/2 open-label study, Lancet, 2021;398(10297):314–324.

120. San-Miguel J, Dhakal B, Yong K, et al. Cilta-cel or Standard Care in Lenalido-mide-Refractory Multiple Myeloma. N Engl J Med 2023. https://doi.org/10.1056/NEJMoa2303379.

121. Munshi NC, Anderson LD, Shah N, et al. Idecabtagene Vicleucel in Relapsed and Refractory Multiple Myeloma. New England Journal of Medicine 2021;384(8):705–16.

122. Rodriguez-Otero P, Ailawadhi S, Arnulf B, et al. Ide-cel or Standard Regimens in Relapsed and Refractory Multiple Myeloma, N Engl J Med, 2023;388 (11):1002–1014.

Chimeric Antigen Receptor T-Cells in Indolent Lymphoma, Mantle Cell Lymphoma, Chronic Lymphocytic Leukemia

Parth S. Shah, MD[a], Caron A. Jacobson, MD[b],*

KEYWORDS

- CAR-T • Lymphoma • Indolent lymphoma • Mantle cell • CLL

KEY POINTS

- Chimeric antigen receptor (CAR)-T-cell therapy is available as a therapeutic option for follicular lymphoma and mantle cell lymphoma.
- Although not approved, CAR-T therapy has shown significant promise in the management of chronic lymphocytic leukemia.
- Bruton tyrosine kinase inhibitor therapy appears to have a positive immunomodulatory effect on T cells for CAR-T therapy.

INTRODUCTION

Indolent B-cell non-Hodgkin lymphomas (B-NHL), chronic lymphocytic leukemia (CLL), and mantle cell lymphoma (MCL) are widely treatable but typically incurable with conventional therapies. The ultimate challenge with these lymphomas is that cure remains elusive, and the impact of the disease on quality and quantity of life is significant; a portion of patients will die from either disease or treatment-associated toxicity, and lymphoma-related mortality remains the most common cause of death.[1] Most patients with indolent B-NHL will enjoy long survival with their disease and may die from other causes; exceptions to this include patients diagnosed at a young age, patients with early relapsing disease within 24 months of frontline chemoimmunotherapy, and patients with disease relapsed multiple times requiring 3 or more lines of therapy.[2,3] CLL with high-risk cytogenetics and mutations as well as progression after Bruton's tyrosine kinase (BTK) inhibitors and venetoclax have a particularly poor

[a] Dartmouth Cancer Center, 1 Medical Center Drive, Lebanon, NH 03750, USA; [b] Dana-Farber Cancer Institute, 450 Brookline Avenue, Boston, MA 02215-5450, USA
* Corresponding author.
E-mail address: Caron_Jacobson@dfci.harvard.edu

Hematol Oncol Clin N Am 37 (2023) 1077–1088
https://doi.org/10.1016/j.hoc.2023.07.002
0889-8588/23/© 2023 Elsevier Inc. All rights reserved.

prognosis.[3] Finally, MCL generally has a shorter overall survival (OS) than either of these diseases, and for high-risk patients including those with complex cytogenetics and *TP53* mutations and all patients that have relapsed after frontline chemoimmunotherapy and BTK inhibitors, response to and survival after available conventional therapies is quite short.[4] It is in these contexts, where options and survival are limited, that CD19-directed CAR T-cell therapy has been explored, specifically in follicular lymphoma (FL) and marginal zone lymphoma (MZL) in the third line and beyond and in MCL following chemoimmunotherapy as well as a BTK inhibitor. This article will explore the results from these trials, their successes as well as their limitations, and new directions to improve cellular therapies and outcomes for these patients.

BACKGROUND
Follicular Lymphoma

FL is a mature B-cell malignancy derived from germinal center B-cells. It is the second most common lymphoma in Western countries and the United States (US) and accounts for 20% to 25% of all lymphoid malignancies. About 80% of FL patients carry the translocation (14; 18) which encodes the BCL2 antiapoptotic protein, which is the hallmark molecular finding in FL.[1] Other genetic and epigenetic abnormalities are associated with the pathogenesis and progression of FL, such as chromatin-modifying mutations (KMT2D, CREEBP, EZH2), immune evasion (TNFRSF14, CREBBP), and transcriptional regulation (STAT6, BCL6, BCL2) among others and that involve T-cell function and tumor microenvironment.[5]

The prognosis of FL improved for patients of all ages after the addition of rituximab to chemotherapy regimens in early 2000.[6] A recent large French–American study showed a 10-year OS of 80% in FL patients treated with rituximab-containing regimens.

However, there remain patients with high-risk FL, with worse outcomes and short OS, including patients that relapse within 2 years of completing therapy (5 year OS: 50%); those with histologic transformation following first-line therapy (5 year OS: 55%); and those who have progressed after 2 prior lines of therapy (5 year OS: 75%; median progression-free survival [PFS]: 17 m).[7–12] The utilization of CD19-directed CAR-T cell therapy holds significant promise in these patient populations (**Table 1**).[13]

Marginal Zone Lymphoma

MZL are rare lymphoid tumors with heterogenous presentation that account for approximately 5% to 15% of all non-Hodgkin's lymphoma (NHL) in the western hemisphere. The main subtypes are extranodal MZL of mucosal-associated lymphoid tissue, the most common type (70% of MZL), followed by splenic MZL and nodal MZL. As seen in FL, MZL patients with early relapse or postoperative day (POD)-24 or with transformation to high-grade lymphoma have inferior OS, and management of these patients continues to be challenging.[14,15]

Mantle Cell Lymphoma

MCL is a rare subtype of NHL of mature B cells characterized by translocation between chromosomes 11 and 14 (t(11;14)), leading to overexpression of *CCND1*. Advanced age, male gender, elevated serum lactate dehydrogenase level, and poor prognostic markers such as increased expression of Ki-67 and the presence of *TP53* mutations, as well as complex karyotype, are associated with poor outcomes.[4] Some MCLs can behave indolently, but many require therapy at diagnosis, and those that do not behave indolently generally require therapy within the first few years following diagnosis. Once these lymphomas either do not respond to or relapse following frontline

Table 1
Clinical trial results for FDA-approved CAR-T therapies for follicular lymphoma

Clinical Trials	CAR T-cell Product	N	Median (Range) Age, Years	Median Prior Lines of Therapy	Toxicities		Response	Survival
ZUMA-5[29]	Axicabtagene ciloleucel	124	60 (53–67)	3 (2–4)	CRS		ORR 94%	3 y PFS 54%
					Any grade	78%	CR 79%	3 y OS 76%
					Grade 3+	15%		
					ICANS			
					Any grade	56%		
					Grade 3+	6%		
ELARA[31]	Tisagenlecleucel	97	57 (49–64)	4 (2–13)	CRS		ORR 86%	2 y PFS 57%
					Any grade	48%	CR 69.1%	2 y OS 88%
					Grade 3+	0%		
					ICANS			
					Any grade	11%		
					Grade 3+	3%		

Abbreviations: CAR, chimeric antigen receptor; CR, complete response; CRS, cytokine release syndrome; ICANS, immune effector cell associated neurologic syndrome; ORR, overall response rate; OS, overall survival; PFS, progression-free survival.

chemoimmunotherapy and then progress through a BTK inhibitor, prognosis is generally poor, and median OS is less than 1 year.[16]

Chronic Lymphocytic Leukemia

CLL is a chronic lymphoproliferative disease characterized by malignant transformation of mature antigen-experienced B lymphocytes and accumulation of monoclonal malignant B cells in peripheral blood, bone marrow, lymph nodes, and spleen. CLL is diagnosed in 191,000 new patients and estimated to cause 61,000 deaths per year worldwide and remains largely incurable with any treatment other than allogeneic stem cell transplantation (alloSCT) despite the advent of new therapies. Most patients with CLL will have a very indolent course, with some never needing therapies and many others dying with CLL rather than from CLL. However, certain high-risk subgroups, including those with del17p and/or mutations in *TP53* as well as those with an unmutated *IGVH*, as well as those who progress following BTK inhibitors and venetoclax, can have limited survival.[17] CAR-T therapy had its earliest success in high-risk CLL and those relapsed multiple times, but treatment of larger cohorts has since been disappointing.[18–20] Efforts to improve T-cell function in these patients have recently yielded encouraging results.[21,22]

CHIMERIC ANTIGEN RECEPTOR T-CELL THERAPY IN INDOLENT B-NON-HODGKIN'S LYMPHOMA

The initial single-institution first-in-human studies of CD19 CAR T-cell therapy included a handful of patients with FL although most patients treated had more aggressive malignancies like B-cell acute lymphoblastic leukemia or large B-cell lymphoma given the lack of definitive alternative options and the concerns about CAR T-cell-related toxicities, including cytokine release syndrome (CRS) and immune effector cell therapy–associated neurotoxicity syndrome (ICANS).[23–26] These patients achieved compete responses (CRs) and prolonged survival at very high rates, with nearly 50% of patients remaining in remission at 5-year follow-up.[27] It made sense then to trial these therapies in FL relapsed multiple times, where CR rates, PFS, and OS are historically poor.[12,28]

The ZUMA-5 study was an open-label, multicenter phase 2 study of axicabtagene ciloleucel (axi-cel), an anti-CD19 CD28z CAR T-cell therapy in relapsed/refractory FL and MZL after 2 or more prior lines of therapy (including an anti-CD20 monoclonal antibody with an alkylating agent).[29] It enrolled and treated 148 patients, including 124 patients with FL and 24 patients with MZL. The first 84 FL patients to reach 12 months of follow-up were considered the pivotal registration cohort, whereas the MZL cohort was considered an exploratory cohort.

Among the pivotal FL cohort and the MZL cohort, the overall response rate (ORR) was 92%, with a CR rate of 76%. In FL, ORR was 94% with a CR rate of 79%, whereas in MZL, ORR was 83% with a CR rate of 65%, with 3 patients deemed unevaluable due to a lack of measurable disease on central radiology review. More important than these high response rates, these responses were durable. At a median follow-up of 17.5 months, the median duration of response (DOR), PFS, and OS were not reached, with over 60% of patients alive and without disease relapse at 18 months. These responses were similar for all high-risk subgroups, including patients with progression of disease within 24 months of chemoimmunotherapy (POD-24). Persistence of CAR T cells did not seem to be necessary for a durable response, as 69% of patients with ongoing response at 18 months had B-cell recovery despite 55% still having gene-marked CAR T cells indicating that these residual CAR T cells were not functional.

The SCHOLAR-5 study examined treatment patterns and outcomes of real-world FL patients on third line of treatment (LoT) or higher, for whom existing data are limited, to establish a historical baseline against which the results of ZUMA-5 were compared.[28] Data were obtained from the retrospective analysis of databases from 7 multinational institutions, as well as the DELTA trial of idelalisib in relapsed/refractory FL. It included adults (≥18 years) with grade 1-3a FL, initiating ≥3rd LoT (n = 128), including 87, 63, and 47 initiating therapy in the third, fourth, and fifth LoT, respectively. Just under one-third of the total patients progressed within 24 months of first-line chemoimmunotherapy (31%), while 28% had prior autologous stem cell transplantation, and 31% were refractory to the previous line of therapy. After applying propensity matching to more closely match the patients enrolled on ZUMA-5, using known prognostic variables, 85 patients from SCHOLAR-5 and 86 patients on ZUMA-5 were compared. The median follow-up was 25.4 and 23.3 months for SCHOLAR-5 and ZUMA-5, respectively. Median OS and PFS were significantly superior on ZUMA-5 compared with SCHOLAR-5 (59.8 m vs not reached; 12.7 m vs not reached).[11]

In diseases like FL and MZL, where survival is long and there are multiple well-tolerated options, safety and tolerability are exceedingly important. While the acute CAR T-cell toxicities such as CRS and ICANS are reversible and manageable, they carry morbidity and mortality risk that have to be balanced with the disease-related risks themselves. For all patients treated on ZUMA-5, the rates of any grade and grade 3 and higher CRS were 82% and 7%, respectively, and median time to CRS onset was 4 days. For patients with FL, these rates were 78% and 6%, respectively, compared with those in patients with MZL, where they were 100% and 8%, respectively. ICANS of any grade occurred in 59% of patients, 56% of patients with FL, and 71% of patients with MZL. ICANS was grade 3 or higher in 19% of patients and 15% and 38% in FL and MZL patients, respectively. In general, toxicities were less frequent, less intense, and more delayed in ZUMA-5 than in the ZUMA-1 trial of axi-cel in large B-cell lymphoma,[30] especially in the FL cohort. Deaths from adverse events occurred in 4 (3%) patients; one of which was multi-organ system failure in the setting of CRS, which was deemed to be treatment-related.

The ELARA study was the open-label, multicenter phase 2 study of tisagenlecleucel, an anti-CD19 4-1BBz CAR T-cell therapy, in relapsed/refractory FL in the third line and beyond, resulting in its approval in this setting.[31] This study treated 97 patients with an ORR of 86% and CR rate of 69%, and responses were comparable among high-risk subgroups like POD-24 and those with bulky disease. At the median follow-up of 9.9 months, responses were ongoing in nearly 70% of patients, and 50% of patients with an initial partial response (PR) had achieved a CR in subsequent follow-up. Unlike with axi-cel, most patients with FL treated with tisa-cel did not have B-cell recovery with short follow-up. CRS occurred in 49% of patients with a median time to onset of 4 days, but all were grade 1 or 2. ICANS occurred in 37% of patients and was of grade 3 or higher in 4%. One patient had grade 4 ICANS that occurred with concurrent HHV6 encephalitis. No patient had prolonged grade 3 or higher neutropenia. Consistent with this favorable toxicity profile, tisagenlecleucel was administered in the outpatient setting in 18% of patients. Among these 17 patients, 11 (65%) required inpatient hospitalization for postinfusion adverse event management. The median length of stay for hospitalization was 4 days, and none of the patients infused in the outpatient setting required intensive care unit care.

As ELARA was a single-arm trial, a comparison was performed to explore tisa-cel outcomes from the ELARA trial with usual care from a real-world cohort using the ReCORD-FL data. ReCORD-FL was a retrospective study involving data from 187 patients with relapsed/refractory FL treated in the third line and beyond at 10 centers across North America and Europe.[10] An indirect treatment comparison was performed for 97 patients from the ELARA trial and 143 patients from the ReCORD-FL study. The line of therapy for which outcomes were assessed was selected or matched between cohorts using propensity score modeling.[32] After baseline factor adjustment via weighting by odds, there was a statistically significantly improvement in CR rate (69.1 vs 37.3%), ORR (85.6 vs 69.1%), 12-month PFS (70.5 vs 51.9%), and 12-month OS (96.6 vs 71.7%) for tisa-cel over standard of care, respectively.

A study of a third anti-CD19 CAR T-cell therapy with a 4-1BB costimulatory domain, lisocabtagene ciloleucel (liso-cel) in relapsed/refractory FL is ongoing, and we await reporting of the results.

CHIMERIC ANTIGEN RECEPTOR T-CELL THERAPY IN MANTLE CELL LYMPHOMA

Unlike indolent B-NHL, patients with relapsed/refractory MCL, especially those relapsing after BTK inhibitors, have a very poor prognosis with a median OS less than 1 year.[4] Available therapies in this setting, like venetoclax and lenalidomide, have low overall and complete response rates with limited durability. Despite the toxicity profile, then, CAR T-cells, if they worked, would meet a critical unmet need in this population as evidenced in recent clinical trials (**Table 2**).

The ZUMA-2 study examined brexucabtagene autoleucel (brexu-cel) in relapsed/refractory MCL after chemoimmunotherapy and a BTK inhibitor.[33,34] Brexu-cel is the same CAR construct as axi-cel, except that there is an extra step during manufacturing to purge the pheresis product of any circulating CD19+ B cells. A total of 74 patients were enrolled in the trial and underwent leukapheresis. Brexu-cel was successfully manufactured for 71 patients (96%) and administered to 68 (92%). Among the first 60 treated patients who had at least 7 months of follow-up, ORR was 93% and CR rate was 67%. Over half of patients with an initial PR or stable disease had a deepening of response over time. Survival estimates at a median follow-up of 36 months include median DOR, PFS, and OS of 28.2 months, 25.8 months, and 46.6 months, respectively.[34] Unlike with axi-cel in FL, most patients with ongoing response at 12m and beyond had ongoing B-cell aplasia. Patients who had received bendamustine within 6 months of trial enrollment had a significantly lower CR rate and likelihood of ongoing response at 18 months. This was associated with a lower peak, as well as area under the curve, CAR T-cell concentrations consistent with a deleterious effect of bendamustine on T-cell function.

CRS occurred in 91% of patients. CRS was grade 3 or higher in 15% of patients; there was no grade 5 CRS. Median time to CRS was 2 days, and all events resolved within a median of 11 days. ICANS occurred in 63% of patients and was grade 3 or higher in 31% of patients. There was no grade 5 ICANS, but one patient did develop reversible grade 4 cerebral edema. Prolonged cytopenias of grade 3 or higher for longer than 90 days occurred in 26% of patients.

ZUMA-2 led to international approvals of brexu-cel for the treatment of relapsed/refractory MCL, and this is currently the only FDA-approved CAR T-cell product in MCL. The first report of brexu-cel in the real-world setting following commercial approval was published by Wang and colleagues.[35]

Of 189 patients who underwent leukapheresis, 168 (89%) received brexu-cel infusion. Of leukapheresed patients, 79% would not have met ZUMA-2 eligibility criteria. Best overall and complete response rates were 90% and 82%, respectively (see **Table 2**). At a median follow-up of 14.3 months after infusion, the estimates for 6- and 12-month PFS were 69% and 59%, respectively. Patients with high-risk MCL had a shorter PFS. Interestingly, patients with recent bendamustine exposure (within

Table 2
CAR T-cell therapies for mantle cell lymphoma

Data Set	CAR T-cell Product	N	Median Prior Lines of Therapy	Toxicities	Response	Survival
ZUMA-2 trial[33,34]	Brexucabtagene autoleucel	74	3 (1–5)	CRS Any grade 91% Grade 3+ 15% ICANS Any grade 63% Grade 3+ 31%	ORR 91% CR 68%	2 y PFS 53% 30 m OS 60%
European Early Access Program[55]	Brexucabtagene autoleucel	39	2 (1–8)	CRS Any grade 91% Grade 3+ 2.6% ICANS Any grade 64% Grade 3+ 36%	ORR 91% CR 79%	1y PFS 51% 1y OS 61%
US CAR T consortium[35]	Brexucabtagene autoleucel	189	3 (1–9)	CRS Any grade 91% Grade 3+ 8% ICANS Any grade 61% Grade 3+ 32%	ORR 89% CR 80%	1 y PFS 59% 1 y OS 75%
Non-approved CAR T-cell for MCL						
TRANSCEND NHL 001[36]	Lisocabtagene maraleucel	41	3 (1–7)	CRS Any grade 50% Grade 3+ 3% ICANS Any grade 28% Grade 3+ 9%	ORR 84% CR 59%	NR

Abbreviations: CAR, chimeric antigen receptor; CR, complete remission; CRS, cytokine release syndrome; ICANS, immune effector cell associated neurologic syndrome; N, number of patients; ORR, overall response rate; OS, overall survival; PFS, progression-free survival.

the last 24 months) also had shorter PFS and OS. Reassuringly, these results compare favorably with those of the ZUMA-2 study.

Liso-cel has been tested in relapsed/refractory MCL in the TRANSCEND NHL-001 study, which was also the pivotal study of liso-cel in relapsed/refractory large B-cell lymphoma leading to its approval in this disease in the third line and beyond. The MCL cohort has not been fully presented or published to date, but among the first 32 patients treated that have been presented, the ORR was 84% and CR rate was 59%.[36] At a median follow-up of 10.9 months for this cohort, the median DOR had not been reached. CRS occurred in 50% of patients and was grade 3 or higher in 3%. ICANS occurred in 34% of patients and was grade 3 or higher in 13%. Prolonged cytopenias beyond day 30 occurred in 34% of patients.

CHIMERIC ANTIGEN RECEPTOR T-CELL THERAPY IN CHRONIC LYMPHOCYTIC LEUKEMIA

As mentioned previously, the first successful reports of CD19 CAR T-cell therapy were in 3 patients with CLL treated with the product that was to become tisagenlecleucel.[37] Not only did these patients have deep responses after progressing through all available lines, but two of these patients have remained in remission for over 10 years at[20,38] last reporting. Despite this early success, larger trials of CAR T cells in CLL have been disappointing, perhaps owing to the negative effect the malignant B-cells have on T-cell function. To test this hypothesis, investigators at the University of Pennsylvania treated mouse models of CLL with autologous CAR T-cells that had resulted in response and lack of response in patients in clinical trials.[39] CAR T cells that led to response in patients led to response in mice, and CAR T cells that were ineffective in patients were ineffective in mice, pointing to a T-cell defect rather than a lymphoma-specific mechanism of resistance. On further analysis, CAR T cells that led to response had a distinct gene expression profile consistent with an early memory phenotype, had higher levels of STAT3 signaling, and had lower expression of PD1 and LAG3 than CAR T cells that did not lead to response. Patients who had received at least 6 months of the BTK inhibitor ibrutinib before T-cell collection were more likely to have these favorable T-cell attributes, leading to a phase 2 clinical trial wherein patients who had less than a CR to 6 months of ibrutinib were enrolled, had T-cells collected, and were treated with a humanized anti-CD19 CAR T-cell product.[21] This trial treated 19 patients, with a median follow-up of 41 months. By iwCLL criteria, the CR rate at 3 months was 44%, and the minimal residual disease (MRD) negativity rate was 72%. At 4 years, the estimated PFS was 70%, and estimated OS was 84%. Rates of any and grade 3 or higher CRS were 100% and 11%, respectively, and rates of any and grade 3 or higher ICANS was 28% and 6%, respectively.

Liso-cel may have more promise in CLL based on the results of the TRANSCEND CLL-004 study, which has been presented but not published to date. In 23 evaluable patients, ORR and CR rate was 82% and 45%, respectively.[40] At 12 months, 50% of patients were in ongoing response. CRS occurred in 74% of patients and was grade 3 or higher in 9%. ICANS occurred in 39% of patients and was grade 3 or higher in 22%. This study also included a cohort of patients treated with a liso-cel and ibrutinib initiated at the time of liso-cel infusion and continued for at least 90 days.[41] Nineteen patients were treated, and the ORR was 95% with a CR rate of 63%. MRD negativity was achieved in the blood and bone marrow in 89% and 79% of patients, respectively. CRS occurred in 74% of patients and was grade 3 or higher in 5%. ICANS occurred in 32% of patients and was grade 3 or higher in 16%. Although promising, the number are too small and follow-up too short to determine if there is a benefit in the addition of ibrutinib for 3+ months at the time of liso-cel infusion. Final results of this study are awaited and expected to be reviewed for consideration of FDA approval in the coming year.

DISCUSSION

As previously discussed, indolent B-NHL-like FL and MZL, MCL, and CLL all represent historically incurable malignancies with conventional therapies outside of alloSCT.[42] With variable natural histories, the need for definitive therapies like alloSCT at the expense of toxicity is considered differently across the diagnoses, with most patients with FL, MZL, and CLL unlikely to need such therapies, while most eligible patients with MCL likely to tolerate the toxicity risk to improve their relatively short OS. However, high-risk FL, MZL, and CLL all represent unmet needs for whom survival is limited and improved therapies are absolutely necessary.[43] It is in these patients, eligible relapsed MCL and high-risk relapsed FL, MZL, and CLL, that a therapy like CD19 CAR T-cell therapy offers a significant improvement over other available therapies, and given the prolonged remissions among the earliest patients with these diseases treated on the first-in-human studies, it is in these patients that the CD19 CAR T-cell therapy may have curative potential.[26,44,45] Unlike alloSCT, which provides life-long immune surveillance, it is unclear what sort of protection CD19 CAR T cells offer over time, and if these CAR T-cells do not persist, the question becomes how might they control disease for 10+ years in some cases and how might they cure these diseases? In order to do so, these CAR T cells must either be effective against a hypothetical lymphoma stem cell, which is expected to be quiescent and therefore resist killing by conventional therapies, or by recruiting host immune cells to provide more permanent protection. Longer follow-up is needed to assess whether a proportion of patients with these diseases are ultimately cured.

Regardless of the answer to this question, what is already known is that despite the remarkable success of these therapies, patients do still relapse. And for these patients, new agents are needed. CD20 bispecifics have proven to be highly effective in these diseases, are available off the shelf, and have a favorable toxicity profile, and thereby are excellent options to sequence either before or after CAR T-cell therapy.[46-50] In addition, exploration of these CAR T-cell therapies in earlier lines of therapy, including in the second line for POD-24 FL and for high-risk MCL patients in an MRD-positive CR, are ongoing. CARs that target multiple or new antigens, including dual-antigen-targeted CARs (ie, CD19/CD20 or CD19/CD22 CARs),[51-53] and anti-ROR1 CAR T-cells could either supplant or be sequenced after CD19 CAR T cells in these diseases, respectively.[54] While the jury is still out as to whether engineered cell therapies can cure these otherwise incurable diseases, there is no doubt that they are extending survival and having an irrefutable positive impact on patient outcomes.

REFERENCES

1. Carbone A, et al. Follicular lymphoma. Nat Rev Dis Primers 2019;5:83.
2. Mohty R, Kharfan-Dabaja MA. CAR T-cell therapy for follicular lymphoma and mantle cell lymphoma. Ther Adv Hematology 2022;13. 20406207221142132.
3. van der Straten L, Hengeveld PJ, Kater AP, et al. Treatment Approaches to Chronic Lymphocytic Leukemia With High-Risk Molecular Features. Frontiers Oncol 2021;11:780085.
4. Jain P, Dreyling M, Seymour JF, et al. High-Risk Mantle Cell Lymphoma: Definition, Current Challenges, and Management. J Clin Oncol 2020;38:4302-16.

5. Kumar E, Pickard L, Okosun J. Pathogenesis of follicular lymphoma: genetics to the microenvironment to clinical translation. Brit J Haematol 2021;194:810–21.

6. Forstpointner R, et al. The addition of rituximab to a combination of fludarabine, cyclophosphamide, mitoxantrone (FCM) significantly increases the response rate and prolongs survival as compared with FCM alone in patients with relapsed and refractory follicular and mantle cell lymphomas: results of a prospective randomized study of the German Low-Grade Lymphoma Study Group. Blood 2004;104:3064–71.

7. Sarkozy C, et al. Cause of Death in Follicular Lymphoma in the First Decade of the Rituximab Era: A Pooled Analysis of French and US Cohorts. J Clin Oncol 2019;37:144–52.

8. Casulo C, et al. Early Relapse of Follicular Lymphoma After Rituximab Plus Cyclophosphamide, Doxorubicin, Vincristine, and Prednisone Defines Patients at High Risk for Death: An Analysis From the National LymphoCare Study. J Clin Oncol 2015;33:2516–22.

9. Batlevi CL, et al. Follicular lymphoma in the modern era: survival, treatment outcomes, and identification of high-risk subgroups. Blood Cancer J 2020;10:74.

10. Salles G, et al. A Retrospective Cohort Study of Treatment Outcomes of Adult Patients With Relapsed or Refractory Follicular Lymphoma (ReCORD-FL). Hemasphere 2022;6:e745.

11. Ghione P, et al. Comparative effectiveness of ZUMA-5 (axi-cel) vs SCHOLAR-5 external control in relapsed/refractory follicular lymphoma. Blood 2022;140:851–60.

12. Casulo C, et al. Treatment patterns and outcomes of patients with relapsed or refractory follicular lymphoma receiving three or more lines of systemic therapy (LEO CReWE): a multicentre cohort study. Lancet Haematol 2022;9:e289–300.

13. Kanters S, et al. Clinical outcomes in patients relapsed/refractory after ≥2 prior lines of therapy for follicular lymphoma: a systematic literature review and meta-analysis. BMC Cancer 2023;23:74.

14. Cheah CY, Zucca E, Rossi D, et al. Marginal zone lymphoma: present status and future perspectives. Haematologica 2022;107:35–43.

15. Zucca E, et al. Marginal zone lymphomas: ESMO Clinical Practice Guidelines for diagnosis, treatment and follow-up. Ann Oncol 2020;31:17–29.

16. Burkart M, Karmali R. Relapsed/Refractory Mantle Cell Lymphoma: Beyond BTK Inhibitors. J Personalized Medicine 2022;12:376.

17. Kipps TJ, et al. Chronic lymphocytic leukaemia. Nat Rev Dis Primers 2017;3:16096.

18. Frey NV, et al. Long-Term Outcomes From a Randomized Dose Optimization Study of Chimeric Antigen Receptor Modified T Cells in Relapsed Chronic Lymphocytic Leukemia. J Clin Oncol 2020;38:2862–71.

19. Turtle CJ, et al. Durable Molecular Remissions in Chronic Lymphocytic Leukemia Treated With CD19-Specific Chimeric Antigen Receptor–Modified T Cells After Failure of Ibrutinib. J Clin Oncol 2017;35:851.

20. Porter DL, et al. Chimeric antigen receptor T cells persist and induce sustained remissions in relapsed refractory chronic lymphocytic leukemia. Sci Transl Med 2015;7:303ra139.

21. Gill S, et al. Anti-CD19 CAR T Cells in Combination with Ibrutinib for the Treatment of Chronic Lymphocytic Leukemia. Blood Adv 2022;6:5774–85.

22. Fraietta JA, et al. Ibrutinib enhances chimeric antigen receptor T-cell engraftment and efficacy in leukemia. Blood 2016;127:1117–27.

23. Porter DL, Levine BL, Michael K, et al. Antigen Receptor–Modified T Cells in Chronic Lymphoid Leukemia. New Engl J Med 2011;365:725–33.

24. Shah NN, et al. Long-Term Follow-Up of CD19-CAR T-Cell Therapy in Children and Young Adults With B-ALL. J Clin Oncol 2021;39:1650–9.

25. Kochenderfer JN, et al. Chemotherapy-Refractory Diffuse Large B-Cell Lymphoma and Indolent B-Cell Malignancies Can Be Effectively Treated With Autologous T Cells Expressing an Anti-CD19 Chimeric Antigen Receptor. J Clin Oncol 2014;33:540–9.

26. Stephen SS, et al. Chimeric Antigen Receptor T Cells in Refractory B-Cell Lymphomas. New Engl J Med 2017;377:2545–54.

27. Chong EA, Ruella M, Schuster SJ, et al. at the U. of. Five-Year Outcomes for Refractory B-Cell Lymphomas with CAR T-Cell Therapy. New Engl J Med 2021;384:673–4.

28. Ghione P, et al. Treatment patterns and outcomes in relapsed/refractory follicular lymphoma: results from the international SCHOLAR-5 study. Haematologica 2022;108:822–32.

29. Jacobson CA, et al. Axicabtagene ciloleucel in relapsed or refractory indolent non-Hodgkin lymphoma (ZUMA-5): a single-arm, multicentre, phase 2 trial. Lancet Oncol 2022;23:91–103.

30. Neelapu SS, et al. Axicabtagene Ciloleucel CAR T-Cell Therapy in Refractory Large B-Cell Lymphoma. New Engl J Medicine 2017;377:2531–44.

31. Fowler NH, et al. Tisagenlecleucel in adult relapsed or refractory follicular lymphoma: the phase 2 ELARA trial. Nat Med 2022;28:325–32.

32. Salles GA, et al. Efficacy comparison of tisagenlecleucel vs usual care in patients with relapsed or refractory follicular lymphoma. Blood Adv 2022;6:5835–43.

33. Wang M, et al. KTE-X19 CAR T-Cell Therapy in Relapsed or Refractory Mantle-Cell Lymphoma. New Engl J Med 2020;382:1331–42.

34. Wang M, et al. Three-Year Follow-Up of KTE-X19 in Patients With Relapsed/Refractory Mantle Cell Lymphoma, Including High-Risk Subgroups, in the ZUMA-2 Study. J Clin Oncol 2023;41:555–67.

35. Wang Y, et al. Brexucabtagene Autoleucel for Relapsed or Refractory Mantle Cell Lymphoma in Standard-of-Care Practice: Results From the US Lymphoma CAR T Consortium. J Clin Oncol 2023;JCO2201797. https://doi.org/10.1200/jco.22.01797.

36. Palomba ML, et al. Safety and Preliminary Efficacy in Patients with Relapsed/Refractory Mantle Cell Lymphoma Receiving Lisocabtagene Maraleucel in Transcend NHL 001. Blood 2020;136:10–1.

37. Kalos M, et al. T Cells with Chimeric Antigen Receptors Have Potent Antitumor Effects and Can Establish Memory in Patients with Advanced Leukemia. Sci Transl Med 2011;3:95ra73.

38. Melenhorst JJ, et al. Decade-long leukaemia remissions with persistence of CD4+ CAR T cells. Nature 2022;602:503–9.

39. Fraietta JA, et al. Determinants of response and resistance to CD19 chimeric antigen receptor (CAR) T cell therapy of chronic lymphocytic leukemia. Nat Med 2018;24:563–71.

40. Siddiqi T, et al. Phase 1 TRANSCEND CLL 004 study of lisocabtagene maraleucel in patients with relapsed/refractory CLL or SLL. Blood 2021;139:1794–806.

41. Wierda WG, et al. Transcend CLL 004: Phase 1 Cohort of Lisocabtagene Maraleucel (liso-cel) in Combination with Ibrutinib for Patients with Relapsed/Refractory (R/R) Chronic Lymphocytic Leukemia/Small Lymphocytic Lymphoma (CLL/SLL). Blood 2020;136:39–40.

42. Kuruvilla J. The role of autologous and allogeneic stem cell transplantation in the management of indolent B-cell lymphoma. Blood 2016;127:2093–100.

43. Matasar MJ, et al. Follicular Lymphoma: Recent and Emerging Therapies, Treatment Strategies, and Remaining Unmet Needs. Oncol 2019;24:e1236–50.

44. Cappell KM, Kochenderfer JN. Long-term outcomes following CAR T cell therapy: what we know so far. Nat Rev Clin Oncol 2023;1–13. https://doi.org/10.1038/s41571-023-00754-1.

45. Cappell KM, et al. Long-Term Follow-Up of Anti-CD19 Chimeric Antigen Receptor T-Cell Therapy. J Clin Oncol 2020;38:3805–15.

46. Budde LE, et al. Safety and efficacy of mosunetuzumab, a bispecific antibody, in patients with relapsed or refractory follicular lymphoma: a single-arm, multicentre, phase 2 study. Lancet Oncol 2022;23:1055–65.

47. Rodgers TD, et al. Early Relapse in First-Line Follicular Lymphoma: A Review of the Clinical Implications and Available Mitigation and Management Strategies. Oncol Ther 2021;9:329–46.

48. Lopedote P, Shadman M. Targeted Treatment of Relapsed or Refractory Follicular Lymphoma: Focus on the Therapeutic Potential of Mosunetuzumab. Cancer Management Res 2023;15:257–64.

49. Phillips T, et al. Improvements in Lymphoma Symptoms and Health-Related Quality of Life in Patients with Relapsed or Refractory Large B-Cell Lymphoma Treated with Subcutaneous Epcoritamab (EPCORE NHL-1). Blood 2022;140:8022–3.

50. Thieblemont C, et al. Epcoritamab, a Novel, Subcutaneous CD3xCD20 Bispecific T-Cell–Engaging Antibody, in Relapsed or Refractory Large B-Cell Lymphoma: Dose Expansion in a Phase I/II Trial. J Clin Oncol 2023;41:2238–47.

51. Yin Y, et al. Parallel CD19/CD20 CAR-Activated T-Cells Are More Effective for Refractory B-Cell Lymphoma In Vitro and In Vivo. Evid-based Compl Alt 2022;2022:1227308.

52. Spiegel JY, et al. CAR T cells with dual targeting of CD19 and CD22 in adult patients with recurrent or refractory B cell malignancies: a phase 1 trial. Nat Med 2021;27:1419–31.

53. Zhang Y, et al. Long-term activity of tandem CD19/CD20 CAR therapy in refractory/relapsed B-cell lymphoma: a single-arm, phase 1–2 trial. Leukemia 2022;36:189–96.

54. Peng H, et al. ROR1-targeting switchable CAR-T cells for cancer therapy. Oncogene 2022;41:4104–14.

55. Iacoboni G, et al. Real-world evidence of brexucabtagene autoleucel for the treatment of relapsed or refractory mantle cell lymphoma. Blood Adv 2022;6:3606–10.

Chimeric Antigen Receptor T Cells in Multiple Myeloma

Parth Shah, MD[a,b,]*, Adam S. Sperling, MD, PhD[b,c]

KEYWORDS

- Multiple myeloma • CAR-T • BCMA • GPRC5D • BiTEs

KEY POINTS

- Chimeric antigen receptor (CAR)-T in multiple myeloma is a rapidly evolving field.
- Unlike most other malignancies, several markers are in advanced stages of clinical investigation in multiple myeloma, with several having a unique side effect profile.
- Alternate sources of CARs such as allogeneic CARs and the use of combination therapy will be critical in optimizing their use in myeloma therapy.

BACKGROUND

Multiple myeloma (MM) is the second most common hematological malignancy with an approximate incidence of up to 8.5 cases per 100,000 persons per year.[1–4] Despite considerable advances in treatment options, including new generations of proteasome inhibitors, immunomodulatory drugs, and monoclonal antibodies, MM remains incurable with most patients relapsing and eventually dying of disease-related complications.[5]

A substantial proportion of patients either do not respond to current therapies or acquire resistance to treatment. Patients who are triple-class or penta-class refractory have an overall survival (OS) of 9.2 and 5.6 months, respectively, highlighting the need for improved therapeutic options for patients with MM.[6] It is well accepted that MM develops in a dysfunctional immune environment, evidenced by the fact that most active anti-MM therapies target the immune microenvironment in addition to neoplastic plasma cells.[7] This includes the immunomodulatory imide drugs (IMiDs), which upregulate IL-2 in T cells, proteosome inhibitors that induce immunogenic cell death, and monoclonal antibodies that promote antibody-dependent cellular toxicity and natural killer (NK)-cell-mediated tumor cell killing.[8] New treatment approaches

[a] Department of Hematology, Dartmouth Cancer Center, 1 Medical Center Drive, Lebanon, NH 03750, USA; [b] Medical Oncology, Dana-Farber Cancer Institute, 450 Brookline Avenue, Boston, MA 02115, USA; [c] Division of Hematology, Brigham and Women's Hospital, 75 Francis Street, Boston, MA 02115, USA
* Corresponding author. 1 Medical Center Drive, Lebanon, NH 03750.
E-mail address: Parth_Shah@DFCI.HARVARD.EDU

Hematol Oncol Clin N Am 37 (2023) 1089–1105
https://doi.org/10.1016/j.hoc.2023.05.008
0889-8588/23/© 2023 Elsevier Inc. All rights reserved.

have continued to focus on immune modulation as a mechanism of anti-MM activity, including the development of antibody–drug conjugates (ADCs),[9] bispecific T-cell engaging antibodies (BiTEs), and chimeric antigen receptor (CAR) T cells. In particular, CAR-T cells and BiTEs have demonstrated high overall and durable responses leading to their recent approvals by the FDA.[10-14]

CAR-T cells are genetically engineered T cells modified ex vivo to express a chimeric receptor constituted by an antigen receptor containing a single-chain variable fragment (scFv) and an intracellular T-cell receptor (TCR) signaling domain.[15] The scFv is the recognition domain directed to target unique antigens on tumor cells. The intracellular domain of the CAR contains signaling components including domains from CD3-zeta (first generation), in addition to a costimulatory domain such as CD28 or 41bb (second generation) or both (third generation).[16] Of note, CAR-T target cell recognition and activation does not require major histocompatibility complex (MHC)-mediated presentation of antigens. During manufacturing, the patient's own T cells or donor-derived T cells, in the case of allogeneic CAR-T, are isolated and genetically modified to express the CAR. Adoptively transferred CAR-T cells are therefore equipped to induce and sustain long-lasting remissions through a synergy of antibody-based target cell recognition and the memory and effector function of T cells.[17] This approach differs from BiTEs, which serve as a molecular bridge bringing tumor cells into close proximity of native T cells and activating them.[18]

Here, we review recent data on targets in MM, approaches to developing cell therapies targeting them and the future outlook for this developing field.[19-22]

Chimeric Antigen Receptor T Sources

CAR-T cells are currently derived from 1 of 2 sources, either autologous or allogeneic T cells.[23] Autologous CARs have the advantage of limited risk of immune rejection, and no risk of inducing graft versus host disease, thus limiting potential toxicity. However, this approach does have several limitations including the ability to harvest T cells of adequate quality and quantity as many patients have been exposed to multiple lines of cytotoxic and anti-lymphocytic therapy that may alter T-cell function and numbers.[24] Also, the relatively long times needed to manufacture cells, often 4 to 6 weeks, can limit use in patients with aggressive or rapidly progressive disease.[25]

Efforts are ongoing to develop novel manufacturing approaches to decrease the time in culture (10–14 days for standard CARs), decrease vein-to-vein time, and potentially improve the quality of the CAR T-cell product by selecting cells with more favorable T-cell phenotypes. These approaches have used shortened ex vivo manufacturing time completed in as little as 2 days with cell expansion occurring in vivo. Preliminary results have demonstrated promising response rates and evidence of selection for CAR T-cell products enriched for stem and central memory phenotypes.[26-28] Whether these approaches will lead to improved outcomes for patients remains to be seen.

Allogenic CAR-T cells represent an off-the-shelf alternative to traditional CAR manufacturing. The potential immunogenicity and the short persistence of the product remain the main challenges to using allogenic CAR-T cells.[29,30] A second issue is the potential for graft versus host disease (GVHD) driven by the infused T cells. A principal driver of GVHD following allogeneic CAR T-cell administration is thought to be the presence of αβ T cells, the cell type mostly commonly used to generate CAR-T cells. Two main strategies have been developed to reduce the risk of GVHD: the selection of virus-specific T cells that do not target host antigens and the genetic ablation of the endogenous TCR locus.[31,32] The use of virus-specific memory T cells during hematopoietic stem cell transplantation was able to control viral infections without occurrence of GVHD.[33,34] A small clinical trial using allogeneic virus-specific T cells expressing the anti-CD19 CAR construct demonstrated that these were safe and capable of anti-tumor activity without clinical manifestation of GVHD. New clinical trials are ongoing using anti-CD19 and anti-CD30 CAR-T cells engineered with Epstein–Barr virus-specific allogeneic T cells.[30] To overcome host recognition and rejection, allogeneic CAR-T manufacturing strategies have used the deletion of antigens like CD52 such that anti-CD52 antibodies can be used during lymphodepletion to selectively remove host T cells.[30]

Targets in Multiple Myeloma

In the ideal world, the target for cell therapies would be expressed at a high level on malignant plasma cells, not be expressed on any normal tissues, and be required for MM cell viability thus limiting the risk of antigen loss. Much work has focused on identifying such targets and most trials for CAR-T in MM have primarily focused on the B-cell maturation antigen (BCMA). BCMA is the target for the 2 FDA-approved CAR T-cell products in MM.[35] It is predominantly expressed on differentiated B cells and has high expression on malignant plasma cells.[19] BCMA, also known as TNF receptor superfamily 17 (TNFRSF17), is a cell surface receptor and functions to promote prosurvival signals upon binding to its ligands—B-cell activator of the TNF family (BAFF) and a proliferation inducing ligand (APRIL)—participating in the proliferation of MM cells.[20] The extracellular domain of BCMA can be cleaved off of the surface of cells by the membrane-bound protease γ-secretase and a soluble portion can thus be shed from MM cells (sBCMA). sBCMA serves as a biomarker of MM tumor burden and shedding may limit therapeutic efficacy by decreasing the concentration of antigen on the membrane of MM cells.[21]

In addition to BCMA, other agents under development target myeloma-specific antigens including G protein-coupled receptor class C group 5 member D (GPRC5D) and Fc receptor homolog 5 (FcRH5) and have shown initial promise in patients with MM, even among those who have previously been exposed to BCMA-targeting drugs.[22] GPRC5D is normally expressed only in the hair follicle and some epithelial cells and is not expressed on normal plasma cells.[36] However, it was identified because of its high expression in neoplastic plasma cells and MM cell lines. Its function in normal skin cells and in neoplastic plasma cells is unknown. Importantly, its expression is independent of BCMA, potentially allowing dual targeting of these antigens.[36,37,38] GPRC5D-based CAR-T cells as well as a BiTEs are undergoing advanced stages of development and are discussed more below.[36,37–39]

FcRH5 is a type I membrane protein that is expressed on B cells and plasma cells and is found on myeloma cells with near 100% prevalence.[40] The function of FcRH5 is unknown, but its expression is higher on neoplastic as compared to normal plasma cells.[41] ADCs and BiTEs have been developed to target this antigen. BFCR4350 A, a humanized bispecific antibody, targets the most membrane-proximal domain of FcRH5 on MM cells and CD3 on T cells. Initial safety and activity data with BFCR4350 A have been encouraging in heavily pretreated myeloma patients.[40,42]

CD138 has been a target of interest in myeloma for many years as it is used as one of the pathologic hallmarks of plasma cells. A CAR-T targeting CD138 demonstrated modest activity but the broad expression of CD138 in epithelial, endothelial, and vascular smooth muscle cells, continues to be a concern in utilization of this target.[43,44]

Although CD19 is expressed in only a subset of patients with MM, the availability of highly active CARs targeting this antigen has led to their use in patients with MM with mixed results.[45] Although there have been reports of deep and durable responses, it is unclear how generalizable this is. Initial efforts to utilize co-infusion of anti-BCMA and anti-CD19 CARs have not demonstrated improved activity over anti-BCMA CARs alone.[46] However, interest still remains in this approach and dual CARs such as GC012 F targeting BCMA and CD19 manufactured in under 36 hours have also made it to early phase clinical trials.[28]

In addition to these well-validated targets, a number of other antigens are being explored in patients with MM.[25] Dual targeting CARs against BCMA and CD38, the antigen targeted by monoclonal antibodies daratumumab and isatuximab, have shown evidence of activity and long-term persistence in initial studies.[22,25] The CARAMABA project is currently utilizing anti-SLAMF7, the antigen targeted by elotuzumab, CARs developed using a sleeping beauty transposon-based manufacturing strategy and is currently recruiting patients.[47] However, preclinical data have looked promising results from the first-in-human study that has not been publicly presented. Kappa and Lambda light chain, which are expressed on the surface of most MM cells, have also been targeted by CAR-T cells in preclinical models and remain a promising approach.[48] Finally, other mature B-cell sell surface molecules such as APRIL are potential targets in MM and CAR-T cells against these targets are being developed.[49,50]

Autologous Chimeric Antigen Receptor T Cells

Several autologous CAR T-cell products have been studied in clinical trials and 2 were recently FDA approved, fundamentally changing the treatment paradigm for patients with relapsed and refractory MM (**Table 1**). Idecabtagene vicleucel (ide-cel, bb2121) is a BCMA-directed CAR T-cell therapy with a humanized scFv and a 41BB costimulatory domain.[13] In the phase 1/2 KaRRMa-1 study, 140 patients with heavily pretreated relapsed and refractory MM were enrolled and 128 patients were infused with ide-cel at doses ranging from 150 to 450 million cells following standard lymphodepletion with fludarabine and cyclophosphamide. With a median follow-up of 13.3 months, 94 of 128 patients (73%) had a response, and 42 of 128 (33%) achieved a complete response (CR) or better. The side effect profile was consistent with other CAR-T products with hematologic adverse events (AE) being most common: neutropenia (91%), anemia (70%), and thrombocytopenia (63%) were the most common events. Cytokine release syndrome (CRS) was reported in 84% of patients with only 7 (5%) being grade 3 or higher. Neurotoxic effects manifested as the immune effector cell-associated neurotoxicity syndrome (ICANS) developed in 18% of patients and were grade 3 in 4 patients (3%). The median time to the onset of CRS was 1 day (range, 1–12), with a median duration of 5 days (range, 1–63). Management of CRS and ICANS included use of IL-6 blocking agents such as tocilizumab in 52% and glucocorticoids in 15% of patients. Three patients (2%) died within 8 weeks of infusion from ide-cel related AEs (bronchopulmonary aspergillosis, gastrointestinal hemorrhage, and CRS). One patient (1%) died between 8 weeks and 6 months from an ide-cel related AE (cytomegalovirus pneumonia).[13] These data led to the FDA-approval of ide-cel in 2021 for patients with MM relapsed after at least 4 prior lines of therapy.

Data from the confirmatory phase 3 randomized KaRMMa-3 trial were recently published.[51] A total of 386 patients with MM relapsed after at least 3 prior lines underwent randomization: 254 to ide-cel and 132 to standard-of-care chemotherapy. At a follow-up of 18.6 months, the median progression-free survival was 13.3 months in the ide-cel group, as compared with 4.4 months in the control group (hazard ratio for disease progression or death, 0.49). The overall response rate (ORR) was 71% in the ide-cel group and in 42% in the standard-regimen group ($P < 0.001$); a complete response occurred in 39% and 5% of patients, respectively. Data on OS are still immature.[51]

Efforts have been made to promote the production of CAR-T cells with favorable characteristic, including increased number of stem and central memory like T cells.

Table 1
Clinical trials of autologous chimeric antigen receptor T cells and their outcomes

	Ide-cel KARMMA[13] (n = 128)	Cilta-cel CARTITUDE-1[12] (n = 97)	bb21217 CRB-4029[54] (n = 69)	P-BCMA 101 PRIME[84] (n = 53)	Orva-cel EVOLVE[85] (n = 62)	CT053[7] (n = 20)	ALLO-715 UNIVERSAL[63,11] (n = 31)	MCARH109 (n = 17)
Phase	II	Ib/II	I	I/II	I/II	I	I	I
Target/Costim	BCMA/41BB	BCMA/4-1BB	BCMA/41BB	BCMA/41BB	BCMA/4-1BB	BCMA/4-1BB	BCMA/4-1BB	GPRC5D/4-1BB
scFv	Chimeric mouse	Chimeric llama	Chimeric mouse	Chimeric mouse	Human	Human	Human	
Specificity	Autologous	Autologous	Autologous - PI3K inhibitor	Autologous—piggyBac	Autologous	Autologous	Allogenic CD52 & TCR Kos	Autologous
No. of infused CAR-T cells	150-450 M	0.75 M/kg	150-450 M	51-1178 M	150-600 M	50-180	40-180 M	24-450 M
Population age, median (range) years of prior lines, median (range)	61 (33-78)	61 (43-78)	62 (33-76)	60 (42-74)	61 (33-77)	55 (39-67)	65 (46-76)	60(38-76)
# of prior lines, median (range)	6 (3-16)	6 (3-18)	6 (3-17)	8 (2-18)	6 (3-18)	4 (2-11)	5 (3-11)	5
Triple-/Penta- refractory	84%/26%	86%/28%	64%/NR	60%/NR	94%/48%	NR	NR	94%/NR
Efficacy	@450 M:							
ORR	82%	98%	60%	50%-75%	92%	100%	50%-75%	44%-90%
CR, rate	39%	80%	28%	NR	36%	35%	NR	35%
PFS, median months	12.1	66%	NR	NR	NR	NR	NR	NR
CRS All grade/grade ≥ 3	96%/6%	95%/5%	70%/4%	17%/0%	89%/3%	79%/0%	45%/0%	88%/5%
Median onset, days (range)	1 (1- 10)	7 (1-12)	2 (1- 20)	NR	2 (1-4)	2 (1-4)	NR	NR
Median duration, days (range)	7 (1-63)	4 (1-97)	4 (1-28)	NR	4 (1-10)	4 (1-8)	NR	NR
Tocilizum ab/steroid use	67%/22%	69%/22%	45%/15%	7%/6%	76%/52%	32%/21%	19/10	53%/24%
ICANS All Grade / Grade 3	@450M: 20% / 6% Rest : 17% / 1%	12% / 9%	16% / 4%	4% / 4%	13% / 3%	NR	11% / 0%	0% / 0%

(continued on next page)

Table 1
(continued)

Median onset, days (range)	2 (1–10)	8 (3–12)	27 (11–108)	7 (2–24)	NR	4 (1–6)	NR	NA	NR
Median duration, days (range)	5 (1– 22)	4 (1–12)	75 (2–160)	2 (1–188)	NR	4 (1–10)	NR	NA	NR

Main reported clinical trials of CAR-T cells in multiple myeloma. Data of efficacy and safety are shown.

Abbreviations: Costim, costimulatory domain; CR, complete remission; CRS, cytokine release syndrome; ICANS, immune effector cell-associated neurotoxicity syndrome; ORR, overall response rate; PFS, progression free survival; scFv, single-chain variable fragment.

The use of PI3K inhibitors has been shown to alter T-cell differentiation in vitro.[52,53] This was the basis of the CRB-402 trial of bb21217, which used the same primary CAR-T construct as in the KaRMMa studies with the addition of a PI3K inhibitor (bb007) during ex vivo culture to enrich the product for memory-like T cells and decrease the proportion of highly differentiated or senescent T cells. Seventy-two patients received bb21217 at doses ranging from 150 to 450 million CAR-T cells with a median follow-up for all patients of 9.0 months. Toxicity and overall response rates were similar to that seen in the KaRMMa-1 study. Analysis of peripheral blood samples collected 15 days post bb21217 infusion demonstrated that patients with higher than the median number of CD8+ CAR-T cells expressing CD27 and CD28 had significantly longer duration of response (DOR) compared to patients with lower than the median values.[54] However, this did not result in improved overall outcomes and development of this product has been stopped.

The CARTITUDE-1 study utilized ciltacabtagene autoleucel (cilta-cel), a CAR T-cell therapy that differs from other products due to the presence of 2 BCMA-targeting single-domain antibodies in its extracellular domain, thus increasing the avidity for BCMA. One-hundred thirteen patients with relapsed and refractory MM were enrolled in this study, 97 of whom received a cilta-cel infusion at the recommended phase 2 dose of 0.75×10^6 CAR + viable T cells per kilogram. Median follow-up was 12.4 months and ORR was 97% with 67% achieving a CR or better. The median time to first response was 1 month and responses deepened over time. The median DOR was not reached (95% CI 15.9—not estimable), nor was the PFS (16.8—not estimable). The 12-month progression-free rate (PFR) was 77% and OS rate was 89%. Fourteen deaths occurred in the study: 6 due to treatment-related AEs, 5 due to progressive disease, and 3 due to treatment-unrelated AEs. CRS occurred in 95% of patients, with 6% grade 3. Median time to CRS onset from cilta-cel infusion was 7 days and median duration was 4 days (excluding 1 patient with 97-day duration). Patients received tocilizumab (67%), corticosteroids (22%), and anakinra (19%). Neurotoxicity after cilta-cel infusion, including ICANS, occurred in 21% of 97 patients, but only 2 patients had grade 3 events.

The median time to ICANS onset was 8 days, and the median duration was 4 days. ICANS resolved in all 16 patients.[12] In a small number of patients, late neurotoxicity following cilta-cel was observed with development of gait disturbance and parkinsonian-like symptoms. The mechanism by which this occurs is unknown but has been hypothesized to be related to low-level expression of BCMA in the substantia nigra.[55] Efforts to prevent this devastating complication have focused on minimizing the degree of CAR-T expansion by minimizing disease burden at the time of infusion. Recent updated data showed that at a median follow-up of 27.7 months, the median PFS and OS were still not reached; 27-month PFS and OS rates were 54.9% and 70.4% (95% CI, 60.1–78.6), respectively.[56] Overall response rates and DOR have clearly been higher with cilta-cel as compared to ide-cel, albeit with increased rates of CRS and ICANS, but the reasons for this remain unclear and are an important area of further investigation. A confirmatory phase 3 study is underway.

Resistance to anti-BCMA therapies has been attributed a number of mechanisms including downregulation of BCMA, mutation or deletion of the TNFRSF17 gene, as well as lack of persistent or activity of the engineered T cells.[57–60] Thus, novel therapies targeting new MM antigens and approaches to overcoming T-cell exhaustion and senescence will be needed in the future to combine with BCMA-targeting agents.[38]

One such approach is the use of CAR-T cells targeting GPRC5D. A phase I trial of a GPRC5D targeting CAR-T cell, MCARH109, enrolled 17 patients with relapsed and refractory MM, some of whom had been previously exposed to anti-BCMA therapy.[37] A response was reported in 71% of the patients in the entire cohort. Importantly, patients who had received prior anti-BCMA therapy also showed responses. At the 450×10^6 CAR T-cell dose, 1 patient had grade 4 CRS and ICANS, and 2 patients had a grade 3 cerebellar disorder of unclear cause. No cerebellar disorders, ICANS of any grade, or CRS of grade 3 or higher occurred in the 12 patients who received doses of 25×10^6 to 150×10^6 cells. As expected, based on the normal tissue expression of GPRC5D, on-target but off-tumor toxic effects included transient rash (18%), dysgeusia (12%), and nail changes (65%), all of which were limited to grade 1 or 2. As compared with the bispecific GPRC5D T-cell engager talquetamab, the frequency and severity of rash and dysgeusia were lower with MCARH109.[37,39]

CD19 CAR-T cells have been utilized in the treatment of myeloma with examples of patient responses leading to the idea of targeting both CD19 and BCMA in the same patients.[45]

Approaches to dual targeting of CAR-T cells are in early stages. GC012 F is an autologous CAR-T therapeutic dual-targeting BCMA and CD19 using a next-day manufacturing platform. Sixteen transplant-eligible newly diagnosed patients with high-risk MM received GC012 F infusion in a phase 1 clinical trial. The ORR was 100% and 87.5% of patients achieved a CR or better with all evaluable patients achieving minimal residual disease (MRD) negativity in all dose levels. Because patients also received standard MM induction therapy prior to CAR-T infusion the role of GC012 F in mediating these responses and the importance of the CD19-targeting component cannot be assessed. Only 25% of patients experienced grade 1 to 2 CRS. No cases of ICANS or other neurotoxicity of any grade were observed.[25,28]

A phase I clinical trial of anti-BCMA chimeric antigen receptor T cells (CAR-T-BCMA) with or without anti-CD19 CAR-T cells (huCART19) in patients with MM with low burden of disease responding to third- or later-line therapy (N = 10) or high-risk patients responding to first-line therapy (N = 20), followed by IMiD maintenance was conducted by the group at UPenn. No high-grade CRS and only one instance of low-grade neurologic toxicity was observed. Data on responses were limited and difficult to interpret; however, these data do provide additional evidence for the safety of administering CAR-T cells in earlier lines of therapy.[46] Multiple efforts are currently underway to provide CAR-T cells to patients at earlier stages in disease treatment including in newly diagnosed patients, possibly as a replacement for autologous transplantation, as consolidation for patients who do not achieve an adequate response to induction and in high-risk patients who relapse quickly after first-line therapy.[61]

Other novel approaches to developing antigen recognition domains have also shown activity and may provide unique methods for making dual-targeting CAR-T cells in the future. CART ddBCMA is an autologous anti-BCMA CAR T-cell therapy with a unique, synthetic binding domain targeting BCMA. Instead of the typical scFv approach, the binding domain is a small stable protein, called a D-Domain, comprising only 73 amino acids. The small size of the domain allows for high expression on the surface of T cells and related technology allowing separate infusion of CAR-T cells and the antigen-specificity domain may provide flexible binding domains with the ability to target multiple antigens. Initial data utilizing CART-ddBCMA in 31 patients showed an ORR of 100%. Ninety percent of patients had CRS, with most cases being low grade. No neurologic side effects were noted.[62]

Allogeneic Chimeric Antigen Receptor T Cells

Allogeneic CAR-T cells have been of great interest given the potential ease of use and rapid availability for patients with aggressive and rapidly progressive disease. To bring

Table 2
Allogeneic chimeric antigen receptor T cells in multiple myeloma

Developer	CAR T-Cell Product	Target Antigen	Allogeneic Technology	Tools and Vectorization	Development Phase and Trial Reference
Allogene Therapeutics	ALLO715	BCMA	TRAC and CD52 KO	TALEN mRNA (KO)	Preclinical
Celyad	CYAD-101	NKG2D	Expression of a TRAC-inhibitory molecule peptide consisting of a truncated form of CD3ζ	Retroviral vector (co-expression of TRAC-inhibitory molecule with CAR)	Phase I in CRC (NCT03692429, alloSHRINK)
Poseida Therapeutics	P-BCMAALL01	BCMA	TRAC and MHC class I KO	CRISPR gRNA and dead Cas9 fused to Clo51 nuclease (Cas-CLOVERTM) (KO)	Preclinical

Abbreviations: AAV6, adeno-associated virus 6; ALL, acute lymphoblastic leukemia; AML, acute myeloid leukemia; BCMA, B-cell maturation protein (also known as TNFRSF17); BPDCN, blastic plasmacytoid dendritic cell neoplasm; CAR, chimeric antigen receptor; CEA, carcinoembryonic antigen; CLL1, C-type lectin-like molecule 1; CRC, colorectal cancer; CTL, cytotoxic T cell; CTLA4, cytotoxic T-lymphocyte-associated antigen 4; EBV, Epstein–Barr virus; gRNA, guide RNA; iPSC, inducible pluripotent stem cell; IND, investigational new drug; KO, knockout; MHC, major histocompatibility complex; MM, multiple myeloma; NHL, non-Hodgkin lymphoma; PDC1, programmed cell death protein 1 (gene); PEBL, protein expression blocker; shRNA, short hairpin RNA; TALEN, transcription activator-like effector nuclease; TCR, T-cell receptor; TI, targeted integration; TRAC, T-cell receptor alpha constant chain; ZFN, zinc-finger nuclease.

these to the clinic a variety of constructs and production modalities are being developed (**Table 2**).

In the UNIVERSAL phase I trial a single dose of ALLO-715 was infused into patients with MM following lymphodepletion with a regimen containing fludarabine, cyclophosphamide and ALLO647, which is an anti-CD52 monoclonal antibody. The lymphodepletion chemotherapy used for this allogeneic CAR-T was significantly more intensive than that used for most autologous CARs with fludarabine being administered at 90 mg/m^2 and cyclophosphamide at 900 mg/m^2. Fifty-three patients were enrolled, all of whom received product. CRS requiring the use of tocilizumab and/or corticosteroids across all patients was 19% and 15%, respectively. ICANS was identified in 11% of patients. The most common grade greater than or equal to 3 AEs were anemia (41.2%), neutropenia (41.2%), lymphopenia (29.4%), and thrombocytopenia (29.4%) which were likely enhanced due to the higher doses of lymphodepletion used in this study. Infectious complications occurred in 56% of patients, 29% of which were grade greater than or equal to 3. Of all infections, viral infections or low-grade viral reactivation were most common, potentially attributable to the use of an anti-CD52 antibody in the lymphodepletion regimen. Among patients who received the highest dose (320 × 10^6 CAR + T cells), responses were highest among those who also received higher doses of lymphodepleting chemotherapy. In this group, the ORR was 80% with 50% achieving a very good partial response or better (VGPR) and 20% achieving a CR.[63]

P-BCMA-ALLO1 is an allogeneic CAR-T manufactured using a nonviral transposon-based integration system that introduces a humanized anti-BCMA CAR producing a highly enriched T stem cell memory product. The endogenous TCR and the beta-2 microglobulin gene are eliminated via use of a Cas-CLOVER site-specific gene editing system to eliminate GVHD and reduce MHC class I expression.[64] Seven patients have been treated with P-BCMAALLO1 with 1 patient achieving a VGPR and 2 patients with a partial response.[65]

Other products have been less successful, including CYAD-101, a NKG2D-based allogeneic CAR-T product that was being evaluated in patients with relapsed and refractory MM. Although initial data suggested activity, this study was paused and the product was discontinued on account of patient deaths related to pulmonary complications.[66]

Early results utilizing allogeneic CAR-T therapy in patients with MM have shown promising results, but limitations related to short persistence and the requirement for intensive lymphodepleting regimens that leave patients susceptible to atypical infections remain major obstacles to their use. Significant work is needed to overcome these challenges, better manage infectious complications, improve persistence and long-term outcomes, and bring these agents to the clinic.

Natural Killer-Based Chimeric Antigen Receptor Cells

NK cells are unique innate immune cells that can manifest rapid and potent cytotoxicity of pathogens and cancer cells without the requirement of prior sensitization or recognition of classical peptide antigens. CAR-transduced NK (CAR-NK) cells may be able to simultaneously improve efficacy and control adverse effects including CRS, neurotoxicity, and GVHD. Moreover, because of the inherent properties of NK cells, allogeneic CAR-NK cells could represent an off-the-shelf product satisfying the clinical demand for large-scale manufacture for cancer immunotherapy attribute to the cytotoxic effect via both NK cell receptor-dependent and CAR-dependent signaling cascades.[25,67,68] Currently, no human data for CAR-NK cells have been reported in patients with MM but preclinical studies have shown promising results for the therapeutic efficacy of NKs expressing anti-BCMA CARs with a soluble form of the tumor necrosis factor-related apoptosis-inducing ligand (sTRAIL).[67] This remains an exciting area for future development.

Induced Pluripotent Stem Cell-Derived Chimeric Antigen Receptor Cells

T cells derived from differentiated induced pluripotent stem cells (iPSCs) may offer a platform to produce a virtually endless number of off-the-shelf allogeneic T cells. Several advances have been made recently in the establishment of systems for iPSC-based CAR T-cell generation including the use of feeder free platforms for differentiating T cells in a sustainable manner for a variety of applications. Phase I clinical data utilizing FT576, an iPSC-derived anti-BCMA CARNK cell that can be combined with daratumumab to promote antibody-directed cellular cytotoxicity, showed activity in patients with relapsed and refractory MM.[69,70]

Dendritic Cell-Based Vaccination for Multiple Myeloma

Tumor vaccines in which patient derived MM cells are fused with autologous dendritic cells (DCs) such that a broad array of tumor antigens are presented in the context of the antigen presenting machinery of the DC fusion partner has shown preliminary evidence of activity in MM. Thirty-six patients with newly diagnosed MM received serial vaccinations with DC/MM fusion cells either prior to or following autologous transplantation. Seventy-eight percent of patients achieved a response of at least VGPR and 47% achieved a CR. Remarkably, 24% of patients who achieved a partial response following transplant converted to CR after vaccination consistent with possible vaccine-mediated effects on residual disease. Significant work is ongoing to develop approaches to potentially improve cell selection to increase antitumor response. In addition, work is ongoing to combine DC vaccines with other immune modulators such as the IMiD drugs to alter the tumor and immune microenvironment.[71–74] There is rationale to combine this approach with CAR T-cell therapy to improve T-cell-mediated killing and promote a bystander effect, and preclinical work is ongoing to test this approach.[75]

Combination Approaches

As discussed above, many of the agents used during standard of care therapy for MM have immune-mediated effects. Thus, combinations of cell therapies with both standard approved agents as well as novel immune modulators represent an exciting opportunity to improve patient outcomes.

Gamma Secretase Inhibitors

Downregulation or biallelic loss of BCMA on MM cells following CAR T-cell therapy is a known mechanism of relapse.[57] The multi-subunit γ-secretase complex (GS), an intramembrane protease, reduces CAR T-cell function via cleavage of BCMA and subsequent shedding of the soluble BCMA (sBCMA) extracellular domain into the circulation. Multiple inhibitors of gamma secretase have been developed, initially as therapies for Alzheimer's disease, and are now being tested for combinatorial efficacy with BCMA-targeting agents.[76] A recent phase 1 first inhuman trial of escalating doses of BCMA targeted CAR-T cells in combination with a GS inhibitor (JSMD194) for patients with relapsed or refractory MM. All 18 treated patients completed the 5-day run-in with JSMD194. The only patient who did not demonstrate an increase in BCMA antibody binding capacity after GS inhibitor run-in had previously received BCMA targeted therapy and BCMA expression at screening was virtually absent. With follow-up of 20 months, the median PFS was 11 months. Among patients without prior exposure to BCMA targeted therapy (n = 11), the median PFS has not been reached, whereas among those previously exposed to BCMA targeted therapy (n = 7), the median PFS was 2 months.[67,77] These GS inhibiting agents may be able to be combined with currently approved anti-BCMA drugs, although the optimal order and timing of dosing, and approaches to managing toxicity have yet to be worked out.

Immunotherapeutic Drugs

Regulation of the T-cell phenotypes post CAR-T Infusion has been thought to significantly affect CAR-T activity and clinical outcomes. Thalidomide analogs, such as lenalidomide, have long been known to alter T-cell function and promote secretion of IL2, thought to mediate their immune modulatory effects.[78] Thus, there is significant rationale for combining thalidomide analogs with other immune targeting therapies. In a study combining lenalidomide with CS1 CAR-T cells, in tumor bearing mice, it was found that lenalidomide potentiated the cytotoxicity and memory maintenance of the CARs along with an increase in Th1 cytokine production and immune synapse formation.[79] Lenalidomide has long been used for post-transplant maintenance in MM and potentially could continue to play a similar immunomodulatory role in the post CAR-T setting.[80] Trials are underway to test the use of thalidomide analogs as maintenance following CAR T-cell infusion. Other combination therapies with bispecific antibodies, CAR-T cells and monoclonal antibodies that lead to immune checkpoint inhibition have also shown promise in preclinical models.[81,82,83] Further studies to evaluate rational combinations of checkpoint inhibitors with anti-MM cell therapies are in development.

SUMMARY

In just a short few years a tremendous amount of work has been done toward developing cell therapies for MM, yielding the first approvals for these therapies and fundamentally changing the course of treatment for patients with relapsed and refractory MM. However, patients still uniformly relapse; thus, continued work is needed to develop rational combinations of therapies to improve outcomes and to develop novel cell therapy approaches that may eventually produce cures for this disease.

CONFLICTS OF INTEREST

P. Shah reports no relevant conflicts of interest. A.S. Sperling reports consulting fees from Adaptive Technologies, Novartis, and Roche.

DISCLOSURE

Dr P. Shah reports no relevant conflicts of interest.

ACKNOWLEDGMENTS

P. Shah was supported by the Holland Leukemia Research Fund. A.S. Sperling was supported by grants from the NCI, United States (K08CA252174) and DOD, United States (CA210827).

REFERENCES

1. Phekoo KJ, et al. A population study to define the incidence and survival of multiple myeloma in a National Health Service Region in UK. Brit J Haematol 2004; 127:299–304.

2. Sant M, et al. Incidence of hematologic malignancies in Europe by morphologic subtype: results of the HAEMACARE project. Blood 2010;116:3724–34.
3. Kazandjian D. Multiple myeloma epidemiology and survival: A unique malignancy. Semin Oncol 2016;43:676–81.
4. Ellington TD, Henley SJ, Wilson RJ, et al. Trends in solitary plasmacytoma, extramedullary plasmacytoma, and plasma cell myeloma incidence and myeloma mortality by racial-ethnic group, United States 2003-2016. Cancer Med-us 2021;10:386–95.
5. Kumar S, et al. Gaps and opportunities in the treatment of relapsed-refractory multiple myeloma: Consensus recommendations of the NCI Multiple Myeloma Steering Committee. Blood Cancer J 2022;12:98.
6. Gandhi UH, et al. Outcomes of patients with multiple myeloma refractory to CD38-targeted monoclonal antibody therapy. Leukemia 2019;33:2266–75.
7. Sperling AS, Anderson KC. Facts and Hopes in Multiple Myeloma Immunotherapy. Clin Cancer Res 2021;27:4468–77.
8. Dhodapkar MV. The immune system in multiple myeloma and precursor states: Lessons and implications for immunotherapy and interception. Am J Hematol 2023;98:S4–12.
9. Lonial S, et al. Belantamab mafodotin for relapsed or refractory multiple myeloma (DREAMM-2): a two-arm, randomised, open-label, phase 2 study. Lancet Oncol 2020;21:207–21.
10. Raje N, et al. Anti-BCMA CAR T-Cell Therapy bb2121 in Relapsed or Refractory Multiple Myeloma. New Engl J Med 2019;380:1726–37.
11. de Donk NWCJV, et al. CARTITUDE-2: Efficacy and Safety of Ciltacabtagene Autoleucel, a B-Cell Maturation Antigen (BCMA)-Directed Chimeric Antigen Receptor T-Cell Therapy, in Patients with Multiple Myeloma and Early Relapse after Initial Therapy. Blood 2021;138:2910.
12. Berdeja JG, et al. Ciltacabtagene autoleucel, a B-cell maturation antigen-directed chimeric antigen receptor T-cell therapy in patients with relapsed or refractory multiple myeloma (CARTITUDE-1): a phase 1b/2 open-label study. Lancet 2021;398:314–24.
13. Munshi NC, et al. Idecabtagene Vicleucel in Relapsed and Refractory Multiple Myeloma. New Engl J Med 2021;384:705–16.
14. Moreau P, et al. Teclistamab in Relapsed or Refractory Multiple Myeloma. New Engl J Med 2022;387:495–505.
15. Levine BL, Miskin J, Wonnacott K, et al. Global Manufacturing of CAR T Cell Therapy. Mol Ther - Methods Clin Dev 2017;4:92–101.
16. Subklewe M, Bergwelt-Baildon M von, Humpe A. Chimeric Antigen Receptor T Cells: A Race to Revolutionize Cancer Therapy. Transfus Med Hemoth 2019;46:15–24.
17. Zhang C, Liu J, Zhong JF, et al. Engineering CAR-T cells. Biomark Res 2017;5:22.
18. Huehls AM, Coupet TA, Sentman CL. Bispecific T-cell engagers for cancer immunotherapy. Immunol Cell Biol 2015;93:290–6.
19. Roex G, et al. Safety and clinical efficacy of BCMA CAR-T-cell therapy in multiple myeloma. J Hematol Oncol 2020;13:164.
20. Novak AJ, et al. Expression of BCMA, TACI, and BAFF-R in multiple myeloma: a mechanism for growth and survival. Blood 2004;103:689–94.
21. Shah N, Chari A, Scott E, et al. B-cell maturation antigen (BCMA) in multiple myeloma: rationale for targeting and current therapeutic approaches. Leukemia 2020;34:985–1005.
22. Wudhikarn K, Mailankody S, Smith EL. Future of CAR T cells in multiple myeloma. Hematology 2020;272–9.

23. Song F, et al. Safety and efficacy of autologous and allogeneic humanized CD19-targeted CAR-T cell therapy for patients with relapsed/refractory B-ALL. J Immunother Cancer 2023;11:e005701.

24. Garfall AL, et al. T-cell phenotypes associated with effective CAR T-cell therapy in postinduction vs relapsed multiple myeloma. Blood Adv 2019;3:2812–5.

25. Manier S, et al. Current state and next-generation CAR-T cells in multiple myeloma. Blood Rev 2022;54:100929.

26. Costa LJ, et al. Results from the First Phase 1 Clinical Study of the B-Cell Maturation Antigen (BCMA) Nex T Chimeric Antigen Receptor (CAR) T Cell Therapy CC-98633/BMS-986354 in Patients (pts) with Relapsed/Refractory Multiple Myeloma (RRMM). Blood 2022;140:1360–2.

27. Sperling AS, et al. Phase I Study of PHE885, a Fully Human BCMA-Directed CAR-T Cell Therapy for Relapsed/Refractory Multiple Myeloma Manufactured in <2 Days Using the T-Charge TM Platform. Blood 2021;138:3864.

28. Du J, et al. Phase I Open-Label Single-Arm Study of BCMA/CD19 Dual-Targeting FasTCAR-T Cells (GC012F) As First-Line Therapy for Transplant-Eligible Newly Diagnosed High-Risk Multiple Myeloma. Blood 2022;140:889–90.

29. Brudno JN, Kochenderfer JN. Off-the-shelf CAR T cells for multiple myeloma. Nat Med 2023;1–2. https://doi.org/10.1038/s41591-022-02195-2.

30. Bedoya DM, Dutoit V, Migliorini D. Allogeneic CAR T Cells: An Alternative to Overcome Challenges of CAR T Cell Therapy in Glioblastoma. Front Immunol 2021;12:640082.

31. Wilkie GM, et al. Establishment and Characterization of a Bank of Cytotoxic T Lymphocytes for Immunotherapy of Epstein-Barr Virus-Associated Diseases. J Immunother 2004;27:309–16.

32. Withers B, et al. Establishment and Operation of a Third-Party Virus-Specific T Cell Bank within an Allogeneic Stem Cell Transplant Program. Biol Blood Marrow Tr 2018;24:2433–42.

33. Cruz CRY, et al. Infusion of donor-derived CD19-redirected virus-specific T cells for B-cell malignancies relapsed after allogeneic stem cell transplant: a phase 1 study. Blood 2013;122:2965–73.

34. Münz C. Redirecting T Cells against Epstein–Barr Virus Infection and Associated Oncogenesis. Cells 2020;9:1400.

35. Frigyesi I, et al. Robust isolation of malignant plasma cells in multiple myeloma. Blood 2014;123:1336–40.

36. Smith EL, et al. GPRC5D is a target for the immunotherapy of multiple myeloma with rationally designed CAR T cells. Sci Transl Med 2019;11.

37. Mailankody S, et al. GPRC5D-Targeted CAR T Cells for Myeloma. New Engl J Med 2022;387:1196–206.

38. Larrea C F de, et al. Defining an Optimal Dual-Targeted CAR T-cell Therapy Approach Simultaneously Targeting BCMA and GPRC5D to Prevent BCMA Escape–Driven Relapse in Multiple Myeloma. Blood Cancer Discov 2020;1:146–54.

39. Chari A, et al. Talquetamab, a T-Cell–Redirecting GPRC5D Bispecific Antibody for Multiple Myeloma. New Engl J Med 2022;387:2232–44.

40. Cohen AD, et al. Initial Clinical Activity and Safety of BFCR4350A, a FcRH5/CD3 T-CellEngaging Bispecific Antibody, in Relapsed/Refractory Multiple Myeloma. Blood 2020;136:42–3.

41. Polson AG, et al. Expression pattern of the human FcRH/IRTA receptors in normal tissue and in Bchronic lymphocytic leukemia. Int Immunol 2006;18:1363–73.

42. Stewart AK, et al. Phase I study of the anti-FcRH5 antibody-drug conjugate DFRF4539A in relapsed or refractory multiple myeloma. Blood Cancer J 2019; 9:17.

43. Tian C, et al. Anti-CD138 chimeric antigen receptor-modified T cell therapy for multiple myeloma with extensive extramedullary involvement. Ann Hematol 2017;96:1407–10.

44. Sun C, et al. Safety and efficacy of targeting CD138 with a chimeric antigen receptor for the treatment of multiple myeloma. Oncotarget 2019;10:2369–83.

45. Garfall AL, et al. Chimeric Antigen Receptor T Cells against CD19 for Multiple Myeloma. New Engl J Med 2015;373:1040–7.

46. Garfall AL, et al. Anti-BCMA/CD19 CAR T cells with early immunomodulatory maintenance for multiple myeloma responding to initial or later-line therapy. Blood Cancer Discov 2022;4:118–33.

47. Prommersberger S, et al. CARAMBA: a first-in-human clinical trial with SLAMF7 CAR-T cells prepared by virus-free Sleeping Beauty gene transfer to treat multiple myeloma. Gene Ther 2021;28:560–71.

48. Ranganathan R, et al. CAR T cells Targeting Human Immunoglobulin Light Chains Eradicate Mature B-cell Malignancies While Sparing a Subset of Normal B Cells. Clin Cancer Res 2021;27:5951–60.

49. Tai Y-T, et al. APRIL and BCMA promote human multiple myeloma growth and immunosuppression in the bone marrow microenvironment. Blood 2016;127: 3225–36.

50. Camviel N, et al. Both APRIL and antibody-fragment-based CAR T cells for myeloma induce BCMA downmodulation by trogocytosis and internalization. J Immunother Cancer 2022;10:e005091.

51. Rodriguez-Otero P, et al. Ide-cel or Standard Regimens in Relapsed and Refractory Multiple Myeloma. New Engl J Med 2023;388:1002–14.

52. Zheng W, et al. PI3K orchestration of the in vivo persistence of chimeric antigen receptor-modified T cells. Leukemia 2018;32:1157–67.

53. Funk CR, et al. PI3Kδ/γ inhibition promotes human CART cell epigenetic and metabolic reprogramming to enhance antitumor cytotoxicity. Blood 2022;139: 523–37.

54. Raje NS, et al. Updated Clinical and Correlative Results from the Phase I CRB-402 Study of the BCMA-Targeted CAR T Cell Therapy bb21217 in Patients with Relapsed and Refractory Multiple Myeloma. Blood 2021;138:548.

55. Oekelen OV, et al. Neurocognitive and hypokinetic movement disorder with features of parkinsonism after BCMA-targeting CAR-T cell therapy. Nat Med 2021; 27:2099–103.

56. Martin T, et al. Ciltacabtagene Autoleucel, an Anti–B-cell Maturation Antigen Chimeric Antigen Receptor T-Cell Therapy, for Relapsed/Refractory Multiple Myeloma: CARTITUDE-1 2-Year FollowUp. J Clin Oncol 2023;41:1265–74.

57. Samur MK, et al. Biallelic loss of BCMA as a resistance mechanism to CAR T cell therapy in a patient with multiple myeloma. Nat Commun 2021;12:868.

58. Friedrich MJ, et al. The pre-existing T cell landscape determines the response to bispecific T cell engagers in multiple myeloma patients. Cancer Cell 2023;41: 711–25.e6.

59. Truger MS, Duell J, Zhou X, et al. Single and double hit events in genes encoding for immune targets before and after T cell engaging antibody therapy in MM. Blood Adv 2021;5:3794–8.

60. Già MCD, et al. Homozygous BCMA gene deletion in response to anti-BCMA CAR T cells in a patient with multiple myeloma. Nat Med 2021;27:616–9.

61. Usmani S, et al. KarMMa-2 Cohort 2a: Efficacy and Safety of Idecabtagene Vicleucel in Clinical High-Risk Multiple Myeloma Patients with Early Relapse after Frontline Autologous Stem Cell Transplantation. Blood 2022;140:875–7.

62. Frigault M, et al. Phase 1 Study of CART-Ddbcma for the Treatment of Subjects with Relapsed and/or Refractory Multiple Myeloma. Blood 2022;140:7439–40.

63. Mailankody S, et al. Allogeneic BCMA-targeting CAR T cells in relapsed/refractory multiple myeloma: phase 1 UNIVERSAL trial interim results. Nat Med 2023;1–8. https://doi.org/10.1038/s41591-02202182-7.

64. Tseng H, et al. Memory Phenotype in Allogeneic Anti-BCMA CAR-T Cell Therapy (P-BCMAALLO1) Correlates with In Vivo Tumor Control. Blood 2021;138:4802.

65. Kocoglu MH, et al. 47P Phase I study to assess the safety and efficacy of P-BCMA-ALLO1: A fully allogeneic CAR-T therapy, in patients with relapsed/refractory multiple myeloma (RRMM). Immunoocology Technology 2022;16:100152.

66. Leivas A, et al. NKG2D-CAR-transduced natural killer cells efficiently target multiple myeloma. Blood Cancer J 2021;11:146.

67. Motais B, Charvátová S, Hrdinka M, et al. Anti-BCMA-CAR NK Cells Expressing Soluble TRAIL: Promising Therapeutic Approach for Multiple Myeloma in Combination with Bortezomib and γ-Secretase Inhibitors. Blood 2022;140:12683–4.

68. Zhang L, Meng Y, Feng X, et al. CAR-NK cells for cancer immunotherapy: from bench to bedside. Biomark Res 2022;10:12.

69. Iriguchi S, et al. A clinically applicable and scalable method to regenerate T-cells from iPSCs for offthe-shelf T-cell immunotherapy. Nat Commun 2021;12:430.

70. Mathavan K, et al. Abstract 4190: Combining dual CAR iPSC-derived immune cells with antibody for multi-antigen targeting to overcome clonal resistance in multiple myeloma. Cancer Res 2022;82:4190.

71. Calmeiro J, et al. Dendritic Cell Vaccines for Cancer Immunotherapy: The Role of Human Conventional Type 1 Dendritic Cells. Pharm Times 2020;12:158.

72. Vasir B, et al. Fusion of dendritic cells with multiple myeloma cells results in maturation and enhanced antigen presentation. Brit J Haematol 2005;129:687–700.

73. Dhodapkar KM, et al. Changes in Bone Marrow Tumor and Immune Cells Correlate with Durability of Remissions Following BCMA CAR T Therapy in Myeloma. Blood Cancer Discov 2022;3:490–501.

74. Rosenblatt J, et al. Vaccination with Dendritic Cell/Tumor Fusions following Autologous Stem Cell Transplant Induces Immunologic and Clinical Responses in Multiple Myeloma Patients. Clin Cancer Res 2013;19:3640–8.

75. Capelletti M, et al. Potent Synergy between Combination of Chimeric Antigen Receptor (CAR) Therapy Targeting CD19 in Conjunction with Dendritic Cell (DC)/Tumor Fusion Vaccine in Hematological Malignancies. Blood 2019;134:3227.

76. Pont MJ, et al. γ-Secretase inhibition increases efficacy of BCMA-specific chimeric antigen receptor T cells in multiple myeloma. Blood 2019;134:1585–97.

77. Cowan AJ, et al. Safety and Efficacy of Fully Human BCMA CAR T Cells in Combination with a Gamma Secretase Inhibitor to Increase BCMA Surface Expression in Patients with Relapsed or Refractory Multiple Myeloma. Blood 2021;138:551.

78. Geng CL, et al. Lenalidomide bypasses CD28 co-stimulation to reinstate PD-1 immunotherapy by activating Notch signaling. Cell Chem Biol 2022;29:1260–72.e8.

79. Wang X, et al. Lenalidomide enhances the function of CS1 chimeric antigen receptor redirected T cells against multiple myeloma. Clin Cancer Res 2017;24:2017, clincanres.0344.

80. Shi X, et al. Anti-CD19 and anti-BCMA CAR T cell therapy followed by lenalidomide maintenance after autologous stem-cell transplantation for high-risk newly diagnosed multiple myeloma. Am J Hematol 2022;97:537–47.
81. Frerichs KA, et al. Efficacy and Safety of Daratumumab Combined With All-Trans Retinoic Acid in Relapsed/Refractory Multiple Myeloma. Blood Adv 2021;5: 5128–39.
82. Wang X, et al. Expanding anti-CD38 immunotherapy for lymphoid malignancies. J Exp Clin Canc Res 2022;41:210.
83. Zah E, et al. Systematically optimized BCMA/CS1 bispecific CAR-T cells robustly control heterogeneous multiple myeloma. Nat Commun 2020;11:2283.
84. Costello CL, Gregory TK, Ali SA, et al. Phase 2 study of the response and safety of p-bcma-101 car-t cells in patients with relapsed/refractory (R/r) multiple myeloma(Mm)(Prime). Blood 2019;134:3184.
85. Mailankody S, Jakubowiak AJ, Htut M, et al. Orvacabtagene autoleucel (Orvacel), a B-cell maturation antigen (Bcma)-directed CAR T cell therapy for patients (Pts) with relapsed/refractory multiple myeloma (Rrmm): update of the phase 1/2 EVOLVE study (Nct03430011). JCO. 2020;38(15_suppl):8504-8504.

Chimeric Antigen Receptor T Cells in Hodgkin and T-Cell Lymphomas

Ibrahim N. Muhsen, MD[a,b,c], LaQuisa C. Hill, MD[a,b,c],
Carlos A. Ramos, MD[a,b,c],*

KEYWORDS

- Chimeric antigen receptor T cells • Hodgkin lymphoma
- T-cell non-Hodgkin lymphoma • CD30 • CD5 • CD7

KEY POINTS

- Chimeric antigen receptor (CAR) T cells have improved outcomes in several lymphoproliferative diseases, including B-cell acute lymphoblastic leukemia and B-cell non-Hodgkin lymphoma (CD19.CAR-T cells) and multiple myeloma (BCMA.CAR-T cells).
- CD30.CAR-T cells have shown safety and promising efficacy in relapsed/refractory (r/r) Hodgkin lymphoma (HL), with early phase clinical trial data supporting CD30 as a potential target for CAR-T cells in HL.
- Efforts to improve the antitumor activity of CD30.CAR-T cells in r/r HL with additional genetic modification or combination treatment (eg, with immune check point inhibitors) are ongoing.
- Several potential targets have been identified for T-cell lymphomas (TCLs), and CAR-T cells targeting broadly expressed antigens, such as CD5 and CD7, are currently being explored as treatment of r/r TCL.
- CAR-T cell use in TCL is still in early development stages, and more research is needed to address potential challenges, including the risks of fratricide, prolonged cellular immunodeficiency, and transduction of malignant T cells.

INTRODUCTION

Chimeric antigen receptor (CAR)-transduced T cells (CAR-T) have been shown to improve outcomes in patients with CD19 and BCMA-positive lymphoproliferative disorders. The identification of viable targets for hematological malignancies other than

[a] Section of Hematology and Oncology, Department of Medicine, Baylor College of Medicine, One Baylor Plaza, Houston, TX 77030, USA; [b] Center for Cell and Gene Therapy, Baylor College of Medicine, Texas Children's Hospital and Houston Methodist Hospital, Houston, TX, USA; [c] Dan L. Duncan Comprehensive Cancer Center, Baylor College of Medicine, Houston, TX, USA
* Corresponding author. Center for Cell and Gene Therapy, 6565 Fannin Street Room A6-080, Houston, TX 77030.
E-mail address: caramos@bcm.edu

Hematol Oncol Clin N Am 37 (2023) 1107–1124
https://doi.org/10.1016/j.hoc.2023.05.017
0889-8588/23/© 2023 Elsevier Inc. All rights reserved.
hemonc.theclinics.com

B-cell non-Hodgkin lymphoma (B-NHL) or acute lymphoblastic leukemia (B-ALL) and multiple myeloma (MM) has, however, lagged behind.

CD30 has been validated as a target for classical Hodgkin lymphoma (HL) given the efficacy of brentuximab vedotin (BV), a CD30 monoclonal antibody (mAb) conjugated with monomethyl auristatin E (an antimitotic agent) in multiple settings, including front-line, consolidation, and salvage.[1–3] Although using a murine idiotype (HRS3) instead of the humanized BV idiotype (cAC10), a CD30-specific CAR was originally designed in Germany in the 1990s[4] and later adapted and optimized at Baylor College of Medicine.[5] Human T cells transduced with this CAR (CD30.CAR-Ts) showed activity in xenograft models of HL. The preclinical activity seen in this and other subsequent studies using anti-CD30 CARs laid the foundation for their evaluation in early phase clinical trials.

CD30 is also expressed in a subset of T-cell lymphomas (TCL), and BV has shown good activity in these disorders, making CD30.CAR-Ts a promising potential therapy in this setting as well. Several early phase studies of CD30.CAR-Ts have also allowed the enrollment of patients with CD30-positive TCLs. The restricted expression of CD30 in normal T cells limits the potential "on-target, off-tumor" effects of CD30.CAR-Ts but also prevents their applicability to a wider variety of T-cell malignancies. Therefore, more universal T-cell markers, such as CD2, CD5, and CD7, are being pursued as potential targets.

Targeting a universal T-cell antigen with a T-cell–derived product raises potential deleterious consequences, however. On one hand, because the target antigens are expressed on the CAR-T cells themselves, they may be susceptible to killing by neighboring CAR-Ts during their manufacture (and after infusion), a phenomenon called fratricide.[6] On the other hand, because culture conditions favor the growth and transduction of T cells, circulating malignant cells may get transduced during the manufacturing process when using autologous peripheral blood mononuclear cells (PBMC), providing a means of tumor escape. Finally, because native and malignant T cells share expression of the antigen being targeted, in vivo long-term persistence of CAR-Ts could lead to T-cell aplasia, resulting in profound immunodeficiency.[7] Consequently, to be successful, any treatment strategy will have to address these potential obstacles.

Herein, the authors review published data on clinical trials using CAR-T cells for HL and TCL. They begin by summarizing the results of targeting CD30 via CAR-T cells in HL and then address targeting CD30, CD5, and CD7 with CAR-Ts in TCL (**Fig. 1**). Current challenges and potential future directions are discussed.

CHIMERIC ANTIGEN RECEPTOR-T CELLS IN HODGKIN LYMPHOMA

Although most of the patients with HL are cured with first-line combination chemotherapy, 10% to 20% will have refractory or recurrent (r/r) disease,[8] which has a poor prognosis. Treatment of r/r HL has included salvage chemotherapy or immunotherapy with possible consolidative autologous stem cell transplant. Adoptive T-cell therapy has also been investigated to improve the outcomes of these patients.[9] One of the earliest examples of adoptive T-cell therapy for HL was the use of Epstein-Barr virus (EBV)-specific T cells (EBVSTs), as a significant portion of HLs are associated with EBV infection and express EBV antigens. EBVSTs have shown activity in several EBV-related diseases, including posttransplant lymphoproliferative disease (PTLD).[9–11] However, this approach has several limitations, including the lack of universal EBV positivity in HL and the intrinsic immunosuppressive potential of HL, which may evade the antitumor activity of native EBVST.[12] Although these

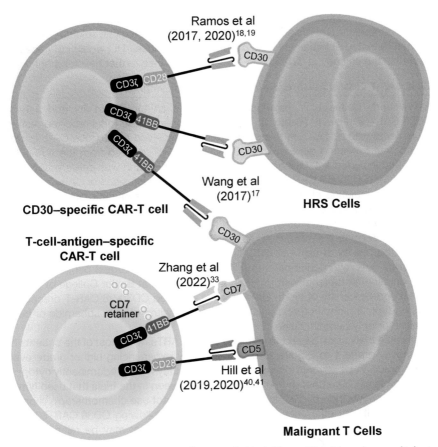

Fig. 1. A summary of the major CAR-T cell targets in Hodgkin and T-cell lymphomas. (Adapted and modified with permission from: Leung WK, Ayanambakkam A, Heslop HE, Hill LC. Beyond CD19 CAR-T cells in lymphoma. Curr Opin Immunol. 2022 Feb; 74:46-52.)

approaches are still being studied and optimized, targeting CD30 via genetically modified T cells has generated considerable interest more recently.

CD30 Expression and Targeting in Hodgkin Lymphoma

CD30 was identified more than 4 decades ago and is a member of the tumor necrosis factor receptor family that is expressed on various immune cells, including some granulocytes and activated B and T lymphocytes. In addition, it is highly expressed by Hodgkin Reed-Sternberg (HRS) cells.[13] The high expression of CD30 in HL has implied a possible role in HL pathogenesis, but data are conflicting. Although some studies have implicated CD30 in ligand-independent activation of the nuclear factor kB (NFkB) pathway, others have suggested that NFkB activation is unrelated to CD30.[14,15] Given the limited expression by other tissues and thus lower potential of "on-target, off-tumor" adverse events, multiple strategies have been developed to target CD30 in HL, including mAbs and antibody-drug conjugates.[13] The success of BV encouraged targeting CD30 with CAR-Ts.

Earlier preclinical studies have demonstrated the ability of anti-CD30 CAR-T cells to lyse HL cell lines expressing CD30.[4,16] The efficacy of these first-generation CAR-Ts, lacking a costimulatory endodomain, was limited but supported the potential efficacy of a CD30-specific CAR. In addition, those studies suggested that soluble CD30, which is often detected at higher levels in patients with advanced HL, would not necessarily decrease the efficacy of CD30.CAR-Ts,[4,5] fostering their further development.

CD30.CAR-T Cells in Relapsed/Refractory Hodgkin Lymphoma

A few early phase trials have investigated the antitumor activity and safety of CD30.CAR-Ts in r/r HL (**Table 1**). The first published phase I trial reported results in 17 patients with r/r HL.[17] In this study, patients received autologous CAR-Ts transduced with a second-generation CD30-specific CAR (derived from the AJ878606.1 mAb) that included a 4-1BB costimulatory endodomain and was delivered by a lentiviral vector (CD30-BB.CAR-T). Patients received 1 or 2 infusions of CAR-Ts after varied lymphodepleting chemotherapy regimens. Two subsequently published studies also used autologous T cells transduced with a CD30-specific CAR, but which was derived from the HRS3 mAb, contained a CD28 costimulatory endodomain, and was delivered via a γ-retrovirus (CD30-28.CAR-T).[18,19] Ramos and colleagues reported the results of using CD30-28.CAR-T in 7 patients with r/r HL without using any lymphodepleting chemotherapy.[18] Subsequently, the largest published study to date enrolled 42 patients with r/r HL in 2 parallel trials at Baylor College of Medicine (BCM) and University of North Carolina who received CD30-28.CAR-T preceded by lymphodepleting chemotherapy using fludarabine with cyclophosphamide or bendamustine or only bendamustine.[19]

All these trials established the safety of CD30.CARTs, with most of the patients having mostly grade 1 to 2 adverse events and few experiencing higher grade events. When grade 3 to 4 adverse events were reported, they were predominantly cytopenias attributable to chemotherapy, as these were only seen in the trials that used lymphodepleting chemotherapy.[17,19] In the study that did not use chemotherapy,[18] patients had no significant difference in their blood counts following CD30.CAR-T infusion, except for a mild decrease in eosinophils, a finding that may be related to CD30 expression by eosinophils. As to events of special interest, the incidence of cytokine release syndrome (CRS) was variable among the studies, ranging from 0 in the trial without chemotherapy to potentially 100%, as Wang and colleagues[17] reported mild febrile illness with fever and chills immediately after CAR infusion in all treated patients. The largest study reported CRS in 24% of patients.[19] All CRS and febrile events were low-grade, self-limited, and did not require any anticytokine therapy. Moreover, none of the studies reported any neurotoxicity. Finally, there was no evidence of excess infectious complications, which was a potential concern with targeting CD30 because this molecule is expressed by activated T cells that play a key role in the control of latent and acute viral infections. Antiviral immunity seemed not to have been compromised in these patients when assessed by virus-specific ELISpot assays on PBMCs before and after CAR-T infusion.[18]

Of note, one of the trials reported a transient, nontender, nonpruritic maculopapular skin rash developing in around half of the treated patients and more frequently in those who received cyclophosphamide.[19] The rash started within 1 week after CAR-T cell infusion and resolved in 1 to 2 weeks without requiring specific therapy. Biopsies of the affected skin showed a nonspecific spongiotic dermatitis with eosinophils, and the finding was postulated to be an "on-target, off-tumor" effect of CD30.CARTs on CD30-expressing cells in the skin.

Apart from safety, these trials showed promising efficacy of the approach. In the study using CD30-BB.CARTs,[17] 6 of the 17 patients with HL had a partial response (PR), corresponding to an overall response rate (ORR) of 39%. The median

Table 1
Summary of the published CD30 CAR-T cells studies

Study	No. of HL Patients	Median Age (Range), y	Patients with Prior BV (%)	LDC	Costimulatory Endodomain (Vector)	Range of CAR-T Cells Doses	Response % (n)	CRS & ICANS % (n)
C. Wang et al,[17] 2017	17	31 (13–55)	4[23]	GEMC (n = 8) Flu + Cy (n = 5) PC (n = 4) Others (n = 4)	4-1BB (Lentivirus)	1.1–2.1 × 10^7 cells/kg	ORR 35%[6] PR 35%[6]	CRS, all grades: 100%[17] CRS, grade ≥3: 0% ICANS, all grades: 0% ICANS, grade ≥3: 0%
Ramos et al,[18] 2017	7	31 (20–65)	5 (71)	None	CD28 (γ-retrovirus)	0.2–2.0 × 10^8 cells/m^2	ORR 29%[2] CR 29%[2 a]	CRS, all grades: 0% CRS, grade ≥3: 0% ICANS, all grades: 0% ICANS, grade ≥3: 0%
Ramos et al,[19] 2021	42	35 (17–69)	38 (90)	Flu + Cy (n = 17) Benda-Flu (n = 17) Benda (n = 8)	CD28 (γ-retrovirus)	0.2–2.0 × 10^8 cells/m^2	ORR 62% (23/37)[b] CR 51% (19/37) PR 11% (4/37)	CRS, all grades: 24%[10] CRS, grade ≥3: 0% ICANS, all grades: 0% ICANS, grade ≥3: 0%

Abbreviations: Benda, bendamustine; BV, brentuximab vedotin; CR, complete response; CRS, cytokine release syndrome; Flu+Cy, fludarabine + cyclophosphamide; GEMC, gemcitabine + epirubicin + mustargen + cyclophosphamide; HL, Hodgkin lymphoma; ICANS, immune effector cell–associated neurotoxicity syndrome; LDC, lymphodepleting chemotherapy; ORR, overall response rate; PC, nab-paclitaxel + cyclophosphamide; PR, partial response.

[a] One patient had no active disease but maintained remission after CAR-T cells.

[b] Thirty-seven patients who had active disease before infusion were included in the ORR calculation.

progression-free survival (PFS) in this study was 14 months. Even without lymphode-pleting chemotherapy, CD30-28.CAR-Ts showed some activity with 1 of 7 patients with HL achieving a complete remission (CR) that lasted more than 36 months and 1 patient maintaining a pretreatment CR for more than 24 months after receiving CAR-Ts.[18] The addition of lymphodepleting chemotherapy was associated with an increased response rate to CD30-28.CAR-Ts, which was likely related to improved in vivo expansion of the cells. Indeed, of the 37 patients who had active disease at the time of CAR-T infusion and received lymphodepleting chemotherapy before CD30-28.CAR-Ts, 23 had a response (ORR 62%) with 19 (51%) achieving CR. Patients who achieved remission had a median PFS of 14.6 months, and 10 of these patients had not had progression at the time of publication, with the longest ongoing CR reported being 25 months. The 1-year overall survival in this patient population was 94%, which is notable given that the patients included in the study were heavily pre-treated, with a median of 7 prior lines of therapy.[19]

An international multicenter phase II trial combining bendamustine and fludarabine lymphodepletion with CD30-28.CAR-Ts (CHARIOT trial, NCT04268706) was open to corroborate the findings of earlier studies. Initial results of the CHARIOT trial, which included 12 heavily pretreated patients (median of 6 lines of therapy), have been presented at the American Society of Hematology (ASH) meeting.[20] Efficacy data were only reported for 5 patients, with an ORR of 100%. Similar larger and comparative studies will be needed to determine the true efficacy of this approach. Ongoing trials of CD30-targeting CAR-T cells are included in **Table 2**.

Challenges and Future Directions

Despite an impressive overall response rate, the duration of responses to CD30.CAR-Ts seems to be shorter than those that have been seen with CD19.CAR-Ts in aggressive NHL, suggesting that additional improvements are needed. Because autologous CAR-T cell products are derived from individuals who usually have been exposed to several rounds of chemotherapy, the biological properties of these products may not be optimal. Hence, ready-made, off-the-shelf T-cell products derived from healthy donors are quite attractive, but the overall treatment strategy will have to be designed in a way that will avoid the potential complications associated with alloreactivity (ie, product rejection and graft-versus-host disease [GVHD]).[21,22] A study treating patients with CD30-positive lymphoma with CD30.CAR-transduced EBVSTs derived from healthy donors is currently ongoing at our center (BESTA trial, NCT04288726). EBVSTs are specific for EBV antigens and therefore should not be alloreactive and cause GVHD. On the other hand, because CD30 is expressed in activated T cells (including alloreactive T cells in the recipient that might mediate rejection), CD30.CAR-Ts may kill alloreactive T cells and thus be protected from rejection. Additional studies will be needed to investigate the safety and efficacy of allogeneic CAR-T cells.[23]

It is worth noting that patients who had received prior CD30 targeting therapy with BV were included in the studies mentioned.[17–19] Although the number of patients is limited, almost half of the patients whose disease had progressed while on BV achieved CR after CD30.CAR-T infusion. In addition, although post-CD30.CAR-T biopsies were obtained in only a small number of patients, CD30 expression was retained in relapsing tumors.[19] These findings suggest that resistance to anti-CD30 treatments is not mediated by antigen loss but that tumor recurrence may be due to insufficient persistence of CAR-Ts within the highly immunosuppressive tumor micro-environment of HL. Improving persistence in this setting is therefore desirable (**Fig. 2**). One possible strategy is to try to augment the efficacy of CD30 CAR-T cells by combining them with an immune checkpoint inhibitor (ICI). CD30.CAR-T cells express

Table 2
Ongoing CD30 clinical trials in Hodgkin lymphoma

Target/Therapy	Identifier[a]	Phase of Study	Type of CAR-T Cells	Institution (Country)	Status[b]
CD30	NCT04288726	I	Allogeneic CD30.CAR-EBVST cells	Baylor College of Medicine (United States)	Recruiting
	NCT02259556	I/II	Autologous CD30.CART cells	Chinese PLA General Hospital (China)	Recruiting
	NCT04653649	I/II	Autologous CD30.CART cells	Fundació Institut de Recerca de l'Hospital de la Santa Creu i Sant Pau (Spain)	Recruiting
	NCT03383965	I	Autologous CD30.CART cells	Immune Cell, Inc. (China)	Recruiting
	NCT02690545	I/II	Autologous CD30.CART	University of North Carolina (United States)	Recruiting
	NCT01192464	I	Autologous CD30.CAR-EBVST cells	Baylor College of Medicine (United States)	Active, not recruiting
	NCT02917083	I	Autologous CD30.CART	Baylor College of Medicine (United States)	Recruiting
	NCT02663297	I	Autologous CD30.CART cells	University of North Carolina (United States)	Active, not recruiting
	NCT04268706	II	Autologous CD30.CART cells	Tessa Therapeutics (Multi-center) (United States)	Active, not recruiting
	NCT04665063	Not reported	Autologous CD30.CART cells	Hebei Senlang Biotechnology Inc., Ltd. (China)	Recruiting
CD30 along with Immune checkpoint inhibitors (ICI)	NCT04134325	I	Autologous CD30.CART cells followed by ICI	University of North Carolina (United States)	Recruiting
	NCT05352828	I	Autologous CD30.CART cells along with ICI	Tessa Therapeutics (multicenter) (United States)	Active, not recruiting
CD30 & CCR4	NCT03602157	I	Autologous CD30.CART cells + CCR4	University of North Carolina (United States)	Recruiting

[a] Listed on clinicaltrials.gov. Search terminology: Hodgkin lymphoma or Hodgkin disease and Chimeric Antigen Receptor or CAR T cells.
[b] Includes studies with active status (both recruiting or not recruiting).

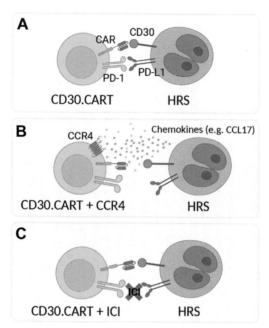

Fig. 2. Different potential strategies of targeting CD30 using CAR-T cells are shown: (*A*) CD30.CARTs, (*B*) CD30.CARTs coexpressing CCR4 (CCL17 receptor), or (*C*) administering it along with immune checkpoint inhibitors (ICI). CCL17 is one of the chemokines secreted by HRS that is thought to attract immunosuppressive effector cells, such as regulatory T cells, to the tumor microenvironment. Expressing CCR4 in CAR-T cells takes advantage of an ordinarily immune inhibitory mechanism. (Figure created with BioRender.com.)

programmed cell death 1 (PD-1) and thus are susceptible to the inhibition by PD-1 ligand. This inhibition could potentially be evaded by administering an ICI before or after CD30 CAR-Ts (eg, NCT04134325) or by producing CAR-T cells that do not express PD-1. Other approaches, still in early phases, include enhancing CD30.CAR-T trafficking to tumors by coexpressing CCR4 (the receptor for CCL17, which is secreted in high amounts by HRS), and additionally targeting the immunosuppressive HL microenvironment using CD19- and CD123-specific CAR-Ts.[9,24–26]

Further studies are also required to optimize other aspects of CAR-T administration, such as defining the optimal lymphodepleting therapy. In addition, work investigating the effects of CD30 CAR-Ts on tumor CD30 expression and clinical predictors of response is needed.[27,28]

CHIMERIC ANTIGEN RECEPTOR-T CELLS IN T-CELL LYMPHOMA

TCLs are a heterogeneous group of neoplasms that, in general, have a worse prognosis when compared with B-cell NHL and HL and for which treatment options (particularly in r/r settings) are limited and exhibit only modest efficacy.[29] The success of adoptive T-cell therapies in B-cell malignancies has led to an interest in applying them in TCL; however, the biology of TCLs creates new challenges, including the potential fratricide and profound immunodeficiency that may be associated with a CAR targeting a universal T-cell antigen.

Several strategies have been exploited to prevent fratricide during CAR-T manufacture, including disrupting gene expression in T cells via CRISPR or other gene editing methods[30,31] or preventing surface expression of the target antigen by inducing its retention in the endoplasmic reticulum.[32,33] In addition, Watanabe and colleagues showed that the expansion of CAR-Ts in the presence of tyrosine kinase inhibitors (ibrutinib and dasatinib) prevents global fratricide while allowing the production of functional CAR-Ts against the universal T-cell marker CD7 without additional cell engineering,[34] suggesting another potential manufacturing method.

Other recent studies have highlighted that a population of T cells that are natively negative for the antigen targeted can be selected in culture after CAR transduction or in vivo after infusion. In vivo expansion of naturally CD7-negative T cells that express a CD7.CAR and are fratricide resistant due to the lack of antigen expression seems to be an important mechanism for CD7.CAR-Ts persistence described by Watanabe and colleagues.[34] In addition, some CARs may spontaneously induce intracellular sequestration or masking of their cognate antigen and thus allow the emergence of an antigen-negative CAR-T population in culture as has been described with CD5.CARs.[35]

Finally, the potential risk of transduction of circulating tumor cells with the CAR needs to be considered. Many of the manufacture protocols include a selection step to try to eliminate any tumor cells in the starting culture or, at a minimum, a screening step to rule out the presence of malignant cells in the final product.

CD30.CAR-T Cells in T-Cell Lymphomas

As CD30 is highly expressed in a subset of TCLs and BV has improved outcomes in these patients,[36] CD30.CAR-Ts are currently being studied in patients with CD30-positive TCL. Although all of the studies discussed in the prior section allowed enrollment of patients with CD30+ TCL, current published results include only 3 patients: 2 with cutaneous anaplastic large cell lymphoma (ALCL) and 1 with systemic ALK-positive ALCL.[17,18] Two patients had at least PR, with the patient with ALK-positive ALCL achieving and maintaining remission for 9 months. The data on using CD30.CARs in TCL are encouraging but CD30 expression is restricted to a small subset of TCLs and thus applicable to a limited group of patients.

CD5.CAR-T Cells in T-Cell Lymphomas

CD5 is a member of the scavenger receptor cysteine-rich superfamily that is expressed on the surface of 85% to 95% of TCLs depending on the disease subtype, with expression otherwise limited to normal T cells, a small subset of B cells (B1a cells), and thymocytes.[6,37] Based on its broad expression across multiple T-cell malignancies, CD5 was identified as a potential therapeutic target, with early studies investigating the use of a murine mAb for treatment of r/r T-cell malignancies (primarily cutaneous TCLs).[38,39] Although the efficacy was marginal, no severe or irreversible toxicities were observed, providing proof of concept that CD5 could be targeted without dire consequences. Nearly 25 years later, researchers at BCM published the first preclinical data using a second-generation CD28-containing CD5.CAR, demonstrating that CD5.CAR-Ts were able to expand and persist in vitro and in vivo with limited fratricide,[35] likely due to intracellular sequestration and degradation of CD5 when it is bound by the CAR in a transduced cell. The CAR-Ts were also able to eliminate T-cell acute lymphoblastic leukemia (T-ALL) in xenograft mouse models. These preclinical results supported the clinical development of CD5.CAR-Ts for CD5-positive T-cell malignancies.

At the time of this writing, there are currently 7 early phase trials registered on Clinicaltrials.gov exploring the use of CD5.CAR-Ts for T-cell malignancies. However, only 4, of which 2 are actively recruiting (USA: BCM; China: Peking University), include

TCLs. Preliminary findings from the BCM trial (NCT030381910) using autologous CD5.CARTs in patients with r/r T-ALL and TCL were encouraging.[40,41] Results of the first 9 treated patients with TCL were presented at the 2021 ASH annual meeting.[42] Disease subtypes included peripheral T-cell lymphoma (PTCL), angioimmunoblastic TCL (AITL), cutaneous TCL, and adult T-cell leukemia/lymphoma. Enrolled patients had been heavily treated, with a median of 5 lines of prior therapy. All received standard lymphodepletion with cyclophosphamide and fludarabine followed by infusion of CD5.CAR-Ts. Responses were seen on all dose levels, in 4 of 9 patients, with 2 CR, 1 PR, and 1 mixed response initially (all prior disease resolved with appearance of one new lesion).[42] Two patients remain alive over 2 years postinfusion. No severe CAR-T–mediated toxicities were observed, with 4 patients experiencing CRS (grade 1–2) and 1 patient having grade 2 neurotoxicity (concurrent with grade 2 CRS). None of the patients had severe infections. Count recovery occurred by day 28 in most patients; however, 3 patients did experience prolonged cytopenias. The safety of CD5.CAR-Ts was also demonstrated in T-ALL patients.[43]

CD7.CAR-T Cells in T-Cell Lymphomas

CD7 is a member of the immunoglobulin superfamily with broad surface expression in T-cell malignancies, including more than 90% of T-ALL. Its expression is, however, variable in TCL depending on the subtype; in AITL and ALCL it exceeds 50%.[6,44] Similar to CD5 mAb, targeting CD7 with a toxin-conjugated mAb showed modest responses, but its use was limited owing to capillary leak syndrome, which was thought to be related to the toxin.[45] In contrast to CD5.CAR, several preclinical studies of CD7.CAR-Ts demonstrated substantial fratricide,[30–32] a major limiting factor for their potential applicability. Several phase I clinical trials using CD7.CAR-Ts to treat T-cell malignancies and exploiting various strategies to avoid fratricide have been published. However, most of the studies currently available primarily include patients with r/r T-ALL, with few studies including TCL patients.[46–48]

Hu and colleagues reported the results of 12 patients (NCT04538599) treated with allogeneic donor-derived CD7-negative CAR-Ts generated with CD7 and TCR/CD3 knockout via CRISPR/Cas9.[47] Four of the patients were categorized as TCL and included 2 patients with T-cell lymphoblastic lymphoma (T-LBL) and 1 patient each with PTCL NOS and EBV+ NK/TCL. The patient with PTCL NOS achieved CR, and a PR was observed in the patient with EBV+ NK/TCL and in 1 patient with T-LBL. Unfortunately, the patient with PTCL NOS developed EBV-associated PTLD ~55 days postinfusion and died of progressive disease despite treatment with rituximab. Most of the patients (83%) developed grade 1 to 2 CRS, but none developed ICANS or GVHD after a median follow-up of 10.5 months.

In an effort to limit the need for gene editing, Lu and colleagues investigated the role of naturally selected CD7-negative T cells in 20 patients with T-ALL (n = 14) or T-LBL (n = 6).[48] Sixteen patients with bone marrow involvement (94%) achieved CR with negative MRD by day 28 postinfusion, whereas 5 of 9 patients with extramedullary disease had an extramedullary CR at a median time of 29 days (range 15–51). CRS occurred in more than 90% of patients, but only one case developed grade 3 CRS. Fourteen patients received subsequent allogenic hematopoietic stem cell transplantation, of which 10 were for remission consolidation. Others have also reported impressive responses in r/r T-ALL with an overall encouraging safety profile.[49]

BCM currently has an ongoing phase I trial (CRIMSON; NCT03690011) that is currently recruiting patients with TCL. The trial uses nonedited autologous CD7.CAR-Ts manufactured in the presence of tyrosine kinase inhibitors, based on the previously

Table 3
Summary of available results from CD5 and CD7 CAR-T cell studies

Study	Total No. TCL Patients (No. Patients)	Median Age (Range), y	Target (CAR Type)	Subtypes of TCL	LDC	Costimulatory Endodomain (Vector)	Range of CAR-T Cells Doses	Responses % (n)	CRS & ICANS % (n)
CD5									
Rouce et al.[42] 2021	9[9]	63 (27–71)	CD5 (Autologous)	PTCL (n = 4) AITL (n = 2) CTCL (n = 2) ATLL (n = 1)	Flu + Cy	CD28 (γ-retrovirus)	$0.1–1.0 \times 10^8$ cells/m^2	ORR 44%[4] CR 33%[3,a] PR 11%[1]	CRS, all grades: 44%[4] CRS, grade ≥3: 0% ICANS, all grades: 11%[1] ICANS, grade ≥3: 0%
Pan et al.[43] 2022	5 (0)	NR	CD5 (donor-derived)	N.A	NR	4-1BB (Lentivirus)	$0.5–1.0 \times 10^6$ cells/kg	ORR 100%[5] CR 100%[5]	CRS 80%[4] CRS, grade ≥3: 0% ICANS, all grades: NR ICANS, grade ≥3: NR
CD7									
Zhang et al.[46] 2023	10[5]	32 (16–69)	CD7 (autologous or donor-derived)	AITL (n = 1) CTCL (n = 1) TLBL (n = 3)	Flu + Cy	4-1BB (Lentivirus)	$1.0–2.0 \times 10^6$ cells/kg	ORR 70% (7/10)[b]	CRS, all grades: 80%[8] CRS, grade ≥3: 10%[1] ICANS, all grades: 0% ICANS, grade ≥3: 0%
Hu et al.[47] 2022	12[4]	34 (8–66)	CD7 (donor-derived)	PTCL, NOS (n = 1) EBV + NK/TCL (n = 1) TLBL (n = 2)	Flu + Cy + Etop	4-1BB (Lentivirus)	2×10^7 cells/kg	ORR 75% (9/12) CR 58% (7/12)[c] PR 17% (2/12)	CRS, all grades: 83%[10] CRS, grade ≥3: 0% ICANS, all grades: 0% ICANS, grade ≥3: 0%

(continued on next page)

Table 3
(continued)

Study	Total No. Patients (No. TCL Patients)	Median Age (Range), y	Target (CAR Type)	Subtypes of TCL	LDC	Costimulatory Endodomain (Vector)	Range of CAR-T Cells Doses	Responses % (n)	CRS & ICANS % (n)
Lu et al,[48] 2022	20[6]	22[3-47]	CD7 (autologous or donor-derived)	TLBL (n = 6)	Flu + Cy	4-1BB (Lentivirus)	$0.5-2.0 \times 10^6$ cells/kg	ORR 95% (19/20) CR 80% (16/20) PR 10% (2/20)	CRS, all grades: 95%[19]; CRS, grade ≥3: 5%[1]; ICANS, all grades: 10%[2]; ICANS, grade ≥3: 0%
Pan et al,[49] 2022	20 (0)	11[2-43]	CD7 (donor-derived)	N.A	Flu + Cy	4-1BB (Lentivirus)	$0.5-1.0 \times 10^6$ cells/kg	ORR 95% (19/20) CR 90% (18/20) PR 5% (1/20)	CRS, all grades: 100%[20]; CRS, grade ≥3: 10%[2]; ICANS all grades: 15%[3]; ICANS, grade ≥3: 0%

Abbreviations: AITL, angioimmunoblastic T-cell lymphoma; ATLL, adult T-cell leukemia/lymphoma; CR, complete response; CRS, cytokine release syndrome; CTCL, cutaneous T-cell lymphoma; Cy-flu, cyclophosphamide+ fludarabine; EBV, Epstein-Barr virus; EBV+ NK/TCL, EBV-associated NK/T-cell lymphomap; Etop, etoposide; ICANS, immune effector cell–associated neurotoxicity syndrome; LDC, lymphodepleting chemotherapy; NOS, not otherwise specified; NR, not reported; ORR, overall response rate; PR, partial response; PTCL, peripheral T-cell lymphoma; TCL, T-cell lymphoma.

a Two AITL and one PTCL achieved CR. ATLL patient achieved PR; result details were provided courtesy of Dr. LaQuisa Hill.

b Details on CR and PR rates were not clear. CTCL patient achieved PR. No individual data were reported about the AITL patient.

c One PTCL, NOS patient achieved CR, and one EBV+ NK/TCL achieved PR.

Table 4
Examples of CAR-T cells clinical trials in T-cell lymphomas

Target[a]	Identifier	Phase of Study	Type of CAR-T Cells	Institution/Sponsor (Country)	Status
CD30	NCT04952584	I	Allogeneic CD30.CAR-EBVST cells	Baylor College of Medicine (United States)	Recruiting
	NCT04083495	II	Autologous CD30.CART cells	University of North Carolina (United States)	Recruiting
	NCT02917083	I	Autologous CD30.CART cells	Baylor College of Medicine (United States)	Recruiting
CD30 & CCR4	NCT03602157	I	Autologous CD30.CART cells + CCR4	University of North Carolina (United States)	Recruiting
CD5	NCT03081910	I	Autologous CD5.CART cells	Baylor College of Medicine (United States)	Recruiting
	NCT04594135	I	CD5.CART cells	iCell Gene Therapeutics/Peking University People's Hospital (China)	Recruiting
CD7	NCT03690011	I	Autologous CD7.CART cells	Baylor College of Medicine (United States)	Recruiting
	NCT05059912	II	CD7.CART cells	The First Affiliated Hospital of Soochow University (China)	Recruiting
	NCT04823091	I	Donor-derived CD7.CART cells	Wuhan Union Hospital (China)	Recruiting
	NCT05290155	I	CD7.CART cells	Shanghai General Hospital (China)	Recruiting
	NCT05377827	I	Allogeneic CD7.CART cells	Washington University School of Medicine (USA)	Not yet recruiting
CD37	NCT04136275	I	Autologous CD37.CART cells	Massachusetts General Hospital (United States)	Recruiting
CD4	NCT04162340	I	Autologous CD4.CART cells	iCell Gene Therapeutics (China)	Recruiting
	NCT04712864	I	Autologous CD4.CART cells	Legend Biotech USA Inc (Multi-center) (United States)	Active, not recruiting
CD147	NCT05013372	Early phase I	CD147.CART cells	Peking University People's Hospital (China)	Not yet recruiting

[a] This table includes examples of studies investigating each target and not inclusive of all the ongoing studies listed on clinicaltrials.gov.

described preclinical work.[34] Preliminary findings include 2 patients with TCL (AITL and CTCL) who achieved a CR and very good PR, respectively (unpublished data). Other studies are ongoing, the results of which are eagerly awaited.

Challenges and Future Directions

Individual subtypes of TCLs are rare and have distinct clinical behaviors posing real challenges to the interpretation of antitumor activity of CAR-Ts in this setting. Longer follow-up and larger studies are needed to confirm the long-term safety and efficacy of CAR-Ts in TCL in general and in each specific type of TCL.

Even if fratricide can be circumvented in culture and in vivo, the profound immunosuppression caused by potential T-cell aplasia is problematic. The studies published to date have not shown that CD5/7.CAR-T cells are associated with a higher rate of severe infectious complications, but fatal post-CD7.CAR-T EBV-related PTLD has been reported in one patient.[47] In an effort to avoid potentially prolonged immunosuppression, several trials are using CAR-T cells in T-cell malignancies as a bridge to allogeneic hematopoietic stem cell transplant (and concurrent immune ablation that should lead to CAR-T eradication) until more data are available on the extent of immunosuppression, infectious complications, as well as the durability of responses. Another potential strategy to ablate CAR-Ts on demand in case of toxicities is the inclusion of a suicide switch, such as an inducible caspase 9, in the CAR construct.[50] An alternative approach takes advantage of the mutually exclusive expression of β-chain constant region types (TRBC1 or TRBC2) in the TCRs of normal T cells versus the expression of a single type of constant region in the TCR of malignant T cells (which are monoclonal). Selectively targeting malignant TRBC1+ T cells will spare native TRBC2+ T cells (and vice-versa), preventing global T-cell aplasia and potentially avoiding severe immunodeficiency.[51]

Although our discussion was limited to the use of CD30, CD5, and CD7-targeting CAR-Ts (**Table 3**), other targets are being investigated, including CD3, CD4, and CCR4 together with CD30.[6,7,52] **Table 4** includes examples of ongoing studies investigating the use of CAR-Ts against different targets in TCL.

SUMMARY

CAR-T cells have improved outcomes in several lymphoproliferative diseases, in particular CD19- and BCMA-positive malignancies. The use of CAR-T cells is likely to expand over the next few decades, with applications to other hematological and solid tumors. CD30.CAR-T cells have promising safety and activity in r/r HL, with early phase clinical trial data supporting CD30 as a therapeutic target for CAR-T cells in this disorder. Clinical data of CAR-T cells for r/r TCLs are much less mature. Malignant T cells widely express CD5 and CD7, which are potential targets for CAR-T cells. However, further research in the treatment of these disorders with CAR-Ts is needed to address potential challenges, including fratricide and cellular immunodeficiency.

CLINICS CARE POINTS

- CAR-Ts targeting CD30 (in HL or TCL) and CD5 or CD7 (in TCL) are currently only available as part of clinical trials.
- CD30.CAR-Ts toxicities are limited compared to other currently FDA-approved CAR-T cells but, despite an impressive overall response rate, the duration of clinical responses in HL

seems to be shorter than those seen with CD19.CAR-Ts in aggressive NHL, suggesting that additional improvements are needed.

- Experience with CD5.CAR-Ts and CD7.CAR-Ts is more limited; these products also appear to be safe in the early post-infusion period, but a main risk of targeting pan-T antigens is the potential for causing long-lasting profound cellular immunodeficiency, which requires effective mitigation strategies.

- Individual subtypes of TCLs are rare and have distinct clinical behaviors posing real challenges to the interpretation of antitumor activity of CAR-Ts in this setting.

CONFLICT OF INTEREST

L.C. Hill has consulted for March Biosciences, is a member of Speakers Bureau for Kite/Gilead, and served on advisory board for Incyte. C.A. Ramos has participated in advisory boards for Novartis, Genentech, and CRISPR Therapeutics and has received research funding from Athenex and Tessa Therapeutics, Singapore. I.N. Muhsen declares no conflict of interest.

ACKNOWLEDGMENTS

This work was supported by National Cancer Institute, United States grants P50 CA126752 and P30 CA125123 and a Specialized Center of Research grant from the Leukemia & Lymphoma Society, United States.

REFERENCES

1. Ansell SM, Radford J, Connors JM, et al. ECHELON-1 Study Group. Overall Survival with Brentuximab Vedotin in Stage III or IV Hodgkin's Lymphoma. N Engl J Med 2022;387(4):310–20.
2. Chen R, Gopal AK, Smith SE, et al. Five-year survival and durability results of brentuximab vedotin in patients with relapsed or refractory Hodgkin lymphoma. Blood 2016;128(12):1562–6.
3. Moskowitz CH, Nademanee A, Masszi T, et al, AETHERA Study Group. Brentuximab vedotin as consolidation therapy after autologous stem-cell transplantation in patients with Hodgkin's lymphoma at risk of relapse or progression (AETHERA): a randomised, double-blind, placebo-controlled, phase 3 trial. Lancet 2015;385(9980):1853–62.
4. Hombach A, Heuser C, Sircar R, et al. An anti-CD30 chimeric receptor that mediates CD3-zeta-independent T-cell activation against Hodgkin's lymphoma cells in the presence of soluble CD30. Cancer Res 1998;58(6):1116–9.
5. Savoldo B, Rooney CM, Di Stasi A, et al. Epstein Barr virus specific cytotoxic T lymphocytes expressing the anti-CD30zeta artificial chimeric T-cell receptor for immunotherapy of Hodgkin disease. Blood 2007;110(7):2620–30.
6. Scherer LD, Brenner MK, Mamonkin M. Chimeric Antigen Receptors for T-Cell Malignancies. Front Oncol 2019;9:126.
7. Safarzadeh Kozani P, Safarzadeh Kozani P, Rahbarizadeh F. CAR-T cell therapy in T-cell malignancies: Is success a low-hanging fruit? Stem Cell Res Ther 2021;12(1):527.
8. Engert A, Plutschow A, Eich HT, et al. Reduced treatment intensity in patients with early-stage Hodgkin's lymphoma. N Engl J Med 2010;363(7):640–52.
9. Ho C, Ruella M, Levine BL, et al. Adoptive T-cell therapy for Hodgkin lymphoma. Blood Adv 2021;5(20):4291–302.

10. Doubrovina E, Oflaz-Sozmen B, Prockop SE, et al. Adoptive immunotherapy with unselected or EBV-specific T cells for biopsy-proven EBV1 lymphomas after allogeneic hematopoietic cell transplantation. Blood 2012;119(11):2644–56.

11. Heslop HE, Slobod KS, Pule MA, et al. Long-term outcome of EBV-specific T-cell infusions to prevent or treat EBV-related lymphoproliferative disease in transplant recipients. Blood 2010;115(5):925–35.

12. Bollard CM, Aguilar L, Straathof KC, et al. Cytotoxic T lymphocyte therapy for Epstein-Barr virus+ Hodgkin's disease. J Exp Med 2004;200(12):1623–33.

13. van der Weyden C.A., Pileri S.A., Feldman A.L., et al., Understanding CD30 biology and therapeutic targeting: a historical perspective providing insight into future directions, Blood Cancer J, 2017;7(9): e603.

14. Horie R, Watanabe T, Morishita Y, et al. Ligandindependent signaling by overexpressed CD30 drives NF-kappaB activation in Hodgkin–Reed–Sternberg cells. Oncogene 2002;21:2493–503, 48.

15. Hirsch B, Hummel M, Bentink S, et al. CD30- induced signaling is absent in Hodgkin's cells but present in anaplastic large cell lymphoma cells. Am J Pathol 2008;172:510–20.

16. Grover NS, Savoldo B. Challenges of driving CD30-directed CAR-T cells to the clinic. BMC Cancer 2019;19(1):203.

17. Wang CM, Wu ZQ, Wang Y, et al. Autologous T Cells Expressing CD30 Chimeric Antigen Receptors for Relapsed or Refractory Hodgkin Lymphoma: An Open-Label Phase I Trial. Clin Cancer Res 2017;23(5):1156–66.

18. Ramos CA, Ballard B, Zhang H, et al. Clinical and immunological responses after CD30-specific chimeric antigen receptor-redirected lymphocytes. J Clin Invest 2017;127(9):3462–71.

19. Ramos CA, Grover NS, Beaven AW, et al. Anti-CD30 CAR-T Cell Therapy in Relapsed and Refractory Hodgkin Lymphoma. J Clin Oncol 2020;38(32):3794–804.

20. Ahmed S, Flinn I, Mei M, et al. Safety and efficacy profile of autologous CD30.CAR-T-Cell therapy in patients with relapsed or refractory classical Hodgkin lymphoma (CHARIOT trial). Blood 2021;138(Supplement 1):3847.

21. Zhao J, Lin Q, Song Y, et al. Universal CARs, universal T cells, and universal CAR-T cells. J Hematol Oncol 2018;11:132.

22. Martínez Bedoya D., Dutoit V. and Migliorini D., Allogeneic CAR-T Cells: An Alternative to Overcome Challenges of CAR-T Cell Therapy in Glioblastoma, Front Immunol, 2021;12:640082.

23. Depil S, Duchateau P, Grupp SA, et al. "Off-the-shelf" allogeneic CAR-T cells: development and challenges. Nat Rev Drug Discov 2020;19:185–99.

24. Ullah F, Dima D, Omar N, et al. Advances in the treatment of Hodgkin lymphoma: Current and future approaches. Front Oncol 2023;13:1067289.

25. Meier JA, Savoldo B, Grover NS. The Emerging Role of CAR T Cell Therapy in Relapsed/Refractory Hodgkin Lymphoma. J Pers Med 2022;12(2):197.

26. Di Stasi A, De Angelis B, Rooney CM, et al. T lymphocytes coexpressing CCR4 and a chimeric antigen receptor targeting CD30 have improved homing and anti-tumor activity in a Hodgkin tumor model. Blood 2009;113(25):6392–402.

27. Marques-Piubelli ML, Kim DH, Medeiros LJ, et al. CD30 expression is frequently decreased in relapsed classic Hodgkin lymphoma after anti-CD30 CAR T-cell therapy. Histopathology 2023. https://doi.org/10.1111/his.14910.

28. Voorhees TJ, Zhao B, Oldan J, et al. Pretherapy metabolic tumor volume is associated with response to CD30 CAR T cells in Hodgkin lymphoma. Blood Adv 2022 Feb 22;6(4):1255–63.

29. Foss FM, Zinzani PL, Vose JM, et al. Peripheral T-cell lymphoma. Blood 2011; 117(25):6756–67.
30. Gomes-Silva D, Srinivasan M, Sharma S, et al. CD7-edited T cells expressing a CD7-specific CAR for the therapy of T-cell malignancies. Blood 2017;130:285–96.
31. Cooper ML, Choi J, Staser K, et al. An "off-the-shelf" fratricide-resistant CAR-T for the treatment of T cell hematologic malignancies. Leukemia 2018;32(9):1970–83.
32. Png YT, Vinanica N, Kamiya T, et al. Blockade of CD7 expression in T cells for effective chimeric antigen receptor targeting of T-cell malignancies. Blood Adv 2017;1:2348–60.
33. Zhang M, Chen D, Fu X, et al. Autologous Nanobody-Derived Fratricide-Resistant CD7-CAR T-cell Therapy for Patients with Relapsed and Refractory T-cell Acute Lymphoblastic Leukemia/Lymphoma. Clin Cancer Res 2022;28(13):2830–43.
34. Watanabe N, Mo F, Zheng R, et al. Feasibility and preclinical efficacy of CD7-unedited CD7 CAR T cells for T cell malignancies. Mol Ther 2023;31(1):24–34.
35. Mamonkin M, Rouce RH, Tashiro H, et al. A T-Cell-Directed chimeric antigen receptor for the selective treatment of T-cell malignancies. Blood 2015;126(8): 983–92.
36. Horwitz S, O'Connor OA, Pro B, et al. ECHELON-2 Study Group. Brentuximab vedotin with chemotherapy for CD30-positive peripheral T-cell lymphoma (ECHELON-2): a global, double-blind, randomised, phase 3 trial. Lancet 2019; 393(10168):229–40.
37. Campana D, van Dongen JJ, Mehta A, et al. Stages of T-cell receptor protein expression in T-cell acute lymphoblastic leukemia. Blood 1991;77(7):1546–54.
38. Bertram JH, Gill PS, Levine AM, et al. Monoclonal antibody T101 in T cell malignancies: a clinical, pharmacokinetic, and immunologic correlation. Blood 1986; 68(3):752–61.
39. LeMaistre CF, Rosen S, Frankel A, et al. Phase I trial of H65-RTA immunoconjugate in patients with cutaneous T-cell lymphoma. Blood 1991;78(5):1173–82.
40. Hill LC, Rouce RH, Smith TS, et al. Safety and anti-tumor activity of CD5 car T-cells in patients with Relapsed/Refractory T-cell malignancies. Blood 2019; 134(Supplement_1):199.
41. Hill L, Rouce RH, Smith TS, et al. CD5 CAR T-Cells for Treatment of Patients with Relapsed/Refractory CD5 Expressing T-Cell Lymphoma Demonstrates Safety and Anti-Tumor Activity. Biol Blood Marrow Transplant 2020;26.
42. Rouce RH, Hill LC, Smith TS, et al. Early Signals of Anti-Tumor Efficacy and Safety with Autologous CD5.CAR T-Cells in Patients with Refractory/Relapsed T-Cell Lymphoma. Blood 2021;138(Supplement 1):654.
43. Pan J, Tan Y, Shan L, et al. Phase I study of donor-derived CD5 CAR T cells in patients with relapsed or refractory T-cell acute lymphoblastic leukemia. J Clin Oncol 2022;40(16_suppl):7028.
44. Wei W, Yang D, Chen X, et al. Chimeric antigen receptor T-cell therapy for T-ALL and AML. Front Oncol 2022;12:967754.
45. Frankel AE, Laver JH, Willingham MC, et al. Therapy of patients with T-cell lymphomas and leukemias using an anti-CD7 monoclonal antibody-ricin A chain immunotoxin. Leuk Lymphoma 1997;26(3–4):287–98.
46. Zhang Y, Li C, Du M, et al. Allogenic and autologous anti-CD7 CAR-T cell therapies in relapsed or refractory T-cell malignancies. Blood Cancer J 2023;13(1):61.
47. Hu Y, Zhou Y, Zhang M, et al. Genetically modified CD7-targeting allogeneic CAR-T cell therapy with enhanced efficacy for relapsed/refractory CD7-positive hematological malignancies: a phase I clinical study. Cell Res 2022 Nov; 32(11):995–1007.

48. Lu P, Liu Y, Yang J, et al. Naturally selected CD7 CAR-T therapy without genetic manipulations for T-ALL/LBL: first-in-human phase 1 clinical trial. Blood 2022; 140(4):321–34.

49. Pan J, Tan Y, Wang G, et al. Donor-Derived CD7 Chimeric Antigen Receptor T Cells for T-Cell Acute Lymphoblastic Leukemia: First-in-Human, Phase I Trial. J Clin Oncol 2021;39(30):3340–51.

50. Di Stasi A, Tey SK, Dotti G, et al. Inducible apoptosis as a safety switch for adoptive cell therapy. N Engl J Med 2011;365(18):1673–83.

51. Maciocia PM, Wawrzyniecka PA, Philip B, et al. Targeting the T cell receptor beta-chain constant region for immunotherapy of T cell malignancies. Nat Med 2017; 23(12):1416–23.

52. Hill L, Lulla P, Heslop HE. CAR-T cell Therapy for Non-Hodgkin Lymphomas: A New Treatment Paradigm. Adv Cell Gene Ther 2019;2(3):e54.

Chimeric Antigen Receptor T Cells in Acute Myeloid Leukemia

Katherine Cummins, MBBS, PhD, FRACP, FRCPA[a],
Saar Gill, MBBS, PhD, FRACP[b],*

KEYWORDS

- Acute myeloid leukemia • Cellular immunotherapy • CAR T cells • CRS
- Myeloablation

KEY POINTS

- Up to 30% of patients with acute myeloid leukemia (AML) who undergo chimeric antigen receptor (CAR) T-cell therapy have evidence of response, although trials are highly heterogeneous. These responses are rarely deep or durable.
- CD123, CD33, and CLL-1 have emerged as the most common targets for CAR T cells in AML.
- CAR T cells against myeloid antigens cause myeloablation as well as cytokine release syndrome, although neurotoxicity is rarely seen.
- Future efforts should focus on AML-specific antigen discovery or engineering, and on further enhancing the activity of CAR T cells.

INTRODUCTION

Chimeric antigen receptor (CAR) T cells are a form of potent antigen-specific immunotherapy. CAR T cells generate impressive rates and depths of remissions in patients with multiply relapsed lymphoid malignancies including B-cell acute lymphoid leukemia (B-ALL),[1–4] aggressive and indolent non-Hodgkin lymphomas,[5–9] and multiple myeloma (MM).[10,11] Recent data also show promising results against T-cell ALL.[12] We and others have demonstrated encouraging preclinical activity of anti-AML activity of CAR T cells directed against CD123, CD33, and other antigens in multiple murine xenograft models[13–17]; yet to date, published reports of the clinical effect of CAR

[a] Peter MacCallum Cancer Centre, University of Melbourne, 305 Grattan Street, Melbourne, VIC 3000, Australia; [b] Division of Hematology-Oncology, University of Pennsylvania Perelman School of Medicine, 8-101 Smilow Center for Translational Research, 3400 Civic Center Boulevard, Philadelphia, PA 19104, USA
* Corresponding author. Smilow Center for Translational Research, Room 8-1013400 Civic Center Boulevard, Building 421, Philadelphia, PA 19104.
E-mail address: saar.gill@pennmedicine.upenn.edu

Hematol Oncol Clin N Am 37 (2023) 1125–1147
https://doi.org/10.1016/j.hoc.2023.06.004
0889-8588/23/© 2023 Elsevier Inc. All rights reserved.

hemonc.theclinics.com

T cells in AML remain scarce and response rates appear low.[18–26] These observations are particularly surprising given the established role of cellular immunotherapy in AML, based on decades of experience with allogeneic stem cell transplantation and donor lymphocyte infusions, in which T cells are an integral component.[27–31]

When CAR T-cell therapy against AML was first conceptualized, it was anticipated that the main clinical challenge would be antigen selection, in view of the shared antigen expression between healthy marrow progenitor cells and malignant blasts. Targets for CART therapy are generally lineage-associated antigens such as CD19 or CD22 for the B-cell malignancies, and CD33 or CD123 for AML. Myeloid antigens that are expressed on AML blasts are also expressed on hematopoietic stem and progenitor cells (HSPC) and some differentiated progeny such as monocytes and granulocytes. Thus, just as potent anti-CD19 CAR T cells lead to prolonged B-cell aplasia, it is anticipated that potent anti-myeloid CAR T cells would lead to myeloid aplasia. This was supported by data from preclinical humanized murine models of CART targeting CD33 or CD123 whereby eradication of AML blasts went hand in hand with eradication of the healthy myeloid compartment.[13,32] Although prolonged B-cell aplasia is relatively benign and easily supported with the administration of immunoglobulin, prolonged myeloid aplasia is more problematic owing to the need for blood and platelet transfusions and the risk of neutropenic infections. This could potentially be circumvented by using CAR T cells as a means to eradicate both malignant and any residual normal hematopoiesis, to be followed by CART deletion and a subsequent rescue allogeneic stem cell transplant to regenerate hematopoietic function. An alternative solution could be to discover and validate novel AML-specific targets, although to date the search for such putative targets is ongoing. Innovative synthetic biology solutions that create AML-specific antigens de novo by combining gene edited hematopoietic cell transplantation with myeloid-directed immunotherapy could solve this problem and remain our favored approach.

In this review article, we will discuss the clinical and preclinical data that support the potential of CAR T cells in AML and related malignancies and speculate on future directions for improvement. We will do this by systematically describing antigen selection, CAR design, choice of effector cell, and clinical trial design. Given the paucity of clinical trial data, we will attempt to synthesize the available preclinical and clinical data, wherever possible, by comparing AML to B-ALL.

BACKGROUND

Approximately 20,000 Americans are diagnosed with AML each year at a median age of diagnosis of 69, and the 5-year survival is approximately 31.7% (https://seer.cancer. gov/statfacts/html/alyl.html accessed May 2, 2023). After decades of incremental gains in acute myeloid leukemia (AML) therapeutics, recent breakthroughs that have led to improvements in clinical outcomes include combination BCL2 antagonism with hypomethylating agents, liposomal chemotherapy, novel targeted therapies, and maintenance therapies.[31,33–38] These advances extend the range of therapeutic options and deliver higher response rates compared with controls in randomized trials, but patients with relapsed/refractory disease continue to have poor outcomes.[37,39] Use of immunotherapy in the form of allogeneic hematopoietic cell transplantation (alloHCT) remains the only modality with the potential to deliver durable remissions.[27–31]

In heavily pre-treated B-ALL, autologous anti-CD19 CAR T cells deliver high rates of complete remissions (62%–93%) that are usually associated with undetectable measurable residual disease (uMRD), occur quickly (within 1 month), and are effective in extramedullary sites including the central nervous system.[3,4,40–43] Six years after the first commercial approval of CART-19 for ALL and with thousands of patients treated worldwide, observations that define patient, disease, and treatment-specific risk factors for success or failure are emerging.[44] These include cytogenetic and molecular features, impact of prior therapy, high disease burden (defined as > 5% marrow blasts) or active extramedullary disease, lower fludarabine exposure as part of the lymphodepleting chemotherapy regimen, or detectable MRD after day 28. Two major patterns of relapse have emerged: antigen-loss relapses may occur early, in the presence of persistently active CART-19, whereas relapses with retention of the targeted antigen typically occur in the setting of failure of CART persistence, best defined functionally as loss of B-cell aplasia by perhaps 6 months after infusion (although this time point is not well defined).

Although B-ALL is a cancer of precursor B cells immediately downstream of the common lymphoid progenitor, AML is thought to arise in very early myeloid progenitors.[45–48] The occurrence of acute leukemias of mixed or ambiguous phenotype, and of acute leukemias that undergo a lineage switch from lymphoid to myeloid (or vice versa) during treatment, indicates a high degree of biological overlap between the 2 diseases.[49] This assertion is further supported by their similar clinical presentations, occasionally overlapping genomics, and by the response to similar classes of drugs.

These observations as well as early preclinical studies on AML therefore led us and other investigators to predict that CAR T cells would be equally active in the AML setting.[13,50] Indeed, in one study we engrafted an ALL cell line or primary patient-derived B-ALL specimens into immunodeficient mice and treated with CAR T cells directed against CD19 or the early hematopoietic marker CD123. We found CART-19 and CART-123 to be equally active in ALL, and showed that CART-123 could be used to treat CD19-negative ALL blasts that occurred in a patient who had earlier received CART-19.[51]

To date, however, available results from trials of CAR T cells in AML have been relatively disappointing. The available clinical data are largely restricted to small case series (**Table 1**) and are further described below. Nonetheless, numerous clinical trials are currently recruiting or shortly to open, and these are outlined in **Table 2**.

CLINICAL CHIMERIC ANTIGEN RECEPTOR T-CELL PLATFORMS IN ACUTE MYELOID LEUKEMIA

LewisY

The first published clinical trial in AML with a CART that showed biological activity sought to target a leukemia-specific antigen. The CAR was designed to target LewisY (LeY), a difucosylated carbohydrate antigen, that is expressed in a range of malignancies, including AML, but with limited expression on healthy tissues.[18] Four patients received CAR T cells transduced with a retroviral vector encoding a CD28-costimulated anti-LeY CAR, after fludarabine-containing lymphodepletion. This therapy was well tolerated, with no cytokine release syndrome (CRS) being observed. Using an aliquot of radiolabeled CAR T cells, the authors demonstrated trafficking to the bone marrow, and in a patient with leukemia cutis CAR T cells were found to infiltrate sites of disease. The best response was a transient cytogenetic remission in a patient with cytogenetic-only MRD at infusion.

CD33

CD33 is a membrane bound glycoprotein that is a member of SIGLEC family, which is present on AML blasts, as well as normal HSPC.[14,58] CD33 is the target of gemtuzumab ozogamicin, an antibody-drug conjugate with an established track record in AML.[59]

Table 1
Chimeric antigen receptor T cell trials in acute myeloid leukemia

Target	Patients Treated	Responses	Toxicity	Comments
CD123				
Donor CART-123[22]	1	PR (?)	CRS gr. 4	
UniCART-123[26]	3	1 PR, 2 CRi	CRS gr. 1 (n = 2) Myelosuppression	Expansion, persistence seen IL-6, TNF, IFN γ detected
CART-123[52]	7 (18 enrolled)	2 MLFS, 1 CRi	CRS gr. 1–2	Peak expansion at day 14 No CD123 loss
UCART-123[53]	16	1 MLFS, 1 CR (uMRD)	CRS in 15/16 including 2 gr.4 and 1 gr.5 CRS	
CD33				
UltraCART-33[54]	24 (10 without and 14 with lymphodepletion)	Objective responses in 30%	Gr. 1 CRS (n = 10), gr. 2 CRS (n = 6), gr. 3 CRS (n = 1). No bone marrow aplasia	Dose-dependent expansion in blood and marrow Persistence up to 7 mo
CART-33[25]	1	PR	CRS, pancytopenia	IL-6, IL-8,TNF, IFN γ detected
CART-33[24]	3	None	CRS (n = 2). ICANS (n = 1)	IL-6, TNF, IFN γ detected
CLL-1 (CLEC12A)				
CART-CLL1[55]	7 (pediatric)	CR in 5/7	Gr. 1–2 CRS (n = 7)	
CART-CLL1[21]	10 (adult)	CR or CRi in 7/10	Low grade CRS (n = 4). High grade CRS (n = 6). Severe pancytopenia (n = 10)	
CART-CLL1[56]	8 (pediatric)	MLFS in 5/8, CRi in 1/8, 1 PR	CRS (n = 8)	Loss of CLL1+ subset in 1 patient
Other				
CART-Lewis Y[18]	4	Cytogenetic response 1/4	None	Trafficking to marrow demonstrated using radiolabeling
NKG2D ligands[57]	12	Objective response in 3/12	Gr. 3–4 CRS (n = 5)	

Abbreviations: CR(i), CR with incomplete count recovery; CR, complete response; CRS, cytokine release syndrome; MLFS, morphologic leukemia-free state; PR, partial response.

Table 2
Currently recruiting and upcoming chimeric antigen receptor T trials in acute myeloid leukemia, April 2023

Intervention	Location	Status	Title	URL
CART-33				
CD33 CAR-T	The first affiliated hospital of medical college of Zhejiang University, Hangzhou, Zhejiang, China	Not yet recruiting	Evaluate the Safety and Efficacy of CD33 CAR-T in Patients With R/R AML	https://ClinicalTrials.gov/show/NCT05473221
Anti-CD33 CAR T cells	Hebei Yanda Lu Daopei Hospital, Langfang, Hebei, China	Not yet recruiting	Anti-CD33 CAR-T Cells for the Treatment of Relapsed/Refractory CD33+ Acute Myeloid Leukemia	https://ClinicalTrials.gov/show/NCT05445765
Anti-CD33 CAR T-cells	City of Hope Medical Center, Duarte, California, United States	Not yet recruiting	CD33-CAR T Cell Therapy for the Treatment of Recurrent or Refractory Acute Myeloid Leukemia	https://ClinicalTrials.gov/show/NCT05672147
Chimeric antigen receptor T cell	Beijing Boren Hospital, Beijing, Beijing, China	Recruiting	Phase I/II Study of Enhanced CD33 CAR T Cells in Subjects With Relapsed or Refractory Acute Myeloid Leukemia	https://ClinicalTrials.gov/show/NCT04835519
CD33CART	Children's Hospital of Los Angeles, Los Angeles, California, United States	Recruiting	Study of Anti-CD33 Chimeric Antigen Receptor-Expressing T Cells (CD33CART) in Children and Young Adults With Relapsed/Refractory Acute Myeloid Leukemia	https://ClinicalTrials.gov/show/NCT03971799
CART-38				
$3 \times 10(6)$ CART-38 cells (dose escalation)	University of Pennsylvania, Philadelphia, Pennsylvania, United States	Not yet recruiting	CART-38 in Adult AML and MM Patients	https://ClinicalTrials.gov/show/NCT05442580

(continued on next page)

Table 2
(continued)

Intervention	Location	Status	Title	URL
CD38 CAR T-cells	The first affiliated hospital of medical college of Zhejiang University, Hangzhou, Zhejiang, China	Recruiting	Clinical Study of CD38 CAR-T Cells in the Treatment of Hematological Malignancies	https://ClinicalTrials.gov/show/NCT05239689
CART-38	The First Affiliated Hospital of Soochow University, Suzhou, Jiangsu, China	Recruiting	CD38-targeted Chimeric Antigen Receptor T Cell (CART) in Relapsed or Refractory Acute Myeloid Leukemia	https://ClinicalTrials.gov/show/NCT04351022
CART-123				
IL3 CAR T-cells	The First Affiliated Hospital, College of Medicine, Zhejiang University, Hangzhou, Zhejiang, China	Not yet recruiting	IL3 CAR-T Cell Therapy for Patients With CD123 Positive Relapsed and/or Refractory Acute Myeloid Leukemia	https://ClinicalTrials.gov/show/NCT04599543
CD123-CAR T	St Jude Children's Research Hospital, Memphis, Tennessee, United States	Recruiting	CD123-Directed Autologous T-Cell Therapy for Acute Myelogenous Leukemia (CATCHAML)	https://ClinicalTrials.gov/show/NCT04318678
CD123 CAR-T cells	Chongqing University Cancer Hospital, Chongqing, Chongqing, China	Recruiting	Safety and Efficacy of CD123-Targeted CAR-T Therapy for Relapsed/Refractory Acute Myeloid Leukemia	https://ClinicalTrials.gov/show/NCT04272125
UCART123v1.2	University of California, San Francisco (UCSF) - Helen Diller Family Comprehensive Cancer Center, San Francisco, California, United States	Recruiting	Study Evaluating Safety and Efficacy of UCART123 in Patients With Relapsed/ Refractory Acute Myeloid Leukemia	https://ClinicalTrials.gov/show/NCT03190278
CART123 cells; cyclophosphamide; fludarabine	Children's Hospital of Philadelphia, Philadelphia, Pennsylvania, United States	Recruiting	CD123 Redirected T Cells for AML in Pediatric Subjects	https://ClinicalTrials.gov/show/NCT04678836

CART-CLL1

CLL1 CAR-T	Not yet recruiting	Evaluate the Safety and Efficacy of CLL1 CAR-T in Patients With R/R AML	https://ClinicalTrials.gov/show/NCT05467202
CLL-1 CAR T cells	Recruiting	Chimeric Antigen Receptor T-cells for The Treatment of AML Expressing CLL-1 Antigen	https://ClinicalTrials.gov/show/NCT04219163
CLL1 CAR T-cells	Recruiting	Clinical Study of CLL1 CAR-T Cells in the Treatment of Hematological Malignancies	https://ClinicalTrials.gov/show/NCT05252572
Anti-CLL1 CART	Recruiting	Anti-CLL1 CAR T-cell Therapy in CLL1 Positive Relapsed/Refractory Acute Myeloid Leukemia (AML)	https://ClinicalTrials.gov/show/NCT04884984
KITE-222 (CART-CLL1)	Recruiting	Study Evaluating the Safety of KITE-222 in Participants With Relapsed/Refractory Acute Myeloid Leukemia	https://ClinicalTrials.gov/show/NCT04789408
Anti-CLL1 CART cells	Recruiting	Clinical Study of Chimeric Antigen Receptor T Lymphocytes (CAR-T) in the Treatment of Myeloid Leukemia	https://ClinicalTrials.gov/show/NCT04923919
CLL1-CD33 cCAR T cells	Recruiting	CLL1-CD33 cCAR in Patients With Relapsed and/or Refractory, High Risk Hematologic Malignancies	https://ClinicalTrials.gov/show/NCT03795779
Dual targeting CART			
CLL1+CD33 CAR-T	Not yet recruiting	Evaluate the Safety and Efficacy of CLL1+CD33 CAR-T in Patients With R/R AML	https://ClinicalTrials.gov/show/NCT05467254

(continued on next page)

Table 2
(continued)

Intervention	Location	Status	Title	URL
Dual CD33-CLL1 CAR-T cells	Department of Hematology, Xinqiao Hospital, Chongqing, Chongqing, China	Not yet recruiting	Dual CD33-CLL1-CAR-T Cells in the Treatment of Relapsed/Refractory Acute Myeloid Leukemia	https://ClinicalTrials.gov/show/NCT05016063
Dual CD33/CLL1 CAR T	Beijing Boren Hospital, Beijing, Beijing, China	Recruiting	Optimized Dual CD33/CLL1 CAR T Cells in Subjects With Refractory or Relapsed Acute Myeloid Leukemia	https://ClinicalTrials.gov/show/NCT05248685
LCAR-AMDR Cells Product	Beijing Gobroad BoRen Hospital, Beijing, Beijing, China	Recruiting	CLL-1/CD33 Targeted LCAR-AMDR Cells in Patients With Relapsed or Refractory Acute Myeloid Leukemia	https://ClinicalTrials.gov/show/NCT05654779
CART-NKG2D				
NKG2D CAR T-cells	The First Affiliated Hospital, College of Medicine, Zhejiang University, Hangzhou, Zhejiang, China	Not yet recruiting	NKG2D CAR-T Cell Therapy for Patients With Relapsed and/or Refractory Acute Myeloid Leukemia	https://ClinicalTrials.gov/show/NCT04658004
CYAD-02 (NKD2G + shRNA)	Mayo Clinic Cancer Center, Jacksonville, Florida, United States	Recruiting	Study in Relapsed/Refractory Acute Myeloid Leukemia or Myelodysplastic Syndrome Patients to Determine the Recommended Dose of CYAD-02	https://ClinicalTrials.gov/show/NCT04167696
CART-CD7				
Anti-CD7 CAR-T		Not yet recruiting	CD7 CAR-T for Patients With r/r CD7+ Hematologic Malignancies	https://ClinicalTrials.gov/show/NCT05454241
WU-CART-007	Washington University School of Medicine, Saint Louis, Missouri, United States	Not yet recruiting	Dose-Escalation and Dose-Expansion Study to Evaluate the Safety and Tolerability of Anti-CD7 Allogeneic CAR T-Cells (WU-CART-007) in Patients With CD7+ Hematologic Malignancies	https://ClinicalTrials.gov/show/NCT05377827

Humanized CD7 CAR-T cells	The First Affiliated Hospital of Soochow University, Suzhou, (Select), China	Recruiting	Humanized CD7 CAR T-cell Therapy for r/r CD7+ Acute Leukemia	https://ClinicalTrials.gov/show/NCT04762485
CD7-specific CAR gene-engineered T cells	Shenzhen Geno-immune Medical Institute, Shenzhen, Guangdong, China	Recruiting	Multi-CAR T Cell Therapy Targeting CD7-positive Malignancies	https://ClinicalTrials.gov/show/NCT04033302
CART-FLT3				
AMG 553	City of Hope National Medical Center, Duarte, California, United States	Not yet recruiting	Study Evaluating the Safety, Tolerability, and Efficacy of FLT3 CAR-T AMG 553 in FLT3-positive Relapsed/Refractory AML	https://ClinicalTrials.gov/show/NCT03904069
Anti-FLT3 CAR-T	The First Affiliated Hospital of Soochow University, Suzhou, Jiangsu, China	Recruiting	Anti-FLT3 CAR T-cell Therapy in FLT3 Positive Relapsed/Refractory Acute Myeloid Leukemia	https://ClinicalTrials.gov/show/NCT05023707
Fludarabine + Cyclophosphamide + TAA05 Cell Injection	Wuhan Union Hospital, Wuhan, Hubei, China	Recruiting	Anti-FLT3 CAR-T Cell (TAA05 Cell Injection) in the Treatment of Relapsed / Refractory Acute Myeloid Leukemia	https://ClinicalTrials.gov/show/NCT05445011
TAA05 cell injection (CART-FLT3)	Anhui Provincial Hospital, Hefei, Anhui, China	Recruiting	TAA05 Cell Injection in the Treatment of Recurrent / Refractory Acute Myeloid Leukemia	https://ClinicalTrials.gov/show/NCT05017883
T cell injection targeting FLT3 chimeric antigen receptor	Union Hospital, affiliated with Tongli Medical College, HuaZhong University of Science and Technology, Wuhan, Hubei, China	Recruiting	TAA05 Injection in the Treatment of Adult Patients With FLT3-positive Relapsed/Refractory Acute Myeloid Leukemia	https://ClinicalTrials.gov/show/NCT05432401
CART against novel antigens				
CAR-T cells against ?IM73	Peking University People's Hospital (PKUPH), Peking, China	Not yet recruiting	Donor-derived CAR-T Cells in the Treatment of AML Patients	https://ClinicalTrials.gov/show/NCT04766840

(continued on next page)

Table 2
(continued)

Intervention	Location	Status	Title	URL
ADGRE2 CAR-T	Mingming Zhang Zhang, Hangzhou, China	Not yet recruiting	Evaluate the Safety and Efficacy of ADGRE2 CAR-T in Patients With R/R AML	https://ClinicalTrials.gov/show/NCT05463640
Anti-siglec-6 (CD33-like) CAR-T cell therapy	Kailin Xu, Xuzhou, Jiangsu, China	Recruiting	Administration of Anti-siglec-6 CAR-T Cell Therapy in Relapsed and Refractory Acute Myeloid Leukemia (rr/AML)	https://ClinicalTrials.gov/show/NCT05488132
CAR-T CD19	Chaim Sheba Medical Center, Ramat Gan, Israel	Recruiting	CAR-T CD19 for Acute Myelogenous Leukemia With t 8:21 and CD19 Expression	https://ClinicalTrials.gov/show/NCT04257175
CI-135 CAR-T cells (or is this CD135 i.e. FLT3????)	Beijing Gaobo Boren Hospital, Beijing, China	Recruiting	Safety and Efficacy Study of CI-135 CAR-T Cells in Subjects With Relapsed or Refractory Acute Myeloid Leukemia	https://ClinicalTrials.gov/show/NCT05266950
B7-H3 target, CAR gene modified gdT cell injection (CD276)	The First Affiliated Hospital , Zhejiang University School of Medicine, Hangzhou, Zhejiang, China	Recruiting	UTAA06 Injection in the Treatment of Relapsed/Refractory Acute Myeloid Leukemia	https://ClinicalTrials.gov/show/NCT05731219
Chimeric antigen receptor T cells (car-t against CD276)	Anhui Provincial Hospital, Hefei, Anhui, China	Recruiting	TAA6 Cell Injection In The Treatment of Patients With Relapsed/Refractory Acute Myeloid Leukemia	https://ClinicalTrials.gov/show/NCT04692948
SC-DARIC33	Seattle Children's Hospital, Seattle, Washington, United States	Recruiting	PLAT-08: A Study Of SC-DARIC33 CAR T Cells In Pediatric And Young Adults With Relapsed Or Refractory CD33+ AML	https://ClinicalTrials.gov/show/NCT05105152
CART-19	The First Affiliated Hospital of Soochow University, Suzhou, Jiangsu, China	Recruiting	CART-19 T Cell in CD19 Positive Relapsed or Refractory Acute Myeloid Leukemia (AML)	https://ClinicalTrials.gov/show/NCT03896854

CD70 CAR T-cells	The first affiliated hospital of Medical College of Zhejiang University, Hangzhou, Zhejiang, China	Recruiting	CD 70 CAR T for Patients With CD70 Positive Malignant Hematologic Diseases	https://ClinicalTrials.gov/show/NCT04662294
Autologous CAR-T cells (CD19/BCMA/CD123/CD7)	Shanghai Pudong Hospital, Fudan University Affiliated Pudong Medical Center, Shanghai, Shanghai, China	Recruiting	Novel CAR-T Cell Therapy in the Treatment of Hematopoietic and Lymphoid Malignancies	https://ClinicalTrials.gov/show/NCT0513612
CAR-NK				
CD123-CAR-NK cells	The Fifth Medical Center of Chinese People's Liberation Army (PLA) General Hospital, Beijing, Beijing, China	Recruiting	Allogenic CD123-CAR-NK Cells in the Treatment of Refractory/ Relapsed Acute Myeloid Leukemia	https://ClinicalTrials.gov/show/NCT05574608
Anti-CD33/CLL1 CAR-NK Cells	Wuxi People's Hospital, Wuxi, Jiangsu, China	Recruiting	Study of Anti-CD33/CLL1 CAR-NK in Acute Myeloid Leukemia	https://ClinicalTrials.gov/show/NCT05215015
NKX101—CAR NK cell therapy	Colorado Blood Cancer Institute, Denver, Colorado, United States	Recruiting	NKX101, Intravenous Allogeneic CAR NK Cells, in Adults With AML or MDS	https://ClinicalTrials.gov/show/NCT04623944
Anti-CD33 CAR NK cells	Department of Hematology, Xinqiao Hospital, Chongqing, Chongqing, China	Recruiting	Anti-CD33 CAR NK Cells in the Treatment of Relapsed/ Refractory Acute Myeloid Leukemia	https://ClinicalTrials.gov/show/NCT05008575
CAR.70/IL15-transduced CB-NK cells	M D Anderson Cancer Center, Houston, Texas, United States	Recruiting	Phase I/II Study of CAR.70-Engineered IL15-transduced Cord Blood-derived NK Cells in Conjunction With Lymphodepleting Chemotherapy for the Management of Relapse/ Refractory Hematological Malignances	https://ClinicalTrials.gov/show/NCT05092451

(continued on next page)

Table 2
(continued)

Intervention	Location	Status	Title	URL
QN-023a	Institute of Hematology & Blood Diseases Hospital, Tianjin, Tianjin, China	Recruiting	Natural Killer(NK) Cell Therapy for Acute Myeloid Leukemia	https://ClinicalTrials.gov/show/NCT05601466
QN-023a	The first affiliated hospital of medical college of Zhejiang University, Hangzhou, Zhejiang, China	Recruiting	Natural Killer (NK) Cell Therapy Targeting CD33 in Acute Myeloid Leukemia	https://ClinicalTrials.gov/show/NCT05665075
Novel strategies				
ARC-T Cells + C123-sepcific adapter (SPRX002)	City of Hope, Duarte, California, United States	Recruiting	Phase I Study of Cell Therapies for the Treatment of Patients With Relapsed or Refractory AML or High-risk MDS	https://ClinicalTrials.gov/show/NCT05457010
Chimeric antigen receptor T cells + peptide specific dendritic cell	Zhujiang Hospital, Southern Medical University, Guangzhou, Guangdong, China	Recruiting	CAR-T Cells Combined With Peptide Specific Dendritic Cell in Relapsed/Refractory Leukemia/MDS	https://ClinicalTrials.gov/show/NCT03291444
PRGN-3006 T Cells (CART33 + mbIL15)	H Lee Moffitt Cancer Center and Research Institute, Tampa, Florida, United States	Recruiting	PRGN-3006 Adoptive Cellular Therapy for Relapsed or Refractory AML or Higher Risk MDS	https://ClinicalTrials.gov/show/NCT03927261
UniCAR02-T (IMP) + TM123	Universitätsklinikum Ulm, Ulm, Baden-Württemberg, Germany	Recruiting	Dose-escalating Trial With UniCAR02-T Cells and CD123 Target Module (TM123) in Patients With Hematologic and Lymphatic Malignancies	https://ClinicalTrials.gov/show/NCT04230265
gdT cell injection targeting B7-H3 chimeric antigen receptor	PersonGen Anke Cellular Therapeutice Co., Ltd., Hefei, Anhui, China	Recruiting	Clinical Study of UTAA06 Injection in the Treatment of Relapsed/Refractory Acute Myeloid Leukemia	https://ClinicalTrials.gov/show/NCT05722171

Investigators in China published a case report of a single patient treated with autologous CART targeting CD33 (CART33)[25]; an adult patient with relapsed CD33+ AML was treated with serial infusions of CART33 and developed a cytokine release syndrome accompanied by detectable CAR product in bone marrow and blood. Although a transient reduction in AML blasts was noted, the patient had disease progression with CD33+ AML blasts. A phase 1 study of a 41BB co-stimulated autologous CART33 enrolled 10 patients with R/R AML, of whom only 3 were able to be infused due to myriad factors including rapid disease progression and manufacturing failures.[24] The patients received a relatively low dose of cells (0.3×10^6 CAR + cells/kg) and while CRS was observed there was no anti-leukemic activity.[24] PRGN-3006 is an autologous CART33 product that undergoes rapid (overnight) manufacturing, thus potentially mitigating the risk of disease progression while awaiting a traditional *ex vivo* expanded product. This product is undergoing evaluation in a phase 1/1b study (NCT03927261). In addition to the benefit of shortened manufacturing time, the construct is engineered to co-express membrane bound IL-15 which enhanced potency in pre-clinical models and also includes a kill switch to enhance safety.[60] Preliminary clinical data described the treatment of 24 patients (20 with AML, 1 with chronic myelomonocytic leukemia, and 3 with myelodysplastic syndrome [MDS]).[54] These patients were heavily pre-treated, with median of 3 prior regimens and 15 had previously undergone allogeneic stem cell transplant (SCT). Patients received up to 1×10^6 CAR T cells/kg, and CRS was observed (grade 1 in 10 patients, grade 2 in 3 patients, and grade 3 in 1 patient). Marrow aplasia was not observed. A dose-dependent expansion of CART-33 was observed in the blood and marrow, and transgene was detectable up to 7 months post-infusion. As expected, in vivo expansion was higher in the 14 patients who received lymphodepletion compared with the 10 patients who did not. One patient achieved a complete remission with incomplete count recovery (CRi) and was successfully bridged to alloSCT, 1 patient experienced a complete response (CR) with partial hematological recovery (CRh) including clearance of pre-existing cytogenetic and molecular abnormalities, and 1 patient with isolated extramedullary leukemia achieved a partial response (PR).

CD123

CD123 is the α-chain of the receptor for the hematopoietic cytokine interleukin 3 (IL-3). CD123 is expressed on the majority of $CD34^+$ hemopoietic progenitor cells, and although its expression is rapidly lost during erythroid and megakaryocytic differentiation, CD123 remains expressed on granulocytic forms through to mature neutrophils, as well as on monocytes and macrophages.[61,62] CD123 is found on a range of hematological malignancies, including AML, blastic plasmacytoid dendritic cell neoplasm (BPDCN), mast cell disorders, MDS, Hodgkin lymphoma, and B-ALL.[51] Interest in CD123 as an immunotherapy target arose from reports that is expressed on putative leukemia stem cells and that it is a marker of chemotherapy resistance.[63] This makes CD123 a particularly attractive target, though on-target off-tumor toxicity is likely to be problematic, including expression on some endothelial cells. A patient with BPDCN who was treated with an anti-CD123 "universal" CART (UCART123, an anti-CD123 CAR T cell with knockout of the T-cell receptor) died from CRS and capillary leak syndrome (CLS) on day 9 post UCART123 infusion.[64] It is unclear if his death was due to CD123 vascular expression, or was multifactorial due to CRS exacerbated by the patient's advanced age and the extent of disease burden at the time of treatment. It is important to note that severe CRS has clinical overlap with CLS. The second patient treated, a younger woman with relapsed / refractory (RR) AML, also developed severe CRS, and the trial was put on hold pending review by the FDA. The second patient survived, and the FDA subsequently allowed the trial to re-open with a log-fold reduction in UCART123 dose, a reduction in lymphodepleting chemotherapy dose and set an upper limit for age of enrollment of 65 years. Updated results from this trial (NCT03190278) were recently presented in abstract form.[53] Sixteen patients have been treated, 8 after fludarabine and cyclophosphamide (FC) and 8 after fludarabine, cyclophosphamide, and alemtuzumab (FCA) conditioning. CRS occurred in 15 of 16 patients (grade 4 in 2 and grade 5 in 1 patient). One patient in the FC cohort achieved morphologic leukemia-free state (MLFS) and one patient in the FCA cohort achieved CR with undetectable MRD. Notably, an additional patient in the FCA cohort scored as SD had a blast reduction from 60% to 5% at day 28. Addition of alemtuzumab to FC conditioning was associated with improved in vivo CAR T-cell expansion.

To mitigate the potential risk of vascular toxicity associated with targeting CD123 with CAR T cells, the first CART123 trial at the University of Pennsylvania was conducted using serial infusions of "bio-degradable" CART123 cells (NCT02623582).[65] Rather than being transduced with lentivirus, which would endow the CAR T-cell population the (usually desirable) capacity of exponential expansion in vivo, these CART123 cells were manufactured by electroporation of mRNA encoding the CAR transgene. Thus, a CART123 cell stimulated by encountering its antigen would have a limited capacity to expand, since CAR mRNA is diluted between daughter T cells after each division. Although there was no measurable anti-leukemic activity responses in this trial, evidence of bioactivity was manifest by fever, CRS, and transient CART123 detection in vivo, without evidence of overt vascular toxicity. The favorable safety data generated by this trial paved the way for a phase 1 trial of lentivirally transduced second-generation CART123 (CD123CAR-41BB-CD3ζ), which has completed recruitment at the University of Pennsylvania (NCT03766126).

The City of Hope National Medical Center opened a CART123 trial in 2015 (NCT02159495), using a lentivirally transduced second-generation CAR (CD123CAR-CD28-CD3ζ-EGFRt), with a flat-dosing strategy and interpatient dose escalation from 5×10^7 CAR $^+$ cells (dose level 1, DL1) to 2×10^8 CAR $^+$ cells (dose level 2, DL2). Interim data have been reported.[52] Seven patients with AML had been treated. One of the 2 patients treated at the lowest dose level achieved a MLFS lasting 70 days, and at recurrence of disease received a second CART123 infusion that reduced the blast count (77.9% to 0.9% by flow cytometry). Of the 5 patients treated at DL2, 1 patient achieved a CRi at day 28, and 1 had a CR at day 84. Three patients had stable disease. No dose-limiting toxicities were reported, and all treatment-related cytopenias had resolved by 12 weeks post-treatment. No CD123-negative relapses have been observed to date, and longer-term data are awaited from this pioneering study that has now completed recruitment.

An alternative approach to deal with the potential for toxicity is the UniCAR platform, in which T cells are transduced with a CD28-costimulated receptor that binds to a soluble adaptor module.[26] The adaptor targeting module confers specificity against a cancer antigen of choice. Three patients with AML were treated with UniCAR123, leading to 1 PR and 2 CRi along with myelosuppression. Notably, myelosuppression was reversible upon withdrawal of the targeting module. This trial was recently updated in abstract form.[66] Fourteen patients have been treated, with CRS in 12. Treatment-related toxicity was rapidly reversible upon discontinuation of adaptor module infusion. Four patients achieved a PR, 2 CRi, and 1 patient with MRD-only disease converted to undetectable MRD.

CLL1 (CLEC12A)

C-type lectin-like molecule-1 (CLL1) was identified as a potential AML target antigen in 2004, and later identified as a likely LCS marker, with CD34+CD38-CLL-1+ cells identified in primary AML samples, with CLL-1 expression subsequently being lost in remission.[67,68] CLL1 is also highly expressed on normal granulocytes and some other myeloid cells. A CLL1-targeting CAR T-cell product has been evaluated in 7 pediatric patients with AML.[55] All patients experienced grade 1–2 CRS and 1 patient had grade 2 immune effector cell associated neurotoxicity syndrome (ICANS). Four patients received a CD28/CD27 co-stimulated product (with an overall response rate [ORR] of 67%) and the other 3 a 41BB co-stimulated product (with an ORR 75%). Four patients achieved a morphologic remission with MRD negativity, and 1 patient a morphologic CR with MRD positivity. One patient was successfully bridged to alloHSCT, 2 non-responding patients died of progressive disease, 1 responding patient subsequently relapsed and died, and 1-year overall survival rate was 57%. In another study, 10 adults were treated with CART-CLL1 and all experienced CRS (4 reported as low grade and 6 as high grade). All 10 experienced severe pancytopenia and 2 patients died of infection in the context of prolonged neutropenia. Of the 10, 7 were said to achieve a CR or CRi. Finally, of 8 children with AML treated with anti-CLL1 CAR T cells, 4 attained MLFS with undetectable MRD, 1 MLFS with detectable MRD, 1 PR, and PR in stable disease but with loss of the CLL1-expressing blast subset.[56]

Natural killer group 2D (NKG2D) ligands

Eight ligands for the natural killer group 2D (NKG2D) receptor are overexpressed on malignant cells and have a role in stimulating anti-tumor immunity, but have limited expression on healthy tissues, providing a potential target for CAR T-cell therapy.[69,70] However, many different types of cellular stress (including inflammation) can upregulate NKG2D ligands on normal tissues, potentially reducing specificity of NKG2D-CARs for malignant tissues due to CAR T-cell induced CRS.[71,72] Autologous first-generation NKG2D-CAR T cells were infused in 7 patients with AML.[73] These engineered cells used the naturally occurring NKG2D receptor as the antigen-binding domain, with endogenous DAP10 expression providing co-stimulation. CART-NKG2D cells were successfully manufactured in all 7 patients, and median infused CAR^+ cells varied across 4 prespecified dose levels (1×10^6, 3×10^6, 1×10^7, 3×10^7) without preceding lymphodepletion. No dose-limiting toxicities were observed. Biological activity in vivo was manifest by cytokine perturbations and CAR-transgene detection, though persistence of the CART population was limited and no objective clinical responses were observed, with all patients requiring subsequent therapies for progressive AML. In a follow-up multicenter dose escalation trial of CART-NKG2D, higher doses of CART-NKG2D were infused (3×10^8, 1×10^9, and 3×10^9).[57] Twelve AML or MDS patients have been treated, of whom 3 had an objective response (2 of whom proceeded to a consolidation alloSCT).

Collectively, clinical trial results in AML across a range of targets and conducted in adults and children show an efficacy signal that is accompanied by a high frequency of CRS and occasionally by profound and protracted myeloablation. These observations will help to guide future efforts in the development of CAR T cells for AML by considering how to increase efficacy while limiting on-target toxicity.

HOW TO REDUCE ON-TARGET TOXICITY

To date, essentially all CAR T-cell targets in hematologic malignancies are lineage-specific: CD19, CD20, or CD22 in B-cell malignances; BCMA or GPRC5D in MM; CD5 or CD7 in T-cell malignancies.[74] Because AML antigens are also expressed on healthy hematopoietic progenitor cells or their mature progeny, potent anti-myeloid antigen CAR T-cell therapy would be expected to result in myeloid aplasia.[75]

Conceptually, there are 4 ways in which CAR T cells could be made more specific to AML: accessing cytoplasmic antigens, discovery of a truly specific membrane-expressed antigen, logic-gated CAR engineering, or creation of a de novo leukemia-specific antigen by a process of subtraction.

Presentation or cross-presentation of intracellular peptide fragments has the potential to stimulate a specific T-cell response to disease-related mutated proteins (neonatigens) or to other tumor-associated antigens [TAA]). Unfortunately, the evidence for naturally occurring neoantigen-specific T cells in AML is scant, and where this has been reported it is limited to particular HLA haplotypes.[76] T cells with specificity for TAA can be expanded by repeated stimulation or can be engineered, and there is clinical evidence for the utility of this approach in preventing relapse after alloSCT when done in patients at high risk for relapse but without active disease.[77,78] Although cytoplasmic proteins are not accessible to CARs, since these are based on antibody-like domains, it is possible to generate targeting domains that are specific for a peptide presented in an major histocompatibility complex (MHC) groove.[79] However, this approach then creates an easy mechanism of escape for AML (downregulation or loss of the relevant MHC molecule), and this is a common escape mechanism in AML relapsing after alloSCT.[80]

Novel target discovery in AML has been attempted using membrane proteomics or glycomics.[81–83] This approach could potentially reveal poorly described proteins, novel post-translational modifications, conformations, or ectopically localized peptides that could serve as AML-specific targets.[84,85]

Logic-gated CARs have been described recently.[86] By integrating data from transcriptomic and proteomic surveys it may be possible to devise systems that are exquisitely tuned to respond to just the right strength of stimulation such that CAR T cells only "fire" upon recognition of malignant cells.[87–89]

A novel approach to mitigate the risk of hematopoietic cell toxicity while still allowing prolonged CART persistence is to first engraft the patient with genetically modified HSPC that lack the shared myeloid antigen. We devised such an approach using Clustered Regularly Interspaced Short Palindromic Repeats (CRISPR)/CRISPR-associated endonuclease (Cas9) to knock out CD33 from HSPC, to be followed by infusion of CART-33. The purpose of the gene editing is create a leukemia-specific antigen by removing CD33 from the surface antigen that is shared by both AML blasts and healthy HSPC, such as CD33, rendering the edited HSPC and their progeny "invisible" to CART33. Following engraftment of these edited (*CD33*KO) cells, the patient may then be treated with CART33 manufactured from the same allogeneic donor. Extensive preclinical data supporting the feasibility of this approach was recently published by our laboratory and others.[15,90,91] Several patients have already received CD33-edited alloSCT followed by an anti-CD33 ADC (NCT04849910). Similar approaches using CRISPR base editing have been recently presented in abstract form for FLT3, CD123, CD117, and CD45.[92,93]

HOW TO INCREASE EFFICACY?

Enormous efforts are under way to further improve CAR T-cell efficacy and persistence, using a variety of creative yet biologically inspired approaches. These have been thoroughly described recently.[74] Of the potentially tractable approaches that could be relatively easily tested in the clinic, 2 broad pathways stand out. The first is combinatorial treatment to increase antigen expression, and the second is an ostensible simple (yet in reality complex, as explained above) progressive dose escalation until efficacy is achieved.

Target density is highly relevant to CAR signaling and hence to downstream CAR T-cell effector functions and proliferation.[94-96] In AML preclinical models, the addition of azacytidine has been shown to increase expression of the immunotherapy target CD123, with a subsequently improved CART-123 anti-tumor function.[97] In AML with mutations in the FLT3 tyrosine kinase, the addition of clinically available FLT3 inhibitors leads to upregulated surface expression of FLT3 and improved activity of anti-FLT3 CAR T cells.[16]

Although it was initially unclear whether there is a dose–response association in CAR T-cell therapy, more recent data from clinical trials in MM and from "real-world" data in pediatric B-ALL now suggest that this is the case.[10,11,98,99] However, the success of this approach is predicated upon the incidence, severity, and reversibility of CAR-associated on- and off-target toxicities. Thus, some of the solutions proposed in the earlier section on toxicity mitigation could initiate a "virtuous cycle" in AML.

SUMMARY

The CAR T-cell platform has been well and truly validated as a relevant therapeutic modality in hematologic malignancies, with sometimes astounding responses in multiply pretreated patients with heavy burdens of ALL, lymphoma, or myeloma. Given that is fundamentally an immune-responsive tumor and despite encouraging preclinical data, it is perhaps surprisingly that AML has lagged behind the other hematologic malignancies. To date, relatively few patients have been treated and the extant results show lower rates and depths of responses compared with B-ALL. A handful of patients who attain CRs have been bridged to salvage alloSCT, with some long-term survivors. The etiology of the poorer than expected responses in AML is as yet unclear, although the high incidence of CRS suggests that investigators have struggled to escalate doses to those that are potentially active. In the absence of truly AML-specific target antigens, myeloablation is an expected on-target toxicity, and this too poses a unique challenge in this disease. Thus, successful efforts to discover or engineer AML-specific antigens or to devise highly specific CAR platforms could also enhance our ability to dose-escalate or to rationally combine with other agents, thus increasing responses while reducing toxicities. AML is a clear area of unmet need, and investigators' ongoing optimism and confidence is reflected in the wide field of new and ongoing clinical trials. We believe that the discovery or engineering of AML-specific targets will provide the necessary breakthroughs that will allow us to capitalize on the proven power of CAR T-cell therapy.

CLINICS CARE POINTS

- CAR T cells have been tested in patients with AML, and there is a clear efficacy signal.
- There is a high incidence of CRS and myelosuppression, and these toxicities likely limit dose escalation.
- Patients with profound myeloablation after AML-directed CAR T-cell therapy have been and, in our opinion, should be salvaged with an alloSCT.

DISCLOSURE

S. Gill has patents related to CAR therapy with royalties paid from Novartis to the University of Pennsylvania. S.G. is a scientific co-founder and holds equity in Interius Biotherapeutics and Carisma Therapeutics. S.G. is a scientific advisor to Carisma,

Cartography, Currus, Interius, Kite, NKILT, Mission Bio, and Vor Bio. K. Cummins has no disclosures.

FUNDING SUPPORT

S. Gill has funding support from the National Institutes of Health, United States, the Leukemia & Lymphoma Society, the Commonwealth of Pennsylvania, the Dresner Research Foundation, the Emerson Collective.

REFERENCES

1. Grupp SA, Kalos M, Barrett D, et al. Chimeric antigen receptor-modified T cells for acute lymphoid leukemia. N Engl J Med 2013;368(16):1509–18.
2. Brentjens RJ, Davila ML, Riviere I, et al. CD19-targeted T cells rapidly induce molecular remissions in adults with chemotherapy-refractory acute lymphoblastic leukemia. Sci Transl Med 2013;5(177):177ra38.
3. Frey NV, Shaw PA, Hexner EO, et al. Optimizing chimeric antigen receptor T-cell therapy for adults with acute lymphoblastic leukemia. J Clin Oncol 2020;38(5):415–22.
4. Shah BD, Ghobadi A, Oluwole OO, et al. KTE-X19 for relapsed or refractory adult B-cell acute lymphoblastic leukaemia: phase 2 results of the single-arm, open-label, multicentre ZUMA-3 study. Lancet 2021;398(10299):491–502.
5. Neelapu SS, Locke FL, Bartlett NL, et al. Axicabtagene Ciloleucel CAR T-Cell Therapy in Refractory Large B-Cell Lymphoma. N Engl J Med 2017;377(26):2531–44.
6. Schuster SJ, Bishop MR, Tam CS, et al. Tisagenlecleucel in adult relapsed or refractory diffuse large B-cell lymphoma. N Engl J Med 2019;380(1):45–56.
7. Abramson JS, Palomba ML, Gordon LI, et al. Lisocabtagene maraleucel for patients with relapsed or refractory large B-cell lymphomas (TRANSCEND NHL 001): a multicentre seamless design study. Lancet 2020;396(10254):839–52.
8. Wang M, Munoz J, Goy A, et al. KTE-X19 CAR T-cell therapy in relapsed or refractory mantle-cell lymphoma. N Engl J Med 2020;382(14):1331–42.
9. Fowler NH, Dickinson M, Dreyling M, et al. Tisagenlecleucel in adult relapsed or refractory follicular lymphoma: the phase 2 ELARA trial. Nat Med 2022;28(2):325–32.
10. Munshi NC, Anderson LD, Shah N, et al. Idecabtagene Vicleucel in Relapsed and Refractory Multiple Myeloma. N Engl J Med 2021;384(8):705–16.
11. Berdeja JG, Madduri D, Usmani SZ, et al. Ciltacabtagene autoleucel, a B-cell maturation antigen-directed chimeric antigen receptor T-cell therapy in patients with relapsed or refractory multiple myeloma (CARTITUDE-1): a phase 1b/2 open-label study. Lancet 2021;398(10297):314–24.
12. Pan J, Tan Y, Wang G, et al. Donor-Derived CD7 Chimeric Antigen Receptor T Cells for T-Cell Acute Lymphoblastic Leukemia: First-in-Human, Phase I Trial. J Clin Oncol 2021;39(30):3340–51.
13. Gill S, Tasian SK, Ruella M, et al. Preclinical targeting of human acute myeloid leukemia and myeloablation using chimeric antigen receptor-modified T cells. Blood 2014;123(15):2343–54.
14. Kenderian SS, Ruella M, Shestova O, et al. CD33-specific chimeric antigen receptor T cells exhibit potent preclinical activity against human acute myeloid leukemia. Leukemia 2015;29(8):1637–47.

15. Kim MY, Yu KR, Kenderian SS, et al. Genetic inactivation of CD33 in hematopoietic stem cells to enable CAR T cell immunotherapy for acute myeloid leukemia. Cell 2018;173(6):1439–53.e19.
16. Jetani H, Garcia-Cadenas I, Nerreter T, et al. CAR T-cells targeting FLT3 have potent activity against FLT3-ITD+ AML and act synergistically with the FLT3-inhibitor crenolanib. Leukemia 2018;32(5):1168–79.
17. Casucci M, Nicolis di Robilant B, Falcone L, et al. CD44v6-targeted T cells mediate potent antitumor effects against acute myeloid leukemia and multiple myeloma. Blood 2013;122(20):3461–72.
18. Ritchie DS, Neeson PJ, Khot A, et al. Persistence and efficacy of second generation CAR T Cell against the LeY Antigen in acute myeloid leukemia. Mol Ther 2013;21(11):2122–9.
19. Zhang H, Gan WT, Hao WG, et al. Successful anti-CLL1 CAR T-cell therapy in secondary acute myeloid leukemia. Front Oncol 2020;10. https://doi.org/10.3389/fonc.2020.00685.
20. Ma YJ, Dai HP, Cui QY, et al. Successful application of PD-1 knockdown CLL-1 CAR-T therapy in two AML patients with post-transplant relapse and failure of anti-CD38 CAR-T cell treatment. Am J Cancer Res 2022;12(2):615–21. Available at: http://www.ncbi.nlm.nih.gov/pubmed/35261791.
21. Jin X, Zhang M, Sun R, et al. First-in-human phase I study of CLL-1 CAR-T cells in adults with relapsed/refractory acute myeloid leukemia. J Hematol Oncol 2022;15(1):88.
22. Yao S, Jianlin C, Yarong L, et al. Donor-derived CD123-targeted CAR T cell serves as a RIC regimen for haploidentical transplantation in a patient with FUS-ERG+ AML. Front Oncol 2019;9:1358.
23. Pemmaraju N, Wilson NR, Senapati J, et al. CD123-directed allogeneic chimeric-antigen receptor T-cell therapy (CAR-T) in blastic plasmacytoid dendritic cell neoplasm (BPDCN): Clinicopathological insights. Leuk Res 2022;121:106928.
24. Tambaro FP, Singh H, Jones E, et al. Autologous CD33-CAR-T cells for treatment of relapsed/refractory acute myelogenous leukemia. Leukemia 2021;35(11):3282–6.
25. Wang QS, Wang Y, Lv HY, et al. Treatment of CD33-directed chimeric antigen receptor-modified T cells in one patient with relapsed and refractory acute myeloid leukemia. Mol Ther 2015;23(1):184–91.
26. Wermke M, Kraus S, Ehninger A, et al. Proof of concept for a rapidly switchable universal CAR-T platform with UniCAR-T-CD123 in relapsed/refractory AML. Blood 2021;137(22):3145–8.
27. Koreth J, Schlenk R, Kopecky KJ, et al. Allogeneic stem cell transplantation for acute myeloid leukemia in first complete remission: systematic review and meta-analysis of prospective clinical trials. JAMA 2009;301(22):2349–61.
28. Li D, Wang L, Zhu H, et al. Efficacy of allogeneic hematopoietic stem cell transplantation in intermediate-risk acute myeloid leukemia adult patients in first complete remission: a meta-analysis of prospective studies. PLoS One 2015;10(7):e0132620.
29. Lancet JE, Uy GL, Newell LF, et al. CPX-351 versus 7+3 cytarabine and daunorubicin chemotherapy in older adults with newly diagnosed high-risk or secondary acute myeloid leukaemia: 5-year results of a randomised, open-label, multicentre, phase 3 trial. Lancet Haematol 2021;8(7):e481–91.
30. Ustun C, Le-Rademacher J, Wang HL, et al. Allogeneic hematopoietic cell transplantation compared to chemotherapy consolidation in older acute myeloid leukemia (AML) patients 60-75 years in first complete remission (CR1): an alliance

(A151509), SWOG, ECOG-ACRIN, and CIBMTR study. Leukemia 2019;33(11): 2599–609.

31. Stone RM, Mandrekar SJ, Sanford BL, et al. Midostaurin plus chemotherapy for acute myeloid leukemia with a FLT3 mutation. N Engl J Med 2017;377(5):454–64.

32. Tasian SK, Kenderian SS, Shen F, et al. Optimized depletion of chimeric antigen receptor T cells in murine xenograft models of human acute myeloid leukemia. Blood 2017;129(17):2395–407.

33. DiNardo CD, Jonas BA, Pullarkat V, et al. Azacitidine and venetoclax in previously untreated acute myeloid leukemia. N Engl J Med 2020;383(7):617–29.

34. Wei AH, Montesinos P, Ivanov V, et al. Venetoclax plus LDAC for newly diagnosed AML ineligible for intensive chemotherapy: a phase 3 randomized placebo-controlled trial. Blood 2020;135(24):2137–45.

35. Lancet JE, Uy GL, Cortes JE, et al. CPX-351 (cytarabine and daunorubicin) Liposome for Injection Versus Conventional Cytarabine Plus Daunorubicin in Older Patients With Newly Diagnosed Secondary Acute Myeloid Leukemia. J Clin Oncol 2018;36(26):2684–92.

36. DiNardo CD, Stein EM, de Botton S, et al. Durable remissions with ivosidenib in IDH1-mutated relapsed or refractory AML. N Engl J Med 2018;378(25):2386–98.

37. Perl AE, Martinelli G, Cortes JE, et al. Gilteritinib or chemotherapy for relapsed or refractory FLT3-mutated aML. N Engl J Med 2019;381(18):1728–40.

38. Wei AH, Dohner H, Pocock C, et al. Oral azacitidine maintenance therapy for acute myeloid leukemia in first remission. N Engl J Med 2020;383(26):2526–37.

39. Ganzel C, Sun Z, Cripe LD, et al. Very poor long-term survival in past and more recent studies for relapsed AML patients: The ECOG-ACRIN experience. Am J Hematol 2018;93(8):1074–81.

40. Laetsch TW, Maude SL, Rives S, et al. Three-year update of tisagenlecleucel in pediatric and young adult patients with relapsed/refractory acute lymphoblastic leukemia in the ELIANA trial. J Clin Oncol 2023;41(9):1664–9.

41. Gardner RA, Finney O, Annesley C, et al. Intent-to-treat leukemia remission by CD19 CAR T cells of defined formulation and dose in children and young adults. Blood 2017;129(25):3322–31.

42. Hay KA, Gauthier J, Hirayama AV, et al. Factors associated with durable EFS in adult B-cell ALL patients achieving MRD-negative CR after CD19 CAR T-cell therapy. Blood 2019;133(15):1652–63.

43. Gardner RA, Shah NN. CAR T-cells for cure in pediatric B-ALL. J Clin Oncol 2023; 41(9):1646–8.

44. Myers RM, Shah NN, Pulsipher MA. How I use risk factors for success or failure of CD19 CAR T cells to guide management of children and AYA with B-cell ALL. Blood 2023;141(11):1251–64.

45. Trumpp A, Haas S. Cancer stem cells: The adventurous journey from hematopoietic to leukemic stem cells. Cell 2022;185(8):1266–70.

46. Paul F, Arkin Y, Giladi A, et al. Transcriptional heterogeneity and lineage commitment in myeloid progenitors. Cell 2015;163(7):1663–77.

47. Zeng AGX, Bansal S, Jin L, et al. A cellular hierarchy framework for understanding heterogeneity and predicting drug response in acute myeloid leukemia. Nat Med 2022;28(6):1212–23.

48. Good Z, Sarno J, Jager A, et al. Single-cell developmental classification of B cell precursor acute lymphoblastic leukemia at diagnosis reveals predictors of relapse. Nat Med 2018;24(4):474–83.

49. Orgel E, Alexander TB, Wood BL, et al. Mixed-phenotype acute leukemia: a cohort and consensus research strategy from the children's oncology group acute leukemia of ambiguous lineage task force. Cancer 2020;126(3):593–601.

50. Mardiros A, Dos Santos C, McDonald T, et al. T cells expressing CD123-specific chimeric antigen receptors exhibit specific cytolytic effector functions and anti-tumor effects against human acute myeloid leukemia. Blood 2013;122(18):3138–48.

51. Ruella M, Barrett DM, Kenderian SS, et al. Dual CD19 and CD123 targeting prevents antigen-loss relapses after CD19-directed immunotherapies. J Clin Invest 2016;126(10):3814–26.

52. Budde LE, Song J, Real MD, et al. Abstract PR14: CD123CAR displays clinical activity in relapsed/refractory (r/r) acute myeloid leukemia (AML) and blastic plasmacytoid dendritic cell neoplasm (BPDCN): Safety and efficacy results from a phase 1 study. Cancer Immunol Res, 8 (4_Supplement), 2020, PR14-PR14.

53. Sallman DA, DeAngelo DJ, Pemmaraju N. Ameli-01: A Phase I Trial of UCART123v1.2, an Anti- CD123 Allogeneic CAR-T Cell Product, in Adult Patients with Relapsed or Refractory (R/R) CD123+ Acute Myeloid Leukemia (AML). In: American Society of Hematology Annual Meeting. ; 2022:2371-2373.

54. Sallman DA, Emariah H, Sweet K. Phase 1/1b Safety Study of Prgn-3006 Ultracar-T in Patients with Relapsed or Refractory CD33-Positive Acute Myeloid Leukemia and Higher Risk Myelodysplastic Syndromes. In: American Society of Hematology Annual Meeting. ; 2022:10313-10315.

55. Pei K, Xu H, Wang P, et al. Anti-CLL1-based CAR T-cells with 4-1-BB or CD28/CD27 stimulatory domains in treating childhood refractory/relapsed acute myeloid leukemia. Cancer Med 2023. https://doi.org/10.1002/cam4.5916.

56. Zhang H, Bu C, Peng Z, et al. Characteristics of anti-CLL1 based CAR-T therapy for children with relapsed or refractory acute myeloid leukemia: the multi-center efficacy and safety interim analysis. Leukemia 2022;36(11):2596–604.

57. Sallman DA, Kerre T, Havelange V, et al. CYAD-01, an autologous NKG2D-based CAR T-cell therapy, in relapsed or refractory acute myeloid leukaemia and myelodysplastic syndromes or multiple myeloma (THINK): haematological cohorts of the dose escalation segment of a phase 1 trial. Lancet Haematol 2023;10(3):e191–202.

58. Ehninger A, Kramer M, Rollig C, et al. Distribution and levels of cell surface expression of CD33 and CD123 in acute myeloid leukemia. Blood Cancer J 2014;4:e218.

59. Hills RK, Castaigne S, Appelbaum FR, et al. Addition of gemtuzumab ozogamicin to induction chemotherapy in adult patients with acute myeloid leukaemia: a meta-analysis of individual patient data from randomised controlled trials. Lancet Oncol 2014;15(9):986–96.

60. Chan T, Ma's X, Carvajal-Borda's F, et al. Preclinical characterization of Prgn-3006 Ultracar-T™ for the treatment of AML and MDS: non-viral, multigenic autologous CAR-T cells administered one day after gene transfer. Blood 2019;134(Supplement_1):2660.

61. Testa U, Fossati C, Samoggia P, et al. Expression of growth factor receptors in unilineage differentiation culture of purified hematopoietic progenitors. Blood 1996;88(9):3391–406.

62. Testa U, Riccioni R, Militi S, et al. Elevated expression of IL-3Rα in acute myelogenous leukemia is associated with enhanced blast proliferation, increased cellularity, and poor prognosis. Blood 2002;100(8):2980–8.

63. Konopleva MY, Jordan CT. Leukemia stem cells and microenvironment: biology and therapeutic targeting. J Clin Oncol 2011;29(5):591–9.

64. Cellectis. Cellectis Reports Clinical Hold of UCART123 Studies. Available at: https://www.cellectis.com/en/press/cellectis-reports-clinical-hold-of-ucart123-studies/. Accessed March 2023.

65. Cummins KD, Frey N, Nelson AM, et al. Treating Relapsed/Refractory (RR) AML with Biodegradable Anti-CD123 CAR Modified T Cells. In: American Society of Hematology Annual Meeting. ; 2017:#1359.

66. Ehninger G, Kraus S, Sala E. Phase 1 Dose Escalation Study of the Rapidly Switchable Universal CAR-T Therapy Unicar-T-CD123 in Relapsed/Refractory AML. In: American Society of Hematology Annual Meeting. ; 2022:2367-2368.

67. Van Rhenen A, Van Dongen GAMS, Kelder A Le, et al. The novel AML stem cell-associated antigen CLL-1 aids in discrimination between normal and leukemic stem cells. Blood 2007;110(7):2659–66.

68. Bakker AQABH, Oudenrijn S Van Den, Feller N, et al. C-type lectin-like molecule-1 : a novel myeloid cell surface marker associated with acute myeloid leukemia. Cancer Res 2004;64:8443–50.

69. Spear P, Barber A, Rynda-Apple A, et al. NKG2D CAR T-cell therapy inhibits the growth of NKG2D ligand heterogeneous tumors. Immunol Cell Biol 2013;91(6):435–40.

70. Spear P, Wu MR, Sentman ML, et al. NKG2D ligands as therapeutic targets. Cancer Immun 2013;13:8.

71. Champsaur M, Lanier LL. Effect of NKG2D ligand expression on host immune responses. Immunol Rev 2010;235(1):267–85.

72. Sheppard S, Ferry A, Guedes J, et al. The paradoxical role of NKG2D in cancer immunity. Front Immunol 2018;9:1808.

73. Baumeister SH, Murad J, Werner L, et al. Phase i trial of autologous CAR T cells targeting NKG2D ligands in patients with AML/MDS and multiple myeloma. Cancer Immunol Res 2019;7(1):100–12.

74. Labanieh L, Mackall CL. CAR immune cells: design principles, resistance and the next generation. Nature 2023;614(7949):635–48.

75. Haubner S, Perna F, Kohnke T, et al. Coexpression profile of leukemic stem cell markers for combinatorial targeted therapy in AML. Leukemia 2019;33(1):64–74.

76. Biernacki MA, Foster KA, Woodward KB, et al. CBFB-MYH11 fusion neoantigen enables T cell recognition and killing of acute myeloid leukemia. J Clin Invest 2020;130(10):5127–41.

77. Lulla PD, Naik S, Vasileiou S, et al. Clinical effects of administering leukemia-specific donor T cells to patients with AML/MDS after allogeneic transplant. Blood 2021;137(19):2585–97.

78. Chapuis AG, Egan DN, Bar M, et al. T cell receptor gene therapy targeting WT1 prevents acute myeloid leukemia relapse post-transplant. Nat Med 2019;25(7):1064–72.

79. Xie G, Ivica NA, Jia B, et al. CAR-T cells targeting a nucleophosmin neoepitope exhibit potent specific activity in mouse models of acute myeloid leukaemia. Nat Biomed Eng 2021;5(5):399–413.

80. Toffalori C, Zito L, Gambacorta V, et al. Immune signature drives leukemia escape and relapse after hematopoietic cell transplantation. Nat Med 2019;25(4):603–11.

81. Mirkowska P, Hofmann A, Sedek L, et al. Leukemia surfaceome analysis reveals new disease-associated features. Blood 2013;121(25):e149–59.

82. Hofmann A, Gerrits B, Schmidt A, et al. Proteomic cell surface phenotyping of differentiating acute myeloid leukemia cells. Blood 2010;116(13):e26–34.

83. Lu C, Glisovic-Aplenc T, Bernt KM, et al. Longitudinal large-scale semiquantitative proteomic data stability across multiple instrument platforms. J Proteome Res 2021;20(11):5203–11.

84. Naik A, Srivastava S, Wiita AP. "Cell surface capture" workflow for label-free quantification of the cell surface proteome. J Vis Exp 2023;(193). https://doi.org/10.3791/64952.

85. Mandal K, Wicaksono G, Yu C. Structural Surfaceomics Reveals an AML-Specific Conformation of Integrin-β2 As an Immunotherapeutic Target. In: American Society of Hematology Annual Meeting. ; 2022:867-868.

86. Hamieh M, Mansilla-Soto J, Riviere I, et al. Programming CAR T cell tumor recognition: tuned antigen sensing and logic gating. Cancer Discov 2023;13(4):829–43.

87. Perna F, Berman SH, Soni RK, et al. Integrating Proteomics and Transcriptomics for Systematic Combinatorial Chimeric Antigen Receptor Therapy of AML. Cancer Cell 2017;32(4):506–19.e5.

88. Haubner S, Mansilla-Soto J, Nataraj S. Target Densities in Malignant and Normal Cells Determine CAR T Cell Efficacy and Off-Target Hematotoxicity. In: American Society of Hematology Annual Meeting. ; 2022:869-870.

89. Haubner S, Mansilla-Soto J, Garcia Angus A. Overcoming Heterogeneity in AML with a Novel or-Gated Hitcar-1XX Platform. In: American Society of Hematology Annual Meeting. ; 2022:865-866.

90. Humbert O, Laszlo GS, Sichel S, et al. Engineering resistance to CD33-targeted immunotherapy in normal hematopoiesis by CRISPR/Cas9-deletion of CD33 exon 2. Leukemia 2019;33(3):762–808.

91. Godwin CD, Laszlo GS, Wood BL, et al. The CD33 splice isoform lacking exon 2 as therapeutic target in human acute myeloid leukemia. Leukemia 2020;34(9):2479–83.

92. Casirati G, Cosentino A, Mucci A. Epitope Engineered Hematopoietic Stem and Progenitor Cells to Enable CAR-T Cell Immunotherapy for Acute Myeloid Leukemia. In: American Society of Hematology Annual Meeting. ; 2022:303-304.

93. Wellhausen N, Rennels AK, Lesch S. Epitope Editing in Hematopoietic Cells Enables CD45-Directed Immune Therapy. In: American Society of Hematology Annual Meeting. ; 2022:862-864.

94. Walker AJ, Majzner RG, Zhang L, et al. Tumor antigen and receptor densities regulate efficacy of a chimeric antigen receptor targeting anaplastic lymphoma kinase. Mol Ther 2017;25(9):2189–201.

95. Fry TJ, Shah NN, Orentas RJ, et al. CD22-targeted CAR T cells induce remission in B-ALL that is naive or resistant to CD19-targeted CAR immunotherapy. Nat Med 2018;24(1):20–8.

96. Spiegel JY, Patel S, Muffly L, et al. CAR T cells with dual targeting of CD19 and CD22 in adult patients with recurrent or refractory B cell malignancies: a phase 1 trial. Nat Med 2021;27(8):1419–31.

97. El Khawanky N, Hughes A, Yu W, et al. Demethylating therapy increases anti-CD123 CAR T cell cytotoxicity against acute myeloid leukemia. Nat Commun 2021;12(1):6436.

98. Raje N, Berdeja J, Lin Y, et al. Anti-BCMA CAR T-cell therapy bb2121 in relapsed or refractory multiple myeloma. N Engl J Med 2019;380(18):1726–37.

99. Stefanski HE, Eaton A, Baggott C, et al. Higher doses of tisagenlecleucel are associated with improved outcomes: a report from the pediatric real-world CAR consortium. Blood Adv 2023;7(4):541–8.

Chimeric Antigen Receptor T-Cell Therapy for Solid Tumors

Jeremiah A. Wala, MD, PhD, Glenn J. Hanna, MD*

KEYWORDS

- Chimeric antigen receptor • Solid tumors • Clinical trials • Cellular engineering
- Tumor microenvironment • Antigen selection

KEY POINTS

- CAR-T therapy in solid tumors is rapidly evolving with over 200 ongoing clinical trials.
- CAR-T therapy in solid tumors raises unique clinical challenges, including dramatic inflammatory responses, that require careful consideration when selecting patients.
- Barriers to CAR-T efficacy in solid tumors include difficulty in trafficking cells to tumors, an immunosuppressive microenvironment, and challenges of finding specific antigen targets.
- Cellular engineering and synthetic biology technologies are being incorporated into new CAR-T products to overcome these challenges.
- Most disease sites have some reported CAR-T trials, although there is considerable heterogeneity and overall limited efficacy to date.

INTRODUCTION

Chimeric antigen receptor (CAR) T-cell studies in the 1990s initially focused on solid tumors,[1,2] and the first human trials of CAR-Ts in 2006 were conducted in patients with ovarian[3] and kidney cancer.[4] Despite this early start in solid tumors, CAR-T cells have made their greatest clinical impact in hematological malignancies. There are currently six FDA-approved CAR-T therapies, with indications in multiple myeloma, acute lymphoblastic leukemia (ALL), and B-cell lymphomas, but none in solid tumors. This review will highlight several challenges specific to CAR-Ts in solid tumors that have slowed their relative clinical development: physical and molecular barriers to trafficking CAR-Ts to tumors, overcoming an immunosuppressive tumor microenvironment (TME), and the difficulty of finding cell surface target antigens without leading to excessive "on-target/off-tumor" toxicity in normal tissue. Over two decades of

Dana-Farber Cancer Institute, 450 Brookline Avenue, Dana Building 2nd Floor, Room 2-140, Boston, MA 02215, USA
* Corresponding author.
E-mail address: glenn_hanna@dfci.harvard.edu

Hematol Oncol Clin N Am 37 (2023) 1149–1168
https://doi.org/10.1016/j.hoc.2023.05.009

hemonc.theclinics.com

research have been focused on clinical, synthetic biology, and cellular engineering approaches to overcome these barriers. As a result, there is a growing literature of pre-clinical studies, completed clinical trials, and now over 200 ongoing trials using CAR-Ts against solid tumors.[5] This review will highlight several of these approaches and briefly summarize the landscape of CAR-T therapy in each of several solid tumor types.

PATIENT SELECTION

Selecting patients for solid tumor CAR-T therapy requires considering the pace of disease progression, patient ability to tolerate both lymphodepletive pre-conditioning and expected inflammatory treatment response, and the logistical requirement of patient access to institutions providing CAR-T clinical trials. Only patients who have progressed through multiple prior lines of therapy are eligible for CAR-Ts, a population that is more likely to have a decreased performance status and symptomatic disease. The process of leukapheresis to harvest cells for CAR-T production further requires adequate bone marrow reserve and sufficient lymphocyte counts (generally an absolute lymphocyte count of at least 0.2×10^9/L).[6] The production of CAR-T cells can take up to six weeks for the required leukapheresis, *ex vivo* transduction of CAR constructs, and CAR-T expansion.[7] Patients with more urgent need for debulking or oncological intervention are ill-suited to wait for CAR-T production, unless a sufficient bridging therapy can be provided.[6] Lymphodepletive pre-conditioning chemotherapy, most commonly with fludarabine and cyclophosphamide infused over a 3-5 day period, is often employed to open an immunological niche for CAR-Ts to expand.[8] Patients are typically hospitalized during this conditioning and for at least several days following CAR-T infusion. The associated costs, factoring in hospitalization, are considerable. As an example, the total treatment cost for tisagenlecleucel was estimated to be around $500,000 per patient in 2018, which has broader public health cost concerns.[9]

CAR-T engagement to both the intended tumor target and from low-level off-tumor antigen expression can lead to a rapid and intense systemic inflammatory response. The two most prevalent manifestations are cytokine release syndrome (CRS) and immune effector cell-associated neurotoxicity syndrome (ICANS). CRS is a systemic inflammatory condition that manifests with fever, malaise, and potentially life-threatening capillary leak hypoxia and hypotension.[10] ICANS manifests with toxic encephalopathy, word-finding difficulty, and seizures and cerebral edema in severe cases.[11] Risk factors for CRS include a higher infusion dose of CAR-Ts, a high disease burden, thrombocytopenia, and the intensity of lymphodepletive chemotherapy.[10,12] Based on retrospective analyses, the FDA has approved the use of the IL-6 inhibitor tocilizumab for severe CRS.[13] ICANS is treated with high-dose corticosteroids and supportive care, whereas tocilizumab may worsen neurological symptoms.[14]

Patients should be counseled about these risks and well-informed of alternative approaches, including best supportive care. A patient's own value judgements about quality and quantity of life are particularly important in considering CAR-T trials, given the extensive time investment required. The oncologist should help patients have measured expectations for CAR-T therapy. For instance, a recent meta-analysis of 22 CAR-T trials in solid tumors identified an overall response rate of 9%.[15] This highlights both real oncological benefit to a minority of patients who may have otherwise limited therapeutic options and the pressing need for new approaches for achieving clinical efficacy.

CHALLENGES TO CHIMERIC ANTIGEN RECEPTOR T-CELLS IN SOLID TUMORS
Trafficking to the tumor

CAR-Ts must be in close physical proximity with their target tumor cells to become activated and deliver cytotoxic perforins and granzymes.[16] In hematological malignancies, CAR-Ts circulate in existing physiologic pathways throughout the blood, lymph nodes, and bone marrow, readily interacting with tumor cells in these compartments. Indeed, the more solid nature of lymphomas may explain in part their relatively lower response rate compared with liquid tumors.[17] In solid tumors, trafficking CAR-Ts to tumor cells requires multiple additional steps: tumor vascular access, extravasation into the tumor microenvironment, overcoming structural and chemokine barriers, and ultimately achieving a sufficient density to maintain effector activity against an immunosuppressive (hypoxic and fibrotic) microenvironment.

In some pre-clinical models, fewer than 2% of adoptively transferred T-cells have been able to infiltrate tumors.[18–20] Physical exclusion of T-cells results from increased density of extra-cellular matrix (ECM) fibronectin and collagen fibers.[21] Tumor-associated macrophages (TAMs) and dendritic cells (DCs) further bind T-cells to slow their transit.[22,23] T-cell migration is controlled by a complex system of chemokine gradients generated by endothelial cells, monocytes, fibroblasts, and tumor cells themselves. Collectively, they down-regulate chemoattractants and "hide" tumors from activated T-cells.[19,24] Finally, hypoxia, nutrient deficiency, and excess cellular waste all serve to exclude effector T-cells and decrease their function.[25]

Synthetic biology efforts to improve CAR-T homing are ongoing, but active clinical trials addressing this issue are relatively limited. In an early pre-clinical model, the chemokine receptor CCR2b was engineered into mesothelin-directed CAR-Ts to improve T-cell tumor infiltration.[26] CD30-directed CAR-Ts have been engineered to express the CCR4 receptor, enhancing cytokine-mediate chemotaxis to Hodgkin's lymphoma tumors.[27] CD70-directed CAR-Ts with a modified IL-8 receptor (CXCR1 or CXCR2) enhance T-cell trafficking and persistence,[28] and are currently being tested in patients with glioblastoma (NCT05366179). Heparanase is an enzyme produced by activated CD4+ T lymphocytes, neutrophils, monocytes, and B lymphocytes to degrade the ECM and allow migration to target tissues.[29] CAR-Ts engineered to produce heparinase have demonstrated increased tumor infiltration in mouse xenograft models.[30]

To assess the ability of CAR-Ts to traffic to their solid tumor targets *in vivo*, CAR-Ts can be labelled prior to infusion to allow for their detection with nuclear imaging. SPECT/CT has been used to localized CAR-Ts engineered to express the human sodium-iodide symporter to take up the radiotracer $^{99m}TcO4^-$.[20] CAR-Ts expressing protein reporters have also been combined with PET imaging, including products expressing PSMA,[31] somatostatin,[32] and an HSV1-tk reporter gene.[33] Radiotracers are useful to differentiate CAR-T-associated inflammation (pseudo-progression) from tumor metabolic activity.[34] These imaging strategies are being employed in several ongoing clinical trials (NCT04420754, NCT05404048).

Direct delivery of CAR-Ts to the tumor can circumvent some of the above trafficking challenges. Early pre-clinical studies in a mouse mesothelioma model identified that mesothelin-directed M28z CAR-Ts delivered via intrapleural injection were able to induce long-term remissions with 30-fold fewer cells than those delivered intravenously.[35] Moreover, this effect was driven not only by increased concentration of CAR-Ts within the tumor, but by an enhanced memory T-cell phenotype marked by a high memory CD4+ T-cell population. The clinical efficacy of this approach was demonstrated in a trial of intrapleural delivery of M28z CAR-Ts in patients with mesothelioma, lung, and breast cancer with pleural involvement.[36] The anatomical location of certain solid tumors also naturally lends itself to regional delivery. Intraventricular delivery in CNS tumors, hepatic artery delivery in liver metastases, intraperitoneal delivery in ovarian cancer, and direct tumor injection in breast and head and neck cancer, are all active regional delivery strategies.[37] As a practical matter, many trials of CAR-Ts employ intratumoral delivery to minimize the risk of systemic toxicity while evaluating localized efficacy.[38]

Overcoming an immunosuppressive tumor micro-environment

Tumor cells are under selective pressure to promote T-cell tolerance, inactivation, and death. Because CAR-Ts are derived from native T-cells, they are vulnerable to the same immunosuppressive tumor microenvironment that provided an immunological niche for the tumor to grow. Tumor cells employ numerous immunosuppressive tactics: upregulating immune checkpoint pathways, altering the function and prevalence of stromal cells, and directly secreting cytokines to abrogate T-cell function.[39] An increasing mechanistic understanding of these pathways, combined with advancements in molecular biology, is leading to new CAR-Ts that can better persist and function within this hostile environment.

Immune checkpoints, including PD-1, CTLA-4, LAG-3, and TIM-3, are cell surface proteins that play a crucial role in regulating T-cell biology by preventing overreaction and promoting self-tolerance.[40] In the TME, T-cells become exhausted and exhibit checkpoint upregulation, leading to tumor tolerance.[41] Tumor cells themselves upregulate PD-L1 and PD-L2 (PD-1 agonists) and secrete anti-inflammatory cytokines such as TGF-β to drive T-cell tolerance.[42,43] One approach to overcome this immunosuppression is through the deletion of the native PD-1 gene during CAR-T transfection. In a mouse xenograft model, CRISPR-Cas9-mediated disruption of PD-1 during CD19-CAR transfection increased tumor clearance from 17% to 100%.[44] A similar approach was used in a pre-clinical mesothelin-directed CAR-T, resulting in strongly augmented cytokine production and cytotoxicity.[45] This CAR-T was tested in a clinical trial of patients with primarily pancreatic and biliary tract cancers, yielding 2/15 patients with stable disease as best response.[46] Numerous other clinical trials of PD-1 knockout CAR-Ts across a range of solid tumors are ongoing.[42]

An alternative approach is to add checkpoint inhibitors at the time of CAR-T infusion.[47] A case report in 2017 described a durable response to the addition of the anti-PD-1 monoclonal antibody pembrolizumab at day 26 after CD-19-directed CAR-T infusion for progressive B-cell lymphoma.[48] A subsequent trial of pembrolizumab for B-cell lymphoma patients refractory to CD19-CAR-Ts resulted in a 25% overall response rate.[49] In solid tumors, a pre-clinical study of GD2-directed CAR-Ts showed that adding pembrolizumab significantly improved T-cell function and reduced T-cell activation-induced cell death.[50] This led to a trial of GD2-directed CAR-Ts in neuroblastoma that included a small arm of three patients who additionally received pembrolizumab.[51] There was one complete response in this arm, although no evidence of increased CAR-T activity in this small cohort. There are ongoing clinical trials using this approach in sarcoma (HER2; NCT04995003) and glioblastoma (EGFR-vIII; NCT03726515 and IL13Rα2; NCT04003649).

The immunosuppressive state of the tumor microenvironment is shaped by an extraordinarily complex network of chemokine-receptor interactions.[39,52] T-helper cells, dendritic cells, macrophages, fibroblasts, and tumors themselves exchange chemokines to steer T-cells towards tolerance and inactivation.[43,53–55] Numerous strategies are being employed in CAR-Ts to redirect these networks to improve CAR-T activity. TGF-β is secreted by tumor cells and is associated with metastasis, neoangiogenesis, and immunosuppression.[43] Several CAR-Ts are targeting this pathway. PSMA-directed CAR-Ts expressing a dominant negative TGF-β isoform (dnTGF-βRII) demonstrated improved persistence and tumor eradication in a mouse model of prostate cancer.[56] A trial of this product in castration-resistant prostate cancer reported a PSA response rate of 30%, including an exceptional 98% PSA reduction in one patient.[57] Unfortunately, this patient also experienced severe CRS secondary to unexpectedly robust CAR-T proliferation and death from concurrent sepsis. Another approach involves a prostate stem cell antigen (PSCA) directed CAR-T engineered with an inverted cytokine receptor fusing the exodomain of the immunosuppressive IL-4 with the activating IL-7 receptor endodomain.[58] Finally, so called "armored" CAR-Ts are engineered to constitutively secrete cytokines, including IL-12,[59] IL-18,[60] IL-15,[56] IL-7,[61] among others,[62] and are being employed in several active trials.

Target selection

The development of clinically active CAR-Ts depends on having the appropriate cell surface target to engage. The primary challenge is identifying a target that has clinical efficacy without leading to unacceptable toxicity. To accomplish this, targets must either be entirely restricted to the tumor itself, a tumor-specific antigen (TSA), or either expressed in low level in normal tissue or on a tissue that can be killed without excessive toxicity, a so-called tumor-associated antigen (TAA).[63] CAR-Ts targeted to the B-cell markers CD19 and CD20 carry a clinically acceptable toxicity-profile because the on-target/off-tumor effect of B-cell aplasia is a generally tolerable condition, save for an increased risk for infections.[64] This therapeutic window is more difficult to achieve in solid tumors, where targeting most lineage markers on tumor surfaces would lead to excessive toxicity to neighboring tissue (eg, lung epithelium, hepatocytes). Cross-reactivity of a HER2-targeted CAR-T to low-level HER2 expression on lung epithelium is thought to have contributed to a high-profile patient death within minutes of receiving CAR-T for metastatic colon cancer early in the clinical development of CAR-T therapy,[65] highlighting the challenge of even low-level off-tumor target expression.

Due to the high mutational burden of many solid tumors (eg, melanoma), targeting a peptide neoantigen could, in-principle, provide an optimal tumor-specific therapeutic window. This approach is the basis behind CARs targeting mutant EGFRvIII.[66] However, because CARs bind to cell-surface molecules, mutations in the 70-80% of proteins that are intracellular are hidden from potential CAR targeting.[67] T-cell-receptor (TCR) engineered cell therapy, which introduces a whole TCR rather than CAR construct, expands the pool of targetable antigens by providing access to intracellular peptides presented on MHC class I molecules.[68] Even so, early immune-based negative selective pressure against neoantigens likely contributes to a low (<3%) frequency of neoantigen presentation in driver genes.[69,70]

High levels of genomic instability in many solid tumors provide ample opportunity for cancer cells to evade CAR-Ts by deleting or mutating the target gene without affecting tumor viability. In hematological malignancies, the most common mechanism of escape for CD19-directed therapy is truncating mutations and copy-number changes leading to loss-of-heterozygosity of CD19.[71] This has been recapitulated in multiple trials in solid tumors.[72,73] Even relative down-regulation of target expression may be sufficient for escape: CAR-T activity is highly dependent on both CAR and tumor-antigen density, and imbalances may lead to insufficient activation.[74] Additionally, genes that are easily modified through epigenetic means, as opposed to mutations or copy-loss, are more prone to escape.[75]

Synthetic biology approaches aim to improve the specificity and scope of CAR targets and thereby reduce toxicity. One approach is dual-targeting, where CARs are engineered to target two different antigens simultaneously.[76] This approach has been applied in pre-clinical models of hepatocellular carcinoma[77] and breast cancer,[78] and was shown to be highly efficacious in a trial for relapsed/refractory B-ALL and diffuse large B-cell lymphoma.[76] Peptide-centric CAR-Ts (PC-CAR-T) target oncogenic peptides displayed by MHC class I molecules similar to a native TCR, but in an HLA-independent manner.[79] In a neuroblastoma mouse model, a PC-CAR-T was used to target an unmutated PHOX2B peptide exclusively expressed by neuroblastoma cells, opening an entirely new class of lineage-restricted intracellular proteins as potential CAR targets.[79] ON-CARs separate the co-stimulatory endodomains onto separate chains that can only be dimerized in the presence of a small molecule, providing an additional tool for controlling CAR-Ts post-infusion in the case of toxicity.[80] SUPRA-CARs use a soluble antigen-binding portion and a universal signal transduction receptor, allowing for more fine-tuned T-cell activation and multiple tumor-antigen recognition.[80]

ADVANCEMENTS IN CHIMERIC ANTIGEN RECEPTOR T-CELL THERAPY BY TUMOR TYPE

The landscape of CAR-T therapy in solid tumors is rapidly evolving–the number of ongoing clinical trials greatly outpaces the available literature of published clinical results. Here we summarize for a non-exhaustive set of disease sites the landscape of completed and ongoing trials, as well as select pre-clinical models. A table of completed or interim reports of clinical efficacy is presented in **Table 1**. Extensive reviews of CAR-T therapy for gastrointestinal tumors[81–84] and cutaneous tumors[85–87] are provided elsewhere.

Head and neck

Head and neck tumors arise from several different tissue types and with widely differing biologic and therapeutic approaches (eg, chemotherapy, immunotherapy, kinase inhibition, hormone therapy). As such, head and neck CAR-T targets are often highly tumor-type specific. For instance, the ongoing trial of GFRα4-directed CAR-T cells[88] is recruiting only in patients with metastatic medullary thyroid cancer (NCT04877613). In anaplastic thyroid cancer, an ongoing trial is targeting ICAM-1 with CAR-T cells engineered to express a somatostatin receptor for post-infusion PET imaging[89] (NCT04420754).

Viral-associated tumors, including Epstein-Barr virus (EBV)-related nasopharyngeal carcinoma and human papillomavirus (HPV)16+ squamous cell carcinoma, provide a therapeutic window through their association with viral non-self-antigens. Viral proteins can be trafficked to the cell surface where they are potential targets for CAR-T therapy, or presented via HLA-mediated display and suitable for TCR-engineered T-cell therapy. In HPV16+ tumors, including head and neck, cervical and vulvar tumors, TCRs targeting the viral E7 protein resulted in a 50% response rate among 12 patients, including in four of eight that were resistant to immunotherapy.[90] However, the follow-up KITE-439 trial based on E7 engineered TCRs towards HPV16 terminated early in development. In nasopharyngeal cancer, several clinical trials using either TCR and CAR-T approaches have been proposed targeting various EBV antigens (LMP1, LMP2, and EBNA1).[91]

Other CAR-T trials in head and neck cancer attempt a range of strategies to overcome the immunosuppressive microenvironment. A preclinical model of head and neck squamous cell carcinoma (HNSCC) used an oncolytic adenovirus system to deliver IL-12 and a PD-L1 blocking antibody to prime tumors before delivering HER2-directed

Table 1
Reported results, including interim results from ongoing trials, of CAR-T therapy among disease sites in this review

Disease Site	Histology	Target	Delivery	NCT	Patients Reported[a]	Results[a]	Reference
Head and neck	Squamous cell carcinoma	panErbB	Multifocal intratumoral	NCT01818323	13	69% DCR	Papa et al,[135] 2018
Head and neck	Thyroid cancer	TSHR	Intravenous	NA	1	PR at 90 days	Ding et al,[136] 2022
CNS	Glioblastoma	EGFRvIII	Intravenous	NCT02209376	10	9 SD (1 long-term non-progressor)	O'Rourke et al[72] 2017
CNS	Glioblastoma	IL13Rα2	Intracranial and intraventricular	NCT02208362	3	1 SD, 1 CR for 7.5 months	Brown et al,[73] 2016 &Brown et al,[137] 2015
CNS	Glioblastoma	HER2	Intravenous	NCT01109095	17	1 PR, 7 SD	Ahmed et al,[138] 2017
CNS	Glioblastoma	EGFRvIII	Intravenous	NCT01454596		No objective responses. Median PFS 1.3 months. 1 Patient with 12.5 month PFS.	Goff et al,[101] 2019
CNS	Neuroblastoma	CD171	Intravenous	NA	11	1 PR	Park et a,[139] 2007
CNS	Neuroblastoma	GD2	Intravenous	NCT00085930	19	1 PR, 3 CR	Louis et a,[140] 2011
CNS	Neuroblastoma	GD2	Intravenous	NCT01822652	11	No objective responses	Heczey et al,[141] 2017
CNS	Neuroblastoma	GD2 (CAR-NK)	Intravenous	NCT03294954	3	1 PR	Heczey et al,[51] 2020
CNS	Neuroblastoma	GD2	Intravenous	NCT02761915	12	No objective responses	Straathof et al,[142] 2020
CNS	Diffuse intrinsic pontine glioma	GD2	Intracerebroventricuar	NCT04196413	4	3 PR	Majzner et al,[96] 2022
Lung	Mesothelioma	Mesothelin	Intrapleural	NCT02414269	27	2 PR, 9 SD	Adusumilli et al,[36] 2021
Lung	Non-small cell lung cancer	EGFR	Intravenous	NCT01869166	11	2 PR, 5 SD	Feng et al,[107] 2016
Sarcoma	HER2-positive sarcoma (primarily osteosarcoma)	HER2	Intravenous	NCT00902044	19	4 SD	Ahmed et al,[111] 2015

(continued on next page)

Table 1
(continued)

Disease Site	Histology	Target	Delivery	NCT	Patients Reported[a]	Results[a]	Reference
Sarcoma	Rhabdomyosarcoma	HER2	Intravenous	NCT00902044	1	Complete response for at least 20 months	Hegde et al,[143] 2020
Genitourinary	Prostate cancer	PSMA	Intravenous	NCT03089203	13	4 PR (>30% PSA reduction). 1 treatment-related death	Narayan et al,[57] 2022
Genitourinary	Prostate cancer	PSMA	Intravenous	NA	5	2 PR	Junghans et al,[118] 2016
Genitourinary	Prostate cancer	PSCA	Intravenous	NCT03873805	12	7 SD (but one PSA decline > 90%)	Dorff et al,[120] 2022
Breast	Triple-negative and ER+	c-Met	Single intratumoral injection	NCT01837602	6	No measurable clinical responses	Tchou et al,[38] 2017
Ovarian	Serous ovarian cancer	MUCT16ecto	Intravenous and intraperitoneal	NCT02498912	18	SD as best response.	O'Cearbhaill et al,[144] 2020

Abbreviations: CR, complete response; DCR, disease control rate; PR, partial response; SD, stable disease.
[a] Includes interim analyses of incomplete trials.

CAR-T cells.[92] This is currently being evaluated in a phase 1 study in a range of tumor types, including HNSCC and salivary gland cancer (NCT03740256). T1E28z is a CAR created with the promiscuous ErbB ligand T1E to simultaneously target a range of ErbB homodimers and heterodimers.[93,94] This is being currently tested in a trial of HNSCC (NCT01818323). Other trials recruiting head and neck patients are targeting antigens found on multiple tumor types, including MUC1, HER2, and EpCAM.

Central nervous system

Central nervous system (CNS) tumors are among the most well-studied disease sites for CAR-T cells, owing to tumor-restricted targets, a paucity of treatment options for relapsed/refractory disease, and a higher proportion of young and otherwise healthy patients (see **Table 1**). The most extensively studied targeted is GD2, a disialoganglioside glycolipid that is overexpressed in neuroblastoma, melanoma, diffuse intrinsic pontine gliomas (DIPG), and medulloblastoma, among other pediatric and adult CNS tumors.[95,96] Preliminary results of a phase 1 trial (NCT04196413) of GD2-CAR-T in H3K27M-mutated DIPG demonstrated a clinical and radiographic response in three out of four patients.[96] Another trial (NCT05298995) is testing iC9-GD2-CAR-T, a third-generation GD2-directed CAR-T engineered with a caspase 9 safety switch in case of excessive toxicity, a particular concern due to expression of GD2 in some normal brain tissue.[97] Other strategies for targeting GD2 include a trial of GD2-directed CAR-Ts engineered with a constitutively active CD34-IL7R* cytokine receptor to provide ligand-free JAK/STAT signaling to improve cell persistence (NCT04099797 [98]) and a trial of anti-GD2 natural-killer CAR-T (CAR-NKT) cells (NCT03294954 [51]).

EGFR variant III (EGFRvIII) is a constitutively active truncated form of EGFR that is frequently overexpressed in glioblastoma, ependymomas, and medulloblastoma, among others.[99] The first trial of EGFRvIII-directed CAR-T cells was conducted in ten patients with glioblastoma.[72] Post-infusion surgical resections in seven patients demonstrated intratumoral CAR-Ts and decreased EGFRvIII expression. In long-term follow-up, one patient survived 36 months after disease recurrence.[100] Another trial of EGFRvIII in glioblastoma yielded a median progression-free survival (PFS) of only 1.3 months and no objective responses.[101] A trial evaluating EGFRvIII-directed CAR-T combined with pembrolizumab in glioblastoma is pending results (NCT03726515).

Other CAR-T targets being investigated in CNS tumors include the co-stimulatory protein B7.H3, the receptor tyrosine kinase HER2, and IL13Rα2. A complete response to IL13Rα2 CAR-Ts in a single patient with glioblastoma was achieved using a single initial intracranial administration followed by weekly intraventricular administrations of CAR-T cells.[73] Recurrence occurred at nonadjacent sites and with evidence of antigen escape with decreased levels of IL13Rα2. A novel approach in glioblastoma is using a chlorotoxin peptide (derived from scorpion venom) as a CAR targeting domain, given its ability to bind to tumor cells.[102]

Lung

The use of CAR-Ts in patients with advanced thoracic malignancies poses unique clinical challenges. On the one hand, patients with significantly reduced lung function secondary to tumor burden, pleural effusions, radiation pneumonitis, or underlying lung disease are ineligible for CAR-T therapy due to the risk of decompensation from CRS. On the other hand, the success of immunotherapy in lung cancer and reports of profound responses to cellular therapy in patients with lung metastases from non-thoracic tumors suggest a potentially favorable tumor environment for cellular therapy.[103]

Mesothelin is a cell-surface protein expressed in several cancers, including mesothelioma, lung adenocarcinoma, ovarian cancer, and pancreatic cancer expression,[104] making it the subject of several CAR-T products.[105] The first mesothelin-directed CAR-T trial reported results in 2013 in three patients with mesothelioma, but was complicated by a case of anaphylaxis leading to cardiac arrest following CAR-T infusion.[106] A subsequent trial enrolled 15 patients, split evenly among mesothelioma, ovarian and pancreatic carcinoma, and demonstrated only one dose-limiting toxicity (grade 4 sepsis) and stable disease as the best response (11/15).[106] This trial used a murine scFv antibody fragment, and the limited clinical efficacy was thought to be related to antibody response to the CAR itself.[105] A trial from the same group with a fully humanized CAR (huCART-meso) is ongoing (NCT03054298).

Receptor tyrosine kinases (RTKs) are promising targets in lung cancer due to both their localization to the cell membrane and the strong dependence of lung cancer to RTK signaling, making escape through RTK downregulation more difficult. A study of EGFR-directed CAR-Ts in non-small cell lung cancer (NSCLC) patients with >50% EGFR expression showed two partial responses in 11 patients.[107] An ongoing EGFR-directed CAR-T trial is using CXCR5-modified CAR-Ts to increase CAR-T persistence (NCT05060796). ROR1 is an RTK expressed in triple-negative breast cancer (TNBC), NSCLC and on normal B-cell-precursors.[108] Due to concerns about bone marrow toxicity, ROR1 CAR-Ts have been modified with synthetic Notch receptors to improve tumor specificity in pre-clinical models.[109] HER2 has recently been demonstrated as an effective target of antibody-drug conjugates in NSCLC.[110] A trial of a combination of CAdVEC, an oncolytic adenovirus, and HER2-directed CAR T cells, is enrolling across solid tumors, including lung cancer (NCT03740256).

Sarcoma

Relapsed or refractory sarcoma remains difficult to treat and has a poor response rate to chemotherapy. The incidence of sarcomas is proportionally higher among children and young adults, a population who may be best suited to tolerate cellular therapy. Although there are a high number of sarcoma subtypes, many sarcomas share cell surface protein expression. This has provided for CAR-T trials that target multiple sarcoma subtypes, easing recruitment concerns and expanding their potential clinical scope.

In a trial of HER2-directed CAR-Ts in 19 patients (16 osteosarcoma, one Ewing sarcoma, one primitive neuroectodermal tumor, one desmoplastic small round cell tumor), four patients achieved stable disease.[111] Multiple other HER2-directed CAR-T trials in sarcoma are ongoing. B7-H3 is overexpressed in tumors such as rhabdomyosarcoma, Ewing sarcoma, and osteosarcoma, and is being tested clinically by the B7-H3-targeting monoclonal antibody enoblituzumab.[112] B7-directed CAR-T trials are also underway in multiple centers for children and young adults with sarcoma (NCT03618381, NCT04897321).

Over 80% of osteosarcomas express the folate receptor.[113] The ENLIGHTen clinical trial is being conducted in patients with osteosarcoma to assess the effectiveness of autologous universal CAR-T cells (NCT05312411). Patients are administered a bispecific small molecule that labels tumor cells with a fluorescein tag for destruction by anti-FITC CAR-Ts. GD2 is a well-characterized candidate target in several tumors, including osteosarcoma and neuroblastoma.[114] An NIH trial is evaluating a third-generation anti-GD2-CAR-T product, engineered with a caspase safety switch in case of clinically unacceptable toxicity, in patients with GD2-positive sarcomas (NCT02107963).

NY-ESO-1 is a cancer/testis antigen expressed in several tumor types, including in 70-80% of synovial sarcomas.[115] Letetresgene autoleucel is an autologous T-cell product with a lentivirally transduced TCR that recognizes HLA-A*02-presented peptides derived from NY-ESO-1. In a study of 50 patients with unresectable, metastatic, or recurrent synovial sarcoma, the objective response rate (ORR) across all doses and lymphodepletion regimens was 33%, including one durable (34 weeks) complete response.[115] Letetresgene autoleucel is also being tested in myxoid/round cell liposarcoma (NCT02992743), with an initial report finding an ORR of 30% across 20 treated patients.[116]

Genitourinary

The most active areas of CAR-T therapy in genitourinary cancer are in prostate and kidney cancers. In prostate cancer, most trials are focused on targeting PSMA, a highly expressed transmembrane protein that is associated with metastatic castration-resistant prostate cancer (mCRPC).[117] As described above, a recent report of PSMA CAR-T therapy in patient with mCRPC reported a response rate of 30% and one treatment-related death.[57] Another trial of PSMA CAR-Ts administered with continuous IL-2 infusion reported partial PSA responses in two-of-five patients.[118] PSCA is also highly expressed on prostate cancer tissue relative to normal tissue.[119] There are no resulted completed trials of PSCA CAR-Ts, but phase 1 trials are currently ongoing, including a recent report indicating an exceptional responder with >90% PSA decline (NCT03873805 [120]).

CAR-T targets in renal cell carcinoma include RTKs (AXL, ROR2, VEGFR2, and c-Met), the glycoprotein MUC1C, the co-stimulatory protein CD70, and the transmembrane enzyme carbonic anhydrase (CaIX).[121] In an ongoing phase I/II trial, patients receive either a ROR2-directed CAR-T (CCT301–59) or an AXL-directed CAR-T (CCT301–38), depending on their staining for these markers by immunohistochemistry (NCT03393936). COBALT-RCC is testing an allogeneic CAR-T product (CTX130) targeting CD70 (NCT03393936). One of the first studies of CAR-Ts in patients targeted CaIX in kidney cancer.[4] This target is now being reevaluated in a trial of CaIX-directed CAR-Ts (NCT04969354).

To-date there have been no completed trials of CAR-Ts in testicular germ cell tumors, although trials are on-going. The carcinoembryonic antigen claudin 6 (CLDN6) is a tight junction protein expressed in nearly all testicular tumors.[122] Preliminary results from a phase 1 trial of BNT-211-01, a claudin-6 directed CAR-T product, reported results from 21 patients (including 13 with testicular cancer) and showed partial response in 7 patients and stable disease in 8 (NCT04503278 [123]). In urothelial cancer, clinical CAR-T progress has also been sparse. There are currently studies of CAR-T products targeting HER2, PSMA, and ROR2 across a range of tumors including bladder cancer, although none that are specific for urothelial tumors.[124]

Breast and ovarian

Despite its prevalence, there are no published completed trials of systemic CAR-T therapy dedicated to breast cancer. However, numerous trials are ongoing. Targets being tested include RTKs (HER2, cMET, ROR1, EGFR), cell surface glycoproteins (MUC1, MSLN, EpCAM, TROP2), and CEA, among others.[125,126] The expression of mesothelin has been shown to correlate with distant metastases and decreased survival in metastatic breast cancer.[127] A trial of regionally delivered mesothelin-directed CAR-T included a single patient with metastatic triple-negative breast cancer (TNBC),[36] and there is an ongoing trial involving 183 patients testing mesothelin CAR-T specifically in mesothelin-expressing breast cancer (NCT02792114). Another trial recruiting specifically breast cancer patients is targeting a tumor-specific cleaved form of MUC1 (MUC1*) with the huMNC2-CAR44 product (NCT04020575). Tn-MUC1 is a cancer-specific MUC1 glycoform with a distinct immune epitope that can be targeted separately from MUC1.[128] A trial of patients with Tn-MUC1 positive cancers, including TNBC and ovarian cancer, is ongoing (NCT04025216). There are also ongoing trials enrolling patients across different disease sites, including breast cancer, targeting HER2, EpCAM, CEA, CD133, GD2, and CD70.

Ovarian cancer was one of the first targets for CAR-T cell therapy, with a trial of five patients receiving folate receptor-directed CAR-T cells reported in 2006.[3] Since this early report, several pre-clinical models have tested CAR-T therapy in ovarian cancer.[129] However, there have been no further completed trials in humans. The currently active trial of PRGN-3005 uses a CAR-T engineered with a safety kill switch, IL-15 receptor, and a CAR targeting the glycoprotein MUC16[130] (NCT03907527). Another active trial is using third-generation CAR-Ts targeting the folate-receptor alpha, with or without cyclophosphamide-based pre-conditioning[131] (NCT03585764). Other current CAR-T trials specifically enrolling in ovarian cancer are targeting B7H3 (NCT05211557), mesothelin (NCT03916679, NCT05372692), and TAG72 (NCT052253630). Many of the trials specific to ovarian cancer patients are employing intraperitoneal CAR-T administration to reduce the risk of systemic toxicity.

SUMMARY

CAR-T therapy in solid tumors is rapidly evolving owing to the explosion of new CAR constructs, target antigens, and cellular engineering technologies. We highlighted only some of the advancements shaping this landscape. New CAR formats including CAR-NKs,[132] CAR-macrophages,[133] and allogeneic CAR-Ts[134] may provide new opportunities for clinical impact. In many disease sites, the number of ongoing clinical trials greatly outnumbers those with reported results. As these trials read out over the next several years, our understanding of the impact of CAR-Ts in solid tumors will greatly expand. Our hope is that these efforts will lead to several candidate CAR-Ts for later-stage clinical testing, advancing towards the goal of achieving an approved CAR-T therapy for widespread clinical use in solid tumors.

CLINICS CARE POINTS

- CAR-T therapy for solid tumors is unproven and is currently only available through clinical trials.
- Delivery of CAR-T therapy in solid tumors usually requires in-patient delivery and early intervention to treat the strong inflammatory response they can produce.
- Management of cytokine release syndrome and immune effector cell-associated neurotoxicity syndrome follows well-established protocols derived from the use of CAR-T therapy in hematological malignancies.
- Patients receiving CAR-Ts must be fit enough to undergo leukapharesis, lymphodepletive chemotherapy and to tolerate waiting several weeks for CAR-T production.

DISCLOSURES

J.A. Wala—no disclosures. G.J. Hanna—relevant disclosures include research support to institution: BMS, Gateway for Cancer Research, Immunitybio, Kite Pharma, KSQ Therapeutics; consulting/honoraria: KSQ Therapeutics.

REFERENCES

1. Gong MC, Latouche JB, Krause A, et al. Cancer patient T cells genetically targeted to prostate-specific membrane antigen specifically lyse prostate cancer cells and release cytokines in response to prostate-specific membrane antigen. Neoplasia N Y N 1999;1(2):123–7.
2. Clay TM, Custer MC, Sachs J, et al. Efficient transfer of a tumor antigen-reactive TCR to human peripheral blood lymphocytes confers anti-tumor reactivity. J Immunol Baltim Md 1950 1999;163(1):507–13.
3. Kershaw MH, Westwood JA, Parker LL, et al. A phase I study on adoptive immunotherapy using gene-modified T cells for ovarian cancer. Clin Cancer Res 2006;12(20 Pt 1):6106–15.
4. Lamers CHJ, Sleijfer S, Vulto AG, et al. Treatment of metastatic renal cell carcinoma with autologous T-lymphocytes genetically retargeted against carbonic anhydrase IX: first clinical experience. J Clin Oncol 2006;24(13):e20–2.
5. Schaft N. The landscape of CAR-T cell clinical trials against solid tumors-a comprehensive overview. Cancers 2020;12(9):2567.
6. Hayden PJ, Roddie C, Bader P, et al. Management of adults and children receiving CAR T-cell therapy: 2021 best practice recommendations of the European Society for Blood and Marrow Transplantation (EBMT) and the Joint Accreditation Committee of ISCT and EBMT (JACIE) and the European Haematology Association (EHA). Ann Oncol 2022;33(3):259–75.
7. Qian S, Villarejo-Campos P, Guijo I, et al. Update for advance CAR-T therapy in solid tumors, clinical application in peritoneal carcinomatosis from colorectal cancer and future prospects. Front Immunol 2022;13. Available at: https://www.frontiersin.org/articles/10.3389/fimmu.2022.841425. Accessed February 2, 2023.
8. Owens K, Bozic I. Modeling CAR T-cell therapy with patient preconditioning. Bull Math Biol 2021;83(5):42.
9. Hernandez I, Prasad V, Gellad WF. Total costs of chimeric antigen receptor T-cell immunotherapy. JAMA Oncol 2018;4(7):994–6.
10. Frey NV, Porter DL. Cytokine release syndrome with novel therapeutics for acute lymphoblastic leukemia. Hematol Am Soc Hematol Educ Program 2016;2016(1): 567–72.
11. Morris EC, Neelapu SS, Giavridis T, et al. Cytokine release syndrome and associated neurotoxicity in cancer immunotherapy. Nat Rev Immunol 2022;22(2): 85–96.
12. Hay KA, Hanafi LA, Li D, et al. Kinetics and biomarkers of severe cytokine release syndrome after CD19 chimeric antigen receptor–modified T-cell therapy. Blood 2017;130(21):2295–306.
13. Le RQ, Li L, Yuan W, et al. FDA approval summary: tocilizumab for treatment of chimeric antigen receptor t cell-induced severe or life-threatening cytokine release syndrome. Oncol 2018;23(8):943–7.
14. Siegler EL, Kenderian SS. Neurotoxicity and cytokine release syndrome after chimeric antigen receptor t cell therapy: insights into mechanisms and novel therapies. Front Immunol 2020;11. Available at: https://www.frontiersin.org/articles/10.3389/fimmu.2020.01973. Accessed February 9, 2023.
15. Hou B, Tang Y, Li W, et al. Efficiency of CAR-T therapy for treatment of solid tumor in clinical trials: a meta-analysis. Dis Markers 2019;2019:3425291.
16. de Saint Basile G, Ménasché G, Fischer A. Molecular mechanisms of biogenesis and exocytosis of cytotoxic granules. Nat Rev Immunol 2010;10(8):568–79.

17. Enblad G, Karlsson H, Loskog ASI. CAR T-cell therapy: the role of physical barriers and immunosuppression in lymphoma. Hum Gene Ther 2015;26(8):498–505.

18. Moon EK, Wang LC, Dolfi DV, et al. Multifactorial T-cell hypofunction that is reversible can limit the efficacy of chimeric antigen receptor-transduced human T cells in solid tumors. Clin Cancer Res 2014;20(16):4262–73.

19. Foeng J, Comerford I, McColl SR. Harnessing the chemokine system to home CAR-T cells into solid tumors. Cell Rep Med 2022;3(3):100543.

20. Emami-Shahri N, Foster J, Kashani R, et al. Clinically compliant spatial and temporal imaging of chimeric antigen receptor T-cells. Nat Commun 2018;9(1):1081.

21. Salmon H, Franciszkiewicz K, Damotte D, et al. Matrix architecture defines the preferential localization and migration of T cells into the stroma of human lung tumors. J Clin Invest 2012;122(3):899–910.

22. Boissonnas A, Licata F, Poupel L, et al. CD8+ tumor-infiltrating T cells are trapped in the tumor-dendritic cell network. Neoplasia 2013;15(1). 85-IN26.

23. Macrophages impede CD8 T cells from reaching tumor cells and limit the efficacy of anti-PD-1 treatment. Proc Natl Acad Sci 2018;115(17):E4041–50.

24. Feig C, Jones JO, Kraman M, et al. Targeting CXCL12 from FAP-expressing carcinoma-associated fibroblasts synergizes with anti–PD-L1 immunotherapy in pancreatic cancer. Proc Natl Acad Sci 2013;110(50):20212–7.

25. Sugiura A, Rathmell JC. Metabolic barriers to T cell function in tumors. J Immunol 2018;200(2):400–7.

26. Moon EK, Carpenito C, Sun J, et al. Expression of a functional CCR2 receptor enhances tumor localization and tumor eradication by retargeted human T cells expressing a mesothelin-specific chimeric antibody receptor. Clin Cancer Res 2011;17(14):4719–30.

27. Di Stasi A, De Angelis B, Rooney CM, et al. T lymphocytes coexpressing CCR4 and a chimeric antigen receptor targeting CD30 have improved homing and antitumor activity in a Hodgkin tumor model. Blood 2009;113(25):6392–402.

28. Jin L, Tao H, Karachi A, et al. CXCR1- or CXCR2-modified CAR T cells co-opt IL-8 for maximal antitumor efficacy in solid tumors. Nat Commun 2019;10(1):4016.

29. Naparstek Y, Cohen IR, Fuks Z, et al. Activated T lymphocytes produce a matrix-degrading heparan sulphate endoglycosidase. Nature 1984;310(5974):241–4.

30. Caruana I, Savoldo B, Hoyos V, et al. Heparanase promotes tumor infiltration and antitumor activity of CAR-redirected T lymphocytes. Nat Med 2015;21(5):524–9.

31. Minn I, Huss DJ, Ahn HH, et al. Imaging CAR T cell therapy with PSMA-targeted positron emission tomography. Sci Adv 2019;5(7):eaaw5096.

32. Vedvyas Y, Shevlin E, Zaman M, et al. Longitudinal PET imaging demonstrates biphasic CAR T cell responses in survivors. JCI Insight 2016;1(19):e90064.

33. Keu KV, Witney TH, Yaghoubi S, et al. Reporter gene imaging of targeted T cell immunotherapy in recurrent glioma. Sci Transl Med 2017;9(373):eaag2196.

34. Wang J, Hu Y, Yang S, et al. Role of Fluorodeoxyglucose positron emission tomography/computed tomography in predicting the adverse effects of chimeric antigen receptor T cell therapy in patients with non-hodgkin lymphoma. Biol Blood Marrow Transplant J Am Soc Blood Marrow Transplant 2019;25(6):1092–8.

35. Adusumilli PS, Cherkassky L, Villena-Vargas J, et al. Regional delivery of mesothelin-targeted CAR T cell therapy generates potent and long-lasting CD4-dependent tumor immunity. Sci Transl Med 2014;6(261):261ra151.

36. Adusumilli PS, Zauderer MG, Rivière I, et al. A phase I trial of regional mesothelin-targeted CAR T-cell therapy in patients with malignant pleural disease, in combination with the anti-PD-1 agent pembrolizumab. Cancer Discov 2021;11(11):2748–63.

37. Cherkassky L, Hou Z, Amador-Molina A, et al. Regional CAR T cell therapy: an ignition key for systemic immunity in solid tumors. Cancer Cell 2022;40(6):569–74.
38. Tchou J, Zhao Y, Levine BL, et al. Safety and efficacy of intratumoral injections of chimeric antigen receptor (CAR) T cells in metastatic breast cancer. Cancer Immunol Res 2017;5(12):1152–61.
39. Liu G, Rui W, Zhao X, et al. Enhancing CAR-T cell efficacy in solid tumors by targeting the tumor microenvironment. Cell Mol Immunol 2021;18(5):1085–95.
40. Qin S, Xu L, Yi M, et al. Novel immune checkpoint targets: moving beyond PD-1 and CTLA-4. Mol Cancer 2019;18(1):155.
41. Wherry EJ. T cell exhaustion. Nat Immunol 2011;12(6):492–9.
42. McGowan E, Lin Q, Ma G, et al. PD-1 disrupted CAR-T cells in the treatment of solid tumors: Promises and challenges. Biomed Pharmacother 2020;121:109625.
43. Massagué J. TGFβ in cancer. Cell 2008;134(2):215–30.
44. Rupp LJ, Schumann K, Roybal KT, et al. CRISPR/Cas9-mediated PD-1 disruption enhances anti-tumor efficacy of human chimeric antigen receptor T cells. Sci Rep 2017;7(1):737.
45. Hu W, Zi Z, Jin Y, et al. CRISPR/Cas9-mediated PD-1 disruption enhances human mesothelin-targeted CAR T cell effector functions. Cancer Immunol Immunother CII 2019;68(3):365–77.
46. Wang Z, Li N, Feng K, et al. Phase I study of CAR-T cells with PD-1 and TCR disruption in mesothelin-positive solid tumors. Cell Mol Immunol 2021;18(9):2188–98.
47. Grosser R, Cherkassky L, Chintala N, et al. Combination immunotherapy with CAR T cells and checkpoint blockade for the treatment of solid tumors. Cancer Cell 2019;36(5):471–82.
48. Chong EA, Melenhorst JJ, Lacey SF, et al. PD-1 blockade modulates chimeric antigen receptor (CAR)-modified T cells: refueling the CAR. Blood 2017;129(8):1039–41.
49. Chong EA, Alanio C, Svoboda J, et al. Pembrolizumab for B-cell lymphomas relapsing after or refractory to CD19-directed CAR T-cell therapy. Blood 2022;139(7):1026–38.
50. Gargett T, Yu W, Dotti G, et al. GD2-specific CAR T cells undergo potent activation and deletion following antigen encounter but can be protected from activation-induced cell death by PD-1 blockade. Mol Ther 2016;24(6):1135–49.
51. Heczey A, Courtney AN, Montalbano A, et al. Anti-GD2 CAR-NKT cells in patients with relapsed or refractory neuroblastoma: an interim analysis. Nat Med 2020;26(11):1686–90.
52. Turner MD, Nedjai B, Hurst T, et al. Cytokines and chemokines: at the crossroads of cell signalling and inflammatory disease. Biochim Biophys Acta BBA - Mol Cell Res 2014;1843(11):2563–82.
53. Peng D, Kryczek I, Nagarsheth N, et al. Epigenetic silencing of TH1-type chemokines shapes tumour immunity and immunotherapy. Nature 2015;527(7577):249–53.
54. Zou W, Machelon V, Coulomb-L'Hermin A, et al. Stromal-derived factor-1 in human tumors recruits and alters the function of plasmacytoid precursor dendritic cells. Nat Med 2001;7(12):1339–46.
55. Poh AR, Ernst M. Targeting macrophages in cancer: from bench to bedside. Front Oncol 2018;8. Available at: https://www.frontiersin.org/articles/10.3389/fonc.2018.00049. Accessed February 10, 2023.
56. Kloss CC, Lee J, Zhang A, et al. Dominant-negative TGF-β receptor enhances PSMA-targeted human CAR T cell proliferation and augments prostate cancer eradication. Mol Ther 2018;26(7):1855–66.

57. Narayan V, Barber-Rotenberg JS, Jung IY, et al. PSMA-targeting TGFβ-insensitive armored CAR T cells in metastatic castration-resistant prostate cancer: a phase 1 trial. Nat Med 2022;28(4):724–34.

58. Mohammed S, Sukumaran S, Bajgain P, et al. Improving chimeric antigen receptor-modified T cell function by reversing the immunosuppressive tumor microenvironment of pancreatic cancer. Mol Ther 2017;25(1):249–58.

59. Yeku OO, Purdon TJ, Koneru M, et al. Armored CAR T cells enhance antitumor efficacy and overcome the tumor microenvironment. Sci Rep 2017;7(1):10541.

60. Avanzi MP, Yeku O, Li X, et al. Engineered tumor-targeted T cells mediate enhanced anti-tumor efficacy both directly and through activation of the endogenous immune system. Cell Rep 2018;23(7):2130–41.

61. Golumba-Nagy V, Kuehle J, Hombach AA, et al. CD28-ζ CAR T cells resist TGF-β repression through IL-2 signaling, which can be mimicked by an engineered IL-7 autocrine loop. Mol Ther J Am Soc Gene Ther 2018;26(9):2218–30.

62. Hawkins ER, D'Souza RR, Klampatsa A. Armored CAR T-cells: the next chapter in t-cell cancer immunotherapy. Biol Targets & Ther 2021;15:95–105.

63. Abbott RC, Cross RS, Jenkins MR. Finding the keys to the CAR: Identifying novel target antigens for T cell redirection immunotherapies. Int J Mol Sci 2020;21(2):515.

64. Wudhikarn K, Palomba ML, Pennisi M, et al. Infection during the first year in patients treated with CD19 CAR T cells for diffuse large B cell lymphoma. Blood Cancer J 2020;10(8):1–11.

65. Morgan RA, Yang JC, Kitano M, et al. Case report of a serious adverse event following the administration of T cells transduced with a chimeric antigen receptor recognizing ERBB2. Mol Ther 2010;18(4):843–51.

66. Ravanpay AC, Gust J, Johnson AJ, et al. EGFR806-CAR T cells selectively target a tumor-restricted EGFR epitope in glioblastoma. Oncotarget 2019;10(66):7080–95.

67. Almeida JG, Preto AJ, Koukos PI, et al. Membrane proteins structures: a review on computational modeling tools. Biochim Biophys Acta Biomembr 2017;1859(10):2021–39.

68. Zhao Q, Jiang Y, Xiang S, et al. Engineered TCR-T cell immunotherapy in anti-cancer precision medicine: pros and cons. Front Immunol 2021;12. Available at: https://www.frontiersin.org/articles/10.3389/fimmu.2021.658753. Accessed February 11, 2023.

69. Yarmarkovich M, Farrel A, Sison A, et al. Immunogenicity and immune silence in human cancer. Front Immunol 2020;11:69.

70. Hartmaier RJ, Charo J, Fabrizio D, et al. Genomic analysis of 63,220 tumors reveals insights into tumor uniqueness and targeted cancer immunotherapy strategies. Genome Med 2017;9(1):16.

71. Orlando EJ, Han X, Tribouley C, et al. Genetic mechanisms of target antigen loss in CAR19 therapy of acute lymphoblastic leukemia. Nat Med 2018;24(10):1504–6.

72. O'Rourke DM, Nasrallah MP, Desai A, et al. A single dose of peripherally infused EGFRvIII-directed CAR T cells mediates antigen loss and induces adaptive resistance in patients with recurrent glioblastoma. Sci Transl Med 2017;9(399):eaaa0984.

73. Brown CE, Alizadeh D, Starr R, et al. Regression of glioblastoma after chimeric antigen receptor T-cell therapy. N Engl J Med 2016;375(26):2561–9.

74. Walker AJ, Majzner RG, Zhang L, et al. Tumor antigen and receptor densities regulate efficacy of a chimeric antigen receptor targeting anaplastic lymphoma kinase. Mol Ther 2017;25(9):2189–201.

75. Wei J, Han X, Bo J, et al. Target selection for CAR-T therapy. J Hematol OncolJ Hematol Oncol 2019;12(1):62.

76. Spiegel JY, Patel S, Muffly L, et al. CAR T cells with dual targeting of CD19 and CD22 in adult patients with recurrent or refractory B cell malignancies: a phase 1 trial. Nat Med 2021;27(8):1419–31.

77. Chen C, Li K, Jiang H, et al. Development of T cells carrying two complementary chimeric antigen receptors against glypican-3 and asialoglycoprotein receptor 1 for the treatment of hepatocellular carcinoma. Cancer Immunol Immunother CII 2017;66(4):475–89.

78. Wilkie S, van Schalkwyk MCI, Hobbs S, et al. Dual targeting of ErbB2 and MUC1 in breast cancer using chimeric antigen receptors engineered to provide complementary signaling. J Clin Immunol 2012;32(5):1059–70.

79. Yarmarkovich M, Marshall QF, Warrington JM, et al. Cross-HLA targeting of intracellular oncoproteins with peptide-centric CARs. Nature 2021;599(7885):477–84.

80. Lanitis E, Coukos G, Irving M. All systems go: converging synthetic biology and combinatorial treatment for CAR-T cell therapy. Curr Opin Biotechnol 2020;65:75–87.

81. Akce M, Zaidi MY, Waller EK, et al. The potential of CAR T cell therapy in pancreatic cancer. Front Immunol 2018;9:2166.

82. Bębnowska D, Grywalska E, Niedźwiedzka-Rystwej P, et al. CAR-T cell therapy—an overview of targets in gastric cancer. J Clin Med 2020;9(6):1894.

83. Li H, Yang C, Cheng H, et al. CAR-T cells for colorectal cancer: target-selection and strategies for improved activity and safety. J Cancer 2021;12(6):1804–14.

84. Rochigneux P, Chanez B, De Rauglaudre B, et al. Adoptive cell therapy in hepatocellular carcinoma: biological rationale and first results in early phase clinical trials. Cancers 2021;13(2):271.

85. Chan IS, Bhatia S, Kaufman HL, et al. Immunotherapy for Merkel cell carcinoma: a turning point in patient care. J Immunother Cancer 2018;6(1):23.

86. Razavi A, Keshavarz-Fathi M, Pawelek J, et al. Chimeric antigen receptor T-cell therapy for melanoma. Expert Rev Clin Immunol 2021;17(3):209–23.

87. Simon B, Uslu U. CAR-T cell therapy in melanoma: A future success story? Exp Dermatol 2018;27(12):1315–21.

88. Bhoj VG, Li L, Parvathaneni K, et al. Adoptive T cell immunotherapy for medullary thyroid carcinoma targeting GDNF family receptor alpha 4. Mol Ther Oncolytics 2021;20:387–98.

89. Vedvyas Y, McCloskey JE, Yang Y, et al. Manufacturing and preclinical validation of CAR T cells targeting ICAM-1 for advanced thyroid cancer therapy. Sci Rep 2019;9(1):10634.

90. Nagarsheth NB, Norberg SM, Sinkoe AL, et al. TCR-engineered T cells targeting E7 for patients with metastatic HPV-associated epithelial cancers. Nat Med 2021;27(3):419–25.

91. Münz C. Redirecting T cells against epstein–barr virus infection and associated oncogenesis. Cells 2020;9(6):1400.

92. Rosewell Shaw A, Porter CE, Watanabe N, et al. Adenovirotherapy delivering cytokine and checkpoint inhibitor augments CAR T cells against metastatic head and neck cancer. Mol Ther J Am Soc Gene Ther 2017;25(11):2440–51.

93. van Schalkwyk MCI, Papa SE, Jeannon JP, et al. Design of a phase I clinical trial to evaluate intratumoral delivery of ErbB-targeted chimeric antigen receptor T-cells in locally advanced or recurrent head and neck cancer. Hum Gene Ther Clin Dev 2013;24(3):134–42.

94. Davies DM, Foster J, Van Der Stegen SJC, et al. Flexible targeting of ErbB dimers that drive tumorigenesis by using genetically engineered T cells. Mol Med Camb Mass 2012;18(1):565–76.

95. Nazha B, Inal C, Owonikoko TK. Disialoganglioside GD2 Expression in Solid Tumors and Role as a Target for Cancer Therapy. Front Oncol 2020;10. Available at: https://www.frontiersin.org/articles/10.3389/fonc.2020.01000. Accessed February 2, 2023.

96. Majzner RG, Ramakrishna S, Yeom KW, et al. GD2-CAR T cell therapy for H3K27M-mutated diffuse midline gliomas. Nature 2022;603(7903):934–41.

97. Sait S, Modak S. Anti-GD2 immunotherapy for neuroblastoma. Expert Rev Anticancer Ther 2017;17(10):889–904.

98. Shum T, Omer B, Tashiro H, et al. Constitutive signaling from an engineered IL-7 receptor promotes durable tumor elimination by tumor redirected T-cells. Cancer Discov 2017;7(11):1238–47.

99. Mimeault M, Batra SK. Complex oncogenic signaling networks regulate brain tumor-initiating cells and their progenies: pivotal roles of wild-type EGFR, EGFRvIII mutant and hedgehog cascades and novel multitargeted therapies. Brain Pathol 2011;21(5):479–500.

100. Durgin JS, Henderson F, Nasrallah MP, et al. Case report: prolonged survival following EGFRvIII CAR T cell treatment for recurrent glioblastoma. Front Oncol 2021;11:669071.

101. Goff SL, Morgan RA, Yang JC, et al. Pilot trial of adoptive transfer of chimeric antigen receptor-transduced t cells targeting EGFRvIII in patients with glioblastoma. J Immunother Hagerstown Md 1997 2019;42(4):126–35.

102. Wang D, Starr R, Chang WC, et al. Chlorotoxin-directed CAR T cells for specific and effective targeting of glioblastoma. Sci Transl Med 2020;12(533):eaaw2672.

103. Leidner R, Sanjuan Silva N, Huang H, et al. Neoantigen T-cell receptor gene therapy in pancreatic cancer. N Engl J Med 2022;386(22):2112–9.

104. Hassan R, Ho M. Mesothelin targeted cancer immunotherapy. Eur J Cancer 2008;44(1):46–53.

105. Klampatsa A, Dimou V, Albelda SM. Mesothelin-targeted CAR-T cell therapy for solid tumors. Expert Opin Biol Ther 2021;21(4):473–86.

106. Maus MV, Haas AR, Beatty GL, et al. T cells expressing chimeric antigen receptors can cause anaphylaxis in humans. Cancer Immunol Res 2013;1(1):26–31.

107. Feng K, Guo Y, Dai H, et al. Chimeric antigen receptor-modified T cells for the immunotherapy of patients with EGFR-expressing advanced relapsed/refractory non-small cell lung cancer. Sci China Life Sci 2016;59(5):468–79.

108. Srivastava S, Furlan SN, Jaeger-Ruckstuhl CA, et al. Immunogenic chemotherapy enhances recruitment of CAR-T cells to lung tumors and improves antitumor efficacy when combined with checkpoint blockade. Cancer Cell 2021; 39(2):193–208.e10.

109. Srivastava S, Salter AI, Liggitt D, et al. Logic-gated ROR1 chimeric antigen receptor expression rescues T cell-mediated toxicity to normal tissues and enables selective tumor targeting. Cancer Cell 2019;35(3):489–503.e8.

110. Li BT, Smit EF, Goto Y, et al. Trastuzumab deruxtecan in HER2-mutant non-small-cell lung cancer. N Engl J Med 2022;386(3):241–51.

111. Ahmed N, Brawley VS, Hegde M, et al. Human epidermal growth factor receptor 2 (HER2) –specific chimeric antigen receptor–modified T cells for the immunotherapy of HER2-positive sarcoma. J Clin Oncol 2015;33(15):1688–96.

112. Thanindratarn P, Dean DC, Nelson SD, et al. Chimeric antigen receptor T (CAR-T) cell immunotherapy for sarcomas: From mechanisms to potential clinical applications. Cancer Treat Rev 2020;82:101934.

113. Yang R, Kolb EA, Qin J, et al. The folate receptor alpha is frequently overexpressed in osteosarcoma samples and plays a role in the uptake of the physiologic substrate 5-methyltetrahydrofolate. Clin Cancer Res 2007;13(9):2557–67.

114. Roth M, Linkowski M, Tarim J, et al. Ganglioside GD2 as a therapeutic target for antibody-mediated therapy in osteosarcoma. Cancer 2014;120(4):548–54.

115. D'Angelo S, Demetri G, Tine BV, et al. 298 Final analysis of the phase 1 trial of NY-ESO-1–specific T-cell receptor (TCR) T-cell therapy (letetresgene autoleucel; GSK3377794) in patients with advanced synovial sarcoma (SS). J Immunother Cancer 2020;8(Suppl 3). https://doi.org/10.1136/jitc-2020-SITC2020.0298.

116. D'Angelo SP, Druta M, Van Tine BA, et al. Primary efficacy and safety of letetresgene autoleucel (lete-cel; GSK3377794) pilot study in patients with advanced and metastatic myxoid/round cell liposarcoma (MRCLS). J Clin Oncol 2022; 40(16_suppl):11500.

117. Perner S, Hofer MD, Kim R, et al. Prostate-specific membrane antigen expression as a predictor of prostate cancer progression. Hum Pathol 2007;38(5):696–701.

118. Junghans RP, Ma Q, Rathore R, et al. Phase I trial of Anti-PSMA designer CAR-T cells in prostate cancer: possible role for interacting interleukin 2-T cell pharmacodynamics as a determinant of clinical response. Prostate 2016;76(14):1257–70.

119. Saeki N, Gu J, Yoshida T, et al. Prostate stem cell antigen (PSCA): a Jekyll and Hyde molecule? Clin Cancer Res 2010;16(14):3533–8.

120. Dorff TB, Blanchard S, Martirosyan H, et al. Phase 1 study of PSCA-targeted chimeric antigen receptor (CAR) T cell therapy for metastatic castration-resistant prostate cancer (mCRPC). J Clin Oncol 2022;40(6_suppl):91.

121. Kim TJ, Lee YH, Koo KC. Current and future perspectives on CAR-T cell therapy for renal cell carcinoma: a comprehensive review. Investig Clin Urol 2022;63(5):486–98.

122. Ushiku T, Shinozaki-Ushiku A, Maeda D, et al. Distinct expression pattern of claudin-6, a primitive phenotypic tight junction molecule, in germ cell tumours and visceral carcinomas. Histopathology 2012;61(6):1043–56.

123. ESMO 2022: BNT211-01: A phase I trial to evaluate safety and efficacy of CLDN6 CAR T cells and CLDN6-encoding mRNA vaccine-mediated in vivo expansion in patients with CLDN6-positive advanced solid tumours. Available at: https://clin.larvol.com/abstract-detail/ESMO%202022/58748707. Accessed February 9, 2023.

124. Zhang Z, Li D, Yun H, et al. CAR-T cells in the treatment of urologic neoplasms: present and future. Front Oncol 2022;12:915171.

125. Yang YH, Liu JW, Lu C, et al. CAR-T cell therapy for breast cancer: from basic research to clinical application. Int J Biol Sci 2022;18(6):2609–26.

126. Gautam N, Elleson KM, Ramamoorthi G, et al. Current state of cell therapies for breast cancer. Cancer J 2022;28(4):301.

127. Tozbikian G, Brogi E, Kadota K, et al. Mesothelin expression in triple negative breast carcinomas correlates significantly with basal-like phenotype, distant metastases and decreased survival. PLoS One 2014;9(12):e114900.

128. Tarp MA, Sørensen AL, Mandel U, et al. Identification of a novel cancer-specific immunodominant glycopeptide epitope in the MUC1 tandem repeat. Glycobiology 2007;17(2):197–209.

129. Zhu X, Cai H, Zhao L, et al. CAR-T cell therapy in ovarian cancer: from the bench to the bedside. Oncotarget 2017;8(38):64607–21.

130. Chan T, Chakiath M, Shepard L, et al. Abstract 6593: PRGN-3005 UltraCAR-T™: multigenic CAR-T cells generated using non-viral gene delivery and rapid manufacturing process for the treatment of ovarian cancer. Cancer Res 2020; 80(16_Supplement):6593.

131. Shah P, Shlansky-Goldberg R, Martin L, et al. 431 First-in-human phase I clinical trial evaluating intraperitoneal administration of MOv19-BBz CAR T cells in patients with alpha folate receptor-expressing recurrent high grade serous ovarian cancer. J Immunother Cancer 2021;9(Suppl 2). https://doi.org/10.1136/jitc-2021-SITC2021.431.

132. Xie G, Dong H, Liang Y, et al. CAR-NK cells: a promising cellular immunotherapy for cancer. EBioMedicine 2020;59. https://doi.org/10.1016/j.ebiom.2020.102975.

133. Klichinsky M, Ruella M, Shestova O, et al. Human chimeric antigen receptor macrophages for cancer immunotherapy. Nat Biotechnol 2020;38(8):947–53.

134. Depil S, Duchateau P, Grupp SA, et al. 'Off-the-shelf' allogeneic CAR T cells: development and challenges. Nat Rev Drug Discov 2020;19(3):185–99.

135. Papa S, Adami A, Metoudi M, et al. A phase I trial of T4 CAR T-cell immunotherapy in head and neck squamous cancer (HNSCC). J Clin Oncol 2018; 36(15_suppl):3046.

136. Ding J, Li D, Liu X, et al. Chimeric antigen receptor T-cell therapy for relapsed and refractory thyroid cancer. Exp Hematol Oncol 2022;11(1):59.

137. Brown CE, Badie B, Barish ME, et al. Bioactivity and safety of IL13Rα2-redirected chimeric antigen receptor CD8+ T cells in patients with recurrent glioblastoma. Clin Cancer Res 2015;21(18):4062–72.

138. Ahmed N, Brawley V, Hegde M, et al. HER2-specific chimeric antigen receptor-modified virus-specific T Cells for progressive glioblastoma: a phase 1 dose-escalation trial. JAMA Oncol 2017;3(8):1094–101.

139. Park JR, DiGiusto DL, Slovak M, et al. Adoptive transfer of chimeric antigen receptor re-directed cytolytic T lymphocyte clones in patients with neuroblastoma. Mol Ther 2007;15(4):825–33.

140. Louis CU, Savoldo B, Dotti G, et al. Antitumor activity and long-term fate of chimeric antigen receptor–positive T cells in patients with neuroblastoma. Blood 2011;118(23):6050–6.

141. Heczey A, Louis CU, Savoldo B, et al. CAR T cells administered in combination with lymphodepletion and PD-1 Inhibition to patients with neuroblastoma. Mol Ther 2017;25(9):2214–24.

142. Straathof K, Flutter B, Wallace R, et al. Antitumor activity without on-target off-tumor toxicity of GD2-chimeric antigen receptor T cells in patients with neuroblastoma. Sci Transl Med 2020;12(571):eabd6169.

143. Hegde M, Joseph SK, Pashankar F, et al. Tumor response and endogenous immune reactivity after administration of HER2 CAR T cells in a child with metastatic rhabdomyosarcoma. Nat Commun 2020;11(1):3549.

144. O'Cearbhaill RE, Park JH, Halton EF, et al. A phase I clinical trial of autologous chimeric antigen receptor (CAR) T cells genetically engineered to secrete IL-12 and to target the MUC16ecto antigen in patients (pts) with MUC16ecto+ recurrent high-grade serous ovarian cancer (HGSOC). In: SGO; 2020. https://sgo.confex.com/sgo/2020/meetingapp.cgi/Paper/16374. Accessed February 24, 2023.

Early and Late Toxicities of Chimeric Antigen Receptor T-Cells

Rebecca Epperly, MD[a], Victoria M. Giordani, MD[b,c],
Lekha Mikkilineni, MD, MA[d,e], Nirali N. Shah, MD, MHSc[b,*]

KEYWORDS

- Chimeric antigen receptor T-cells • Cytokine release syndrome
- Immune effector cell-associated neurotoxicity syndrome • Cytopenia
- Bone marrow dysfunction • Infectious complications

KEY POINTS

- Unified approaches to monitoring, diagnosis, and treatment have improved the clinical management of cytokine release syndrome and neurotoxicity.
- With increased use, new patterns of established toxicities are emerging, including rare presentations of neurotoxicity and hemophagocytic lymphohistiocytosis-like inflammatory disorders.
- As the pool of CAR T-cell recipients increases, delayed effects including prolonged cytopenias, bone marrow dysfunction, infections, and neuropsychiatric toxicities are being identified.
- As extended follow-up becomes available and indications for CAR T-cell therapy increase, ongoing systematic evaluation will be necessary to identify and treat a range of acute and delayed toxicities.

INTRODUCTION

Managing inflammatory toxicities related to chimeric antigen receptor (CAR) T-cells is an essential component to facilitate its use as an important therapeutic and allow for its widespread implementation. Although the earliest efforts focused on identifying and aligning the field on cytokine release syndrome (CRS) and neurotoxicity as the

[a] Department of Bone Marrow Transplantation and Cellular Therapy, St. Jude Children's Research Hospital, 262 Danny Thomas Place, MS 1130, Memphis, TN 38105, USA; [b] Pediatric Oncology Branch, Center for Cancer Research (CCR), National Cancer Institute (NCI), NIH, Building 10, Room 1W-3750, 9000 Rockville Pike MSC 1104, Bethesda, MD 20892, USA; [c] Pediatric Hematology/Oncology, Johns Hopkins Hospital, Baltimore, MD, USA; [d] Blood and Marrow Transplantation & Cellular Therapy, Stanford University, Palo Alto, CA, USA; [e] Stanford School of Medicine, 300 Pasteur Drive, Room H0101, Stanford, CA 94305, USA
* Corresponding author. 9000 Rockville Pike, Building 10, 1W-5750, Bethesda, MD 20892.
E-mail address: nirali.shah@nih.gov

Hematol Oncol Clin N Am 37 (2023) 1169–1188
https://doi.org/10.1016/j.hoc.2023.05.010
0889-8588/23/Published by Elsevier Inc.

hemonc.theclinics.com

most critical adverse events to mitigate, study of subacute and delayed toxicities (eg, cytopenias) and other end-organ toxicities has led to important insights affecting potential therapy. Additionally, because most initial experiences were based on CD19 targeting, with the rapidly evolving field and novel antigen targeting across a spectrum of diseases, new toxicities are emerging. In this section, we provide an overview of the current state of CAR T-cell associated toxicities, distinguishing between early and later toxicities (**Fig. 1**), and highlight key areas of ongoing efforts and future directions.

EARLY TOXICITIES OF CHIMERIC ANTIGEN RECEPTOR T-CELLS
Cytokine Release Syndrome and Immune Effector Cell–associated Neurotoxicity Syndrome

The most notable and most studied CAR T-cell–related toxicities include CRS and immune effector cell–associated neurotoxicity syndrome (ICANS). Defined as a systemic inflammatory response to CAR T-cell expansion and proliferation, CRS can be serious and life-threatening and typically begins with fever.[1-3] Several clinical and biological markers are used to identify CRS and ICANS, and a consensus grading system developed by the American Society for Transplantation and Cellular Therapy (ASTCT) is now available to characterize severity of the syndromes across CAR T-cell constructs.[4]

The set of grading criteria for CRS—which includes parameters of fever, hypotension, and hypoxia—serves as an objective assessment tool and provides a useful benchmark for toxicity profiling across trials. Factors associated with high-grade CRS include high tumor burden[5] and CAR T-cell dose.[6] Onset and time to peak CRS depend on the CAR T-cell product and dose and can also vary by underlying disease and conditioning regimen used.[2]

As several recent reviews provide an excellent overview with detailed guidance on management of CRS and ICANS,[7,8] the main principles are discussed here. Although mild CRS can be self-limiting with patients requiring supportive care (eg, acetaminophen for fevers), severe CRS may require monitoring and intensive care unit admission for the management of end-organ dysfunction. The recent shift in paradigm for preemptive or even prophylactic use of cytokine-directed and inflammatory-directed therapies (eg, corticosteroids and interleukin [IL]-6-signaling blockade) for risk mitigation has generally improved the tolerability of CRS, particularly in patients at high-risk

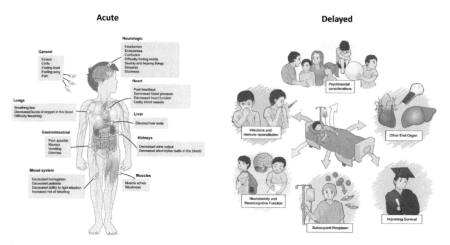

Fig. 1. Considerations related to acute and delayed toxicities following CAR T-cell infusion. (Figures courtesy of NIH Medical Arts.)

for toxicity and/or with underlying comorbidities. The influence of early intervention and influence on CAR T-cell efficacy remain under study.[9] To date, there is evidence to support that tocilizumab does not affect CAR T-cell proliferation, efficacy, and persistence when used for moderate-to-severe CRS[10] or as preemptive therapy to prevent severe CRS.[11] Tocilizumab is generally well tolerated with rapid bioavailability and minimal adverse effects. Corticosteroids are generally recommended as second line of treatment following tocilizumab because there are conflicting data for impact on CAR T-cell function.[12] Currently there are no guidelines identifying the choice of corticosteroid, timing of administration, and optimal use with other immunosuppressive agents.[13]

ICANS, the second most common CAR T-cell–associated toxicity, is thought to be due to disruption of the blood–brain barrier leading to elevated inflammatory cytokines and CAR T-cells in the cerebrospinal fluid.[14] The signs and symptoms of ICANS remain heterogenous and include altered mental status, aphasia, seizure, headache, encephalopathy, and cerebral edema.[11] The ASTCT consensus grading criteria for ICANS incorporates the following features in assessing severity: Immune Effector Cell-Associated Encephalopathy (ICE) score/Cornell Assessment of Pediatric Delirium (CAPD) score, depressed level of consciousness, seizure, motor findings (tremors/myoclonus), and elevated intracranial pressure/cerebral edema.[4] ICE (adults) and CAPD (children aged ≤12 years and patients with global development delay[15]) screening tools provide rapid methods to capture neurocognitive changes at the bedside. The onset and duration of ICANS may vary between CAR constructs. Prevention, treatment, and management of ICANS are not well defined; however, corticosteroids and antiseizure agents are the current mainstay of management.[16] The risk factors for severe ICANS are also less well defined; however, most recent data show that severity of CRS, younger age, preexisting underlying neurological disease, CAR T-cell product, and disease characteristics play an important role in the development of ICANS.[17] Brain imaging is often recommended to distinguish ICANS from other CNS lesions, although this is an area of ongoing efforts.[18]

Cases of refractory CRS that do not resolve with IL-6 receptor blockade or corticosteroids are particularly challenging. To date siltuximab (anti-IL-6 antibody),[19,20] anakinra (IL-1 receptor antagonist),[21] and etanercept (tumor necrosis factor alpha [TNFα] inhibitor)[22] have demonstrated some efficacy in refractory CRS in limited cases. Other cytokine inhibition therapies are being explored and include ruxolitinib and itacitinib (Janus kinase inhibitors),[23] dasatinib (tyrosine kinase inhibitor),[24] and emapalumab (interferon [IFN] gamma inhibitor).[25] Corticosteroid-refractory ICANS is particularly challenging. Intrathecal hydrocortisone may be a potential alternative agent[26] and remains under study. The use of immunosuppressive agents to address CRS/ICANS may be associated with an increased rate of infectious complications.[27,28]

Advancements in CAR T-cell therapies have allowed for the development of tools to predict CRS and ICANS severity. Identifying patients at increased risk of CAR T-cell–related toxicities remains of central importance. Several models are currently being validated and include models such as CAR-HEMATOTOX and EASIX. The former is a rapid and easy scoring system that uses hematological parameters to identify patients at risk of poorer outcomes.[29] The latter uses inflammatory biomarkers such as C-reactive protein and lactate dehydrogenase in a formula to evaluate the degree of endothelial damage.[30]

Rare/Unique Presentations of Neurotoxicity

Beyond typical manifestations of ICANS, emerging atypical neurotoxicity syndromes manifesting as movement disorders and myelopathy have been recently reported, necessitating practitioners to be adept at early recognition of new sequelae of neuro-toxicity that may emerge with novel CAR T-cell constructs.

Five percent of patients treated with ciltacabtagene autoleucel (cilta-cel), an anti-B-cell maturation antigen (BCMA) CAR T-cell therapy on the CARTITUDE-1 study, were reported to have movement and neurocognitive treatment-emergent adverse events (MNTs).[31] Patients with MNTs had normal to near normal ICE scores at the time of MNT presentation and commonly had MNT symptoms occur after recovery from CRS and/or more typical presentation of ICANS.[31] Patients with MNTs exhibited pathology of movement (eg, ataxia, cogwheel rigidity, parkinsonism, motor dysfunction), and/or cognitive and personality changes.[31] Patients who experienced MNTs had at least 2 variables identified as risk factors: high tumor burden at baseline, grade ≥ 2 CRS or any grade ICANS and high CAR T-cell expansion/persistence. After reviewing initial cases of movement disorders on trial, new strategies to select and treat patients before cell infusion were implemented, including providing preinfusion bridging therapy to patients with high tumor burden, early treatment of CRS and ICANS and extended monitoring for MNTs beyond day 100.[31] With implementation of these strategies, CARTITUDE investigators report a reduction in MNTs from 5% to less than 1% across all trials.[31] CARTITUDE investigators identified evidence of BCMA expression in the caudate of brains, potentially highlighting an on-target, off-tumor effect of anti-BCMA therapy.[32] Long-term surveillance across antimyeloma CAR T-cell trials as well as all CAR T-cell trials should include high degree of suspicion for the potential emergence of MNTs.

Patients with new onset paresis and paralysis after CD19-directed CAR T-cell therapy have been reported in several case reports.[33–36] In all cases, patients had a post-CAR T-cell infusion course marked by typical CRS and/or ICANS. Patients began to have symptoms of lower extremity weakness, which, in some cases, progressed to paralysis with ascension to upper extremities.[33–36] Patients were treated with anti-IL-6 therapy in addition to high-dose corticosteroid therapy; one patient expired from infectious complications[33] while remaining patients had varying degrees of recovery.[34–36] Two of the reported cases were associated with a robust expansion of CAR $^+$ T-cells.[34,36] One case highlighted the patients' initial markedly elevated IL-6, TNF-alpha, and IL-10 levels at baseline, potentially highlighting a baseline inflammatory state preinfusion.[34]

Hematologic Toxicities

Coagulopathy is observed in multiple clinical trials using CD19 CAR T-cells, particularly in patients with more severe CRS/ICANS (eg, grade ≥ 3).[37–39] This observation highlights the effects of cytokines on endothelial cells, on the coagulation cascade, and on the fibrinolytic system. Overall, several cytokines, most notably, IL-6, IL-1, IFN-γ, and TNF-α, provoke an inflammatory response that promotes a procoagulant state in patients with CRS. In the procoagulant state, endothelial cells release several factors that foster platelet aggregation, and downregulation of anticoagulant proteins. These cytokines also affect platelet function by inducing increased production and degranulation, which in turn continue to "nourish" a hypercoagulable state by activating factors important in the coagulation cascade.[40] In this context, patients with severe CRS are at risk of both disseminated intravascular coagulopathy[40] and at increased risk of venous thrombotic events.[41]

Hypofibrinogenemia is, to date, the most clinically significant laboratory abnormality in CRS-associated coagulopathy and is associated with an increased incidence of bleeding requiring close monitoring and replacement. It can manifest in the context of severe CRS with hemophagocytic lymphohistiocytosis (HLH)-like manifestations.

The onset and duration of coagulopathy are less well defined and vary greatly among trials.

Cardiovascular Toxicities

Cardiovascular (CV) toxicity from CAR T-cell therapy has been described in early phase clinical trials as well as in real-world experience with currently approved products.[10,42–44] With CRS, cell infusion is analogous to CV toxicity that occurs during sepsis with CAR T-cell–induced immune activation leading to a cascade of inflammatory cytokines that have direct and indirect effects on the CV system.[43,45] Endothelial dysfunction and expression of procoagulant factors promote capillary leakage, leading to hypotension and tachycardia with the potential for hemodynamic instability and multiorgan dysfunction.[45] Although specific mechanisms have not been elucidated, IL-6 and TNF-α are thought to be key mediators of myocardial pathologic conditions. TNF-α and IL-6 have been shown in preclinical models to reduce left-ventricular ejection fraction (LVEF) and mean arterial pressure.[46] QT prolongation and arrhythmias such as atrial fibrillation have been reported after cell-infusion.[47] Importantly, most cases of cardiac toxicity, even severe manifestations, have been reversible in the literature. Screening patients for therapy suitability and/or cardiac optimization may mitigate CV toxicity after infusion. In early phase trials, patients were not treated if they had evidence of impaired ejection fraction or CV comorbidity including arrhythmia or current myocardial infarction (MI). Pretherapy screening should include a detailed CV history including past CV events such as known arrythmias, anthracycline use, chest radiation, and past MI. Baseline assessment is recommended before therapy including history, clinical examination, electrocardiogram and echocardiography, and cardiac biomarkers for patients who have a heightened risk for CV toxicity.[43,45] The early recognition of CRS and neurological toxicity is important to screen for concurrent CV toxicity because there may be overlap in timing of these syndromes as outlined in a recent retrospective study.[48] For severe CV toxicity, anti-IL-6 agents as well as corticosteroid therapy may provide mitigation by decreasing the severity of CRS; however, certain parameters such as reduced LVEF may take months to reverse.[49]

Pulmonary Toxicities

Pulmonary toxicities following CAR T-cell therapies include respiratory failure, cough, pleural effusion, and dyspnea.[50] Although this entity is less well defined, one study reported an association between severe pulmonary toxicities and increased risk of mortality.[51] Associated risks factors for pulmonary toxicity include severe CRS and elevated baseline lactate dehydrogenase level before lymphodepletion. The onset of symptoms can occur anytime within the first 30 days postinfusion. The most common manifestation of pulmonary toxicity is hypoxia and was noted to occur in the first 10 days at a higher incidence in patients with CRS compared with those who did not have CRS.[51] Interestingly, new development or worsening of pleural effusions, ground glass opacities, in addition to hypoxia, have occurred in patients with leukemic involvement of the pleura, independent of disease status pre–CAR T-cell therapy.[52] Similar pulmonary toxicities are described in patients with lymphomatous malignancy in case reports.[53]

Other Acute End-organ Toxicities

As the landscape of CAR T-cell immunotherapy evolves, diagnosis and management of acute toxicities beyond CRS and ICANS demand astute clinical assessment of affected organ systems to improve CAR T-cell tolerance and safety. In that context, **Table 1** highlights organ system dysfunction observed post–CAR T-cell therapy.

Table 1
Acute end-organ toxicities related to CAR T-cells

Cardiac[a–e]	Hematologic[f–h]
• Hypotension	• Venous thromboembolic events
• Hypertension	• Disseminated intravascular coagulation
• Tachycardia	• Coagulopathy
• Cardiogenic shock	• Anemia
• Arrythmias	• Thrombocytopenia
• Left ventricular systolic dysfunction	• Neutropenia
• Heart failure	• Lymphopenia
• Myocardial infarction	• B-cell aplasia
• Cardiomyopathy	• Hemophagocytic lymphohistiocytosis/ Macrophage
• Pericardial diseases	activating syndrome
Pulmonary[i]	**Hepatic[j]**
• Hypoxia	• Elevated Hepatic Enzymes
• Tachypnea	• Portal Vein Thrombosis
• Dyspnea	• Acute fulminant hepatic failure
• Pneumonitis	• Hyperbilirubinemia
• Pulmonary edema	
• Respiratory failure	
• Adult respiratory distress syndrome	
Musculoskeletal	**Gastrointestinal[j]**
• Elevated creatine kinase	• Diarrhea
• Myalgia	• Pancreatitis
	• Constipation
	• Perianal fistula
	• Esophagitis
	• Vomiting
Ophthalmologic/Ocular[k]	**Psychiatric[j]**
• Vison changes	• Anxiety
• Vision impairment	• Insomnia
• Floaters	• Depression
• Photopsia	
Renal[j,l–n]	
• Adrenal insufficiency	
• Renal insufficiency	
• Electrolyte disturbance	

[a] Nenna A, Carpenito M, Chello C, et al. Cardiotoxicity of Chimeric Antigen Receptor T-Cell (CAR-T) Therapy: Pathophysiology, Clinical Implications, and Echocardiographic Assessment. Int J Mol Sci 2022;23(15). https://doi.org/10.3390/ijms23158242.
[b] Hanna KS, Kaur H, Alazzeh MS, et al. Cardiotoxicity Associated With Chimeric Antigen Receptor (CAR)-T Cell Therapy for Hematologic Malignancies: A Systematic Review. Cureus 2022;14(8):e28162. DOI: 10.7759/cureus.28162.
[c] Patel NP, Doukas PG, Gordon LI, Akhter N. Cardiovascular Toxicities of CAR T-cell Therapy. Curr Oncol Rep 2021;23(7):78. DOI: 10.1007/s11912-021-01068-0.
[d] Ganatra S, Redd R, Hayek SS, et al. Chimeric Antigen Receptor T-Cell Therapy-Associated Cardiomyopathy in Patients With Refractory or Relapsed Non-Hodgkin Lymphoma. Circulation 2020;142(17):1687-1690. DOI: 10.1161/CIRCULATIONAHA.120.048100.
[e] Lee DW, Kochenderfer JN, Stetler-Stevenson M, et al. T cells expressing CD19 chimeric antigen receptors for acute lymphoblastic leukaemia in children and young adults: a phase 1 dose-escalation trial. Lancet 2015;385(9967):517-528. DOI: 10.1016/S0140-6736(14)61403-3.
[f] Martin-Rojas RM, Gomez-Centurion I, Bailen R, et al. Hemophagocytic lymphohistiocytosis/ macrophage activation syndrome (HLH/MAS) following treatment with tisagenlecleucel. Clin Case Rep 2022;10(1):e05209. https://doi.org/10.1002/ccr3.5209.
[g] Lichtenstein DA, Schischlik F, Shao L, et al. Characterization of HLH-like manifestations as a CRS variant in patients receiving CD22 CAR T cells. Blood 2021;138(24):2469-2484. https://doi.org/10.1182/blood.2021011898.

[h] Taneja A, Jain T. CAR-T-OPENIA: Chimeric antigen receptor T-cell therapy-associated cytopenias. EJHaem 2022;3(Suppl 1):32-38. https://doi.org/10.1002/jha2.350.

[i] Goldman A, Maor E, Bomze D, et al. Adverse Cardiovascular and Pulmonary Events Associated With Chimeric Antigen Receptor T-Cell Therapy. J Am Coll Cardiol 2021;78(18):1800-1813. https://doi.org/10.1016/j.jacc.2021.08.044.

[j] Wudhikarn K, Pennisi M, Garcia-Recio M, et al. DLBCL patients treated with CD19 CAR T cells experience a high burden of organ toxicities but low nonrelapse mortality. Blood Adv 2020;4(13):3024-3033. https://doi.org/10.1182/bloodadvances.2020001972.

[k] Mumtaz AA, Fischer A, Lutfi F, et al. Ocular adverse events associated with chimeric antigen receptor T-cell therapy: a case series and review. Br J Ophthalmol 2022. https://doi.org/10.1136/bjophthalmol-2021-320814.

[l] Gutgarts V, Jain T, Zheng J, et al. Acute Kidney Injury after CAR-T Cell Therapy: Low Incidence and Rapid Recovery. Biol Blood Marrow Transplant 2020;26(6):1071-1076. DOI: 10.1016/j.bbmt.2020.02.012.

[m] Ahmed G, Bhasin-Chhabra B, Szabo A, et al. Impact of Chronic Kidney Disease and Acute Kidney Injury on Safety and Outcomes of CAR T-Cell Therapy in Lymphoma Patients. Clin Lymphoma Myeloma Leuk 2022;22(11):863-868. DOI: 10.1016/j.clml.2022.07.007.

[n] Farooqui N, Sy-Go JPT, Miao J, et al. Incidence and Risk Factors for Acute Kidney Injury After Chimeric Antigen Receptor T-Cell Therapy. Mayo Clin Proc 2022;97(7):1294-1304. DOI: 10.1016/j.mayocp.2022.05.018.

Although the underlying pathophysiology is not well understood, prompt intervention should be considered and initiated.

Infectious Disease-Related Complications

Infections remain a critical complication from CAR T-cell therapy. Patients may have reduced immunity before cell infusion due to underlying malignancy, earlier therapy, and chronic B-cell depletion.[54,55] Similar rates of infections are seen in pediatric and adult populations receiving CAR T-cells.[54,55] The use of lymphodepleting (LD) chemotherapy can result in a weakening of the mucosal barrier and acute cytopenias with resultant neutropenia and lymphopenia during the peri–CAR T-cell infusion period.[55] Following CAR T-cell therapy, bacterial infections are the predominant type of infectious complication followed by viral and fungal infections.[55–58] As diarrhea can occur during CRS, practitioners should routinely test for infectious causes including testing for Clostridium difficile.[57] Fungal infections occur rarely and usually in patients who have a history of recent fungal infections.[57] Special attention should be given to patients with leukemia and those who have a history of chronic corticosteroid use and/or prolonged neutropenia because they may be at an increased risk of fungal infections. Several factors may place patients at higher risk of infections post–CAR T-cell therapy including more lines of earlier antitumor therapy, higher CAR T-cell dose, high-grade CRS, immunosuppression use, and presence and duration of neutropenia.[55,57,58] To limit infectious complications, a detailed infectious history of each patient should be obtained including earlier antibiotic use and potential resistance patterns and earlier periods of neutropenia posttherapy. Earlier therapy history should be closely evaluated in conjunction with baseline serum lymphocyte and immunoglobulin measurements.[55,57] Infectious disease specialists should be consulted early in advance of any complications that may develop after therapy, particularly in patients at high-risk of infectious complications. Although bacterial and fungal prophylaxis is not routinely recommended, except in patients at high-risk for these infections (eg, previous history of invasive fungal infection, prolonged neutropenia after chemotherapy), viral prophylaxis with an antiherpes agent is generally administered to most patients for the prevention of herpes infections.[57,58] Patients treated with CD19 and BCMA-targeted CAR T-cells may have B-cell depletion or dysfunction from underlying malignancy or earlier therapy and will continue to have B-cell depletion after therapy due to an on-target/off-tumor effect,[55] and thus, immunoglobulins should be measured after therapy at defined intervals.[27,54]

Hemophagocytic lymphohistiocytosis-like Toxicities

HLH-like toxicities, as evident by new onset cytopenias, hepatic transaminase elevations, hypofibrinogenemia, and coagulopathies with or without evidence for active hemophagocytosis—are increasingly being recognized as a rare but potentially life-threatening toxicity that can be associated with fatal complications. Occurring across a host of CAR T-cell constructs and antigen targets, HLH-like complications may be a manifestation of severe CRS (eg, symptoms overlap with CRS onset),[59–65] more delayed HLH-like toxicities (eg, after apparent resolution of CRS) are also increasingly being recognized.[60,66,67] These later manifestations, newly termed as immune effector cell (IEC)–associated HLH-like syndrome (IEC-HS) likely warrant a unique treatment approach—particularly when CRS targeted therapies (eg, tocilizumab) has been optimized. With the primary goal to raise awareness of these toxicities and ultimately improve outcomes, a recent ASTCT consensus statement provides a new framework to foster recognition, grading, treatment, and further study of this rare but complex CAR T-cell–associated toxicity. (Article in review) Further study, which will shed important insights into the overlap among HLH-like toxicities, infections, and cytopenias, is ongoing.

DELAYED TOXICITIES OF CHIMERIC ANTIGEN RECEPTOR T-CELLS

As CAR T-cell therapy is increasingly integrated into the care of patients with hematologic malignancies and early-phase investigations continue across a range of cancer types, it is important to monitor for delayed effects—particularly as patients strive to use CAR T-cells for long-term durable remission. This is essential both to provide care to CAR T-cell recipients and to establish a comprehensive risk profile to guide future therapeutic use (**Table 2**).

Bone Marrow Dysfunction

Bone marrow recovery after CAR T-cell therapy for B-cell malignancies exhibits a biphasic pattern, with most patients recovering in the first month after treatment but a small portion continuing to experience severe neutropenia, ongoing need for red blood cell and/or platelet transfusion support, or low bone marrow cellularity for months to years after treatment.[8,28,68] In adult CD19 CAR T-cell recipients, 16% of patients with ongoing complete remission in the absence of myelodysplastic syndrome continued to require platelet and/or red blood cell transfusion support more than 90 days from CAR T-cell infusion[68] and 9% still experienced grade 3 to 4 neutropenia at 1 year.[28] Additional investigation is needed to understand the interplay between CAR T-cells and the bone marrow microenvironment, which will be key in determining treatment-related risk factors for prolonged bone marrow dysfunction. Management of prolonged bone marrow dysfunction centers on supportive care and evaluation of other contributory causes, with patients receiving transfusion and growth factor support (eg, granulocyte colony stimulating factor [G-CSF] and thrombopoietin receptor agonists) as clinically warranted.[7,69,70] Patients with a history of earlier hematopoietic stem cell transplant (HSCT) have experienced improved bone marrow function after receiving a CD34+ selected hematopoietic progenitor cell boost from their earlier HSCT donor when needed to restore poor marrow function.[7,71,72] Due to concern for on-target off-tumor hematologic toxicity and characteristics of underlying disease, most acute myelogenous leukemia (AML) and T-cell-ALL CAR T-cell studies are

Table 2
Delayed toxicities related to chimeric antigen receptor T-cells

Delayed Toxicities	Monitoring and Therapeutic Considerations
Bone marrow dysfunction	• Subset of patients experience prolonged cytopenias *Tx: platelet/RBC transfusions, growth factors, stem cell boost*
Delayed infections/immune reconstitution	• Viral respiratory infections most common, usually mild • Bacterial and fungal infections can occur, most often in patients with prolonged cytopenias • Subset of patients may respond to subsequent vaccination *Tx: immune globulin replacement, consider vaccination*
Neuropsychiatric/neurocognitive	• Mood disorders and cognitive impairments reported *Additional evaluation needed to delineate from prior tx effects*
Systemic toxicities and other organ systems	• Cardiac and renal toxicities resolve for most patients in acute period but some late events have occurred • Immune-related systemic events rarely reported *Need for systemic, prospective surveillance to further define*
Subsequent malignancies	• Overall occurrence is low to date
Quality of life indices	• Initial treatment-related declines recover in most • Favorable profile in comparison to auto/allo HSCT

Abbreviations: Tx, treatment; RBC, red blood cell; HSCT, hematopoietic stem cell transplant.

designed as a bridge to allogeneic HSCT,[73,74] which will limit the ability to analyze the ongoing impact on bone marrow function.

Immune Reconstitution and Hypogammaglobulinemia

Determinants of posttreatment immune reconstitution are multifactorial, including effects of LD chemotherapy and on-target off-tumor toxicities. A biphasic distribution of total leukocyte and neutrophil recovery has been observed, with most patients recovering at 1-month after infusion but a subset having ongoing leukopenia and neutropenia after several months.[29,39] T-cell recovery after CAR T-cell treatment is led by CD8+ cells, with a lag in CD4+ recovery and a low CD4+/CD8+ ratio persisting even beyond 1-year postinfusion.[27,28,75] B-cell-lymphopenia and hypogammaglobulinemia are hallmarks of B-cell-targeted CAR T-cell therapies.[76] The duration of B-cell aplasia is extremely variable, at times lasting months to years, and has been identified as a surrogate for CAR T-cell persistence.[27,77–79] Immunoglobulin-replacement strategies are institution-dependent but in general target IgG levels 400 or greater to 500 mg/dL with intravenous preparations or 1000 mg/dL or greater with subcutaneous preparations.[77,80] For some adult patients, immunoglobulin replacement is discontinued despite persistent B-cell aplasia and hypogammaglobulinemia in the absence of recurrent infections but the safety of this practice has not been established in pediatric patients.[8]

Vaccination/Vaccine Response

There is evidence of preserved antiviral antibodies after CD19-targeted CAR T-cell treatment in adults mediated by preserved plasma cell-dependent response.[81] Ongoing immune globulin supplementation limits posttreatment evaluation of antiviral responses in pediatric patients, and these cannot be directly extrapolated from adult data given lower pretreatment plasma cell mass.

Antibody-based response to posttreatment vaccination in adult patients is variable, with 30% demonstrating response to influenza vaccination,[82] independent of hypogammaglobulinemia or B/T-cell counts. Responses to severe acute respiratory syndrome coronavirus 2 (SARS-CoV-2) vaccination in CAR T-cell recipients ranged from 7% to 40% and were significantly lower than in HSCT patients.[83,84] Although there is a potential benefit to pursuing post-CAR vaccination for a subgroup of patients, overall responses are inferior to immunocompetent patients.

Delayed Infections

Although the highest infection density occurs in the first month after CAR T-cell treatment, CAR T-cell recipients do experience delayed infections.[55,85,86] In adult patients receiving CD19-targeted CAR T-cell therapy, the most common infections beyond 90 days were viral respiratory tract infections, the majority of which were mild.[68,87-89] However, CAR T-cell recipients developing SARS-CoV-2 infection even months after treatment are at an increased risk for severe disease and prolonged viral shedding, which is associated with the degree of lymphopenia.[76,90] Although the evidence to date is primarily related to CD19-targeted CAR T-cell therapies, late viral infections are also emerging after treatment with BCMA CAR T-cells.[91] Reactivation of herpesviruses has been reported in the late post-CAR T-cell period, although the incidence is unknown due to variable screening practices.[68,92,93] Bacterial infections become less common with increased time from CAR T infusion and decrease in severity. Late fungal infections are rare but have been reported particularly in patients with prolonged bone marrow dysfunction.[71,76,94]

Neuropsychiatric/Neurocognitive Effects

There is currently limited information on delayed neurologic toxicities and the neuropsychiatric influence of CAR T-cell therapy. Observed neuropsychiatric events in patients treated on CAR T-cell studies include new or worsening mood disorders; new neurologic findings include cerebrovascular events, dementia, and peripheral neuropathy.[68,95] In adult patients treated with CD19 CAR T-cell therapy who were followed for patient-reported neuropsychiatric outcomes, 47% reported depression, anxiety, or cognitive difficulty and 18% scored significantly below the general population mean in global mental health indices.[96] Because many patients undergoing CAR T-cell treatment have earlier exposure to other potentially neurotoxic therapies that may have delayed effects, including chemotherapy, radiation, and HSCT,[97] understanding the influence of CAR T-cell therapy will require comprehensive monitoring over time.

Other Organ-specific and Systemic Toxicities

Rare delayed immune-related events (ie, dermatitis, pneumonitis, colitis) have been observed in CAR T-cell recipients, either alone or in combination with checkpoint inhibition, but have not been directly attributed to CAR T-cell therapy.[98,99] Additional delayed events reported in CAR T-cell recipients include cardiac, both cerebrovascular and heart failure,[95] and ongoing renal dysfunction.[95] Notably, most patients with acute cardiac or renal toxicity after CAR T-cell treatment experience recovery to baseline.[95] Systematic data collection in long-term follow up including details of prior exposures, paralleling work done in HSCT survivors, will be key in identifying the ongoing influence of CAR T-cell therapy in additional domains, including endocrine, growth, and metabolism.[100-102]

Quality of Life and Patient-Reported Outcomes

Incorporating patient-reported outcomes (PROs) and quality-of-life (QOL) indices will be key to establish the potential long-term benefits of pursuing CAR T-cell therapy and to identify additional delayed impact. Adult patients receiving BCMA-targeted CAR T-cells reported overall favorable efficacy and toxicity profiles outweighing experienced side effects.[103,104] Patients followed longitudinally report an expected decline in quality of life during CAR T-cell treatment, although the degree of decline and time to recovery were more favorable in CAR T-cell-treated patients than allogeneic or autologous HSCT patients.[105] QOL impact is prolonged in patients who experienced severe CRS or neurotoxicity.[106] A randomized phase 3 study of CD19-targeted CAR T-cell therapy compared with standard of care for relapsed/refractory large B-cell lymphoma favored CAR T-cell therapy in PROs.[107] In a pediatric cohort, QOL improvements were noted 3 months post–CAR T-cell infusion.[108] Because measures of symptom burden and quality of life vary across evaluation tools, further work is needed to establish the optimal platform for monitoring quality of life in CAR T-cell patients and integrating this data in real-time to identify predictors of clinical outcomes.[98,99]

Subsequent Malignancies

Although rare, subsequent malignancies have been observed in patients who received CAR T-cell therapy. In adult populations, nonmelanoma skin cancer and myelodysplastic syndrome have been the most common, with other solid tumors also reported.[68,87,109] In pediatric patients, subsequent neoplasms are uncommon and include AML/MDS and rare solid tumors.[110] Given exposure to earlier therapies, the potential for genetic cancer predisposition, and expected age-related malignancy risks, there is not yet enough data to establish whether CAR T-cell therapy adds to subsequent malignancy risk in this population.

ADDITIONAL CONSIDERATIONS AND FUTURE DIRECTIONS
Toxicity Considerations in Nonresponders and/or with Relapse

Despite the remarkable efficacy of CAR T-cells in patients with B-cell malignancies, for those patients experiencing nonresponse or relapse, outcomes remain poor.[111–113] Particularly relevant to toxicity, for patients with both CAR T-cell expansion and concurrent disease progression, toxicities may be further heightened as inflammatory toxicities from CAR T-cell expansion may be amplified as underlying disease is concurrently progressing (eg, worsening of cytopenias). Considering early restaging in those where disease progression is of concern may serve to guide more optimal management in these circumstances—particularly where it may become necessary to provide disease-directed therapy even at the expense of preserving CAR T-cell efficacy.

Unique Toxicity Considerations of Novel Chimeric Antigen Receptor T-cell Approaches

As CAR T-cell therapies expand, previously unseen toxicities are also developing. As mentioned, BCMA-targeting and parkinsonism-related toxicities were newly identified with implementation of this unique CAR T-cell targeting. Additionally, although on-target, off-tumor targeting of normal B-cells and subsequent B-cell aplasia is an anticipated and tolerable effect, myeloid antigen targeting of stem cells presents a unique challenge that may necessitate a tandem hematopoietic stem cell transplant for salvage of bone marrow aplasia.[114] The experience with engineered T-cell receptor targeting of melanoma associated antigen (MAGE)-A3 and cardiac toxicity that ensued from targeting of titin, an unrelated peptide,[115] further demonstrated the potential of un-predictable off-target toxicities with novel adoptive cell therapy targeting. The develop-ment of tumor inflammation-associated neurotoxicity related to CAR T-cell targeting of central nervous system tumors also warrants special attention, particularly as local anti-inflammatory strategies to optimize outcomes may be preferred over systemic ap-proaches.[116] Finally, the emergence of dual targeting, as a method to overcome anti-gen escape, as a mechanism of resistance to CAR T-cells[117] requires close attention to evaluate for potential of synergistic toxicities—while ensuring that dual targeting functionality is achieved. Importantly, for those with relapse following CAR T-cells, rein-fusions of the same construct and/or use of a novel CAR T-cell construct are increas-ingly being used—raising additional considerations of toxicity—particularly with residual CAR T-cell toxicities from the earlier construct (eg, delayed cytopenias) or the impact of multiple infusions of genetically modified T-cells.

Late Effects

As CAR T-cells are increasingly used, achieving long-term durable remission re-mains a clear goal. Accordingly, close study of late effects is imperative as CAR T-cells are used for curative intent, particularly in children who may live many years and will advance through various stages of growth and development. Although PROs and QOL measures were previously mentioned, they remain a cornerstone for study of late effects, particularly to understand long-term outcomes in patients who may not be receiving as intense or prolonged therapy or in whom stem cell transplantation was potentially able to be avoided. Similarly, considerations of overall growth, endocrinopathies, and cognitive function are imperative for long-term follow-up. Additionally, there is little known about fertility outcomes following CAR T-cells, and futher study is needed, particularly as recent preclinical data from murine models with checkpoint inhibitors has demonstrated an impact on oocyte number and quality.[118,119] A recent publication highlights key considerations impor-tant to fertility following CAR T-cells and outlines areas for future research.[120]

SUMMARY

As commercial utilization of CAR T-cells become more widely available and novel approaches continue to be developed, the number of patients receiving CAR T-cells will exponentially increase. Thus, optimizing management of more well-established toxicities alongside recognition of rare adverse events and develop-ment of treatment strategies will remain imperative—particularly as more CAR T-cells start to become more established for use in earlier stages. For patients in whom CAR T-cells may be used to achieve a long-term durable remission, study of delayed and late toxicities will become necessary and establishing this founda-tion is critical to future research efforts. Finally, acknowledging that different CAR T-cell constructs and targets will be associated with unique and potentially delayed toxicities, further study to identify the biologic underpinnings of novel toxicities will be needed.

CLINICS CARE POINTS

- CAR T-cells are a highly effective form of immunotherapy; however, early inflammatory toxicities of CRS and ICANS can be severe and potentially life-threatening.

- Preemptive and early mitigation strategies are now available to potentially reduce the severity of acute toxicities and impact on end-organ function.

- Although there is less known about delayed toxicities and late effects of CAR T-cells, this is an area where further study is needed—particularly concerning long-term risk of infection, neurocognitive function, and hematologic toxicities (eg, cytopenias).

DISCLOSURES

All authors contributed to this study. N.N.S. receives royalties from Cargo, Inc and has participated in Advisory Boards for Sobi and VOR.

DISCLAIMER

The content of this publication neither necessarily reflect the views of policies of the Department of Health and Human Services nor does mention of trade names, commercial products, or organizations imply endorsement by the US Government.

ACKNOWLEDGMENTS

This study was supported in part by the Intramural Research Program of the National Institutes of Health, National Cancer Institute,United States, Center for Cancer Research and the Warren Grant Magnuson Clinical Center. All funding was provided by the NIH Intramural Research Program (ZIA BC 011923). Figure was generated by NIH Medical Arts.

REFERENCES

1. Riegler LL, Jones GP, Lee DW. Current approaches in the grading and management of cytokine release syndrome after chimeric antigen receptor T-cell therapy. Therapeut Clin Risk Manag 2019;15:323–35.
2. Frey N, Porter D. Cytokine Release Syndrome with Chimeric Antigen Receptor T Cell Therapy. Biol Blood Marrow Transplant 2019;25(4):e123–7.
3. Brudno JN, Kochenderfer JN. Recent advances in CAR T-cell toxicity: Mechanisms, manifestations and management. Blood Rev 2019;34:45–55.
4. Lee DW, Santomasso BD, Locke FL, et al. ASTCT Consensus Grading for Cytokine Release Syndrome and Neurologic Toxicity Associated with Immune Effector Cells. Biol Blood Marrow Transplant 2019;25(4):625–38.
5. Hay KA, Hanafi LA, Li D, et al. Kinetics and biomarkers of severe cytokine release syndrome after CD19 chimeric antigen receptor-modified T-cell therapy. Blood 2017;130(21):2295–306.
6. Yan Z, Zhang H, Cao J, et al. Characteristics and Risk Factors of Cytokine Release Syndrome in Chimeric Antigen Receptor T Cell Treatment. Front Immunol 2021;12:611366.
7. Santomasso BD, Nastoupil LJ, Adkins S, et al. Management of Immune-Related Adverse Events in Patients Treated With Chimeric Antigen Receptor T-Cell Therapy: ASCO Guideline. J Clin Oncol 2021;39(35):3978–92.
8. Maus MV, Alexander S, Bishop MR, et al. Society for Immunotherapy of Cancer (SITC) clinical practice guideline on immune effector cell-related adverse events. J Immunother Cancer 2020;8(2). https://doi.org/10.1136/jitc-2020-001511.
9. Schubert ML, Schmitt M, Wang L, et al. Side-effect management of chimeric antigen receptor (CAR) T-cell therapy. Ann Oncol 2021;32(1):34–48.
10. Maude SL, Frey N, Shaw PA, et al. Chimeric antigen receptor T cells for sustained remissions in leukemia. N Engl J Med 2014;371(16):1507–17.

11. Gardner RA, Ceppi F, Rivers J, et al. Preemptive mitigation of CD19 CAR T-cell cytokine release syndrome without attenuation of antileukemic efficacy. Blood 2019;134(24):2149–58.

12. Neelapu SS, Tummala S, Kebriaei P, et al. Chimeric antigen receptor T-cell therapy - assessment and management of toxicities. Nat Rev Clin Oncol 2018;15(1): 47–62.

13. Dholaria BR, Bachmeier CA, Locke F. Mechanisms and Management of Chimeric Antigen Receptor T-Cell Therapy-Related Toxicities. BioDrugs 2019; 33(1):45–60.

14. Xiao X, Huang S, Chen S, et al. Mechanisms of cytokine release syndrome and neurotoxicity of CAR T-cell therapy and associated prevention and management strategies. J Exp Clin Cancer Res 2021;40(1):367.

15. Brown BD, Tambaro FP, Kohorst M, et al. Immune Effector Cell Associated Neurotoxicity (ICANS) in Pediatric and Young Adult Patients Following Chimeric Antigen Receptor (CAR) T-Cell Therapy: Can We Optimize Early Diagnosis? Front Oncol 2021;11:634445.

16. Sterner RC, Sterner RM. Immune effector cell associated neurotoxicity syndrome in chimeric antigen receptor-T cell therapy. Front Immunol 2022;13:879608.

17. Gust J, Hay KA, Hanafi LA, et al. Endothelial Activation and Blood-Brain Barrier Disruption in Neurotoxicity after Adoptive Immunotherapy with CD19 CAR-T Cells. Cancer Discov 2017;7(12):1404–19.

18. Wallet F, Sesques P, Devic P, et al. CAR-T cell: Toxicities issues: Mechanisms and clinical management. Bull Cancer 2021;108(10S):S117–27.

19. Patel S, Cenin D, Corrigan D, et al. Siltuximab for First-Line Treatment of Cytokine Release Syndrome: A Response to the National Shortage of Tocilizumab. Blood 2022;140(Supplement 1):5073–4.

20. Narkhede M, Di Stasi A, Bal S, et al. Interim Analysis of Investigator-Initiated Phase 2 Trial of Siltuximab in Treatment of Cytokine Release Syndrome and Immune Effector Cell Associated Neurotoxicity Related to CAR T-Cell Therapy. Transplant Cell Ther 2023;29(2):S133–4.

21. Ferreros P, Trapero I. Interleukin Inhibitors in Cytokine Release Syndrome and Neurotoxicity Secondary to CAR-T Therapy. Diseases 2022;10(3). https://doi. org/10.3390/diseases10030041.

22. Zhang L, Wang S, Xu J, et al. Etanercept as a new therapeutic option for cytokine release syndrome following chimeric antigen receptor T cell therapy. Exp Hematol Oncol 2021;10(1):16.

23. Huarte E, O'Connor RS, Peel MT, et al. Itacitinib (INCB039110), a JAK1 Inhibitor, Reduces Cytokines Associated with Cytokine Release Syndrome Induced by CAR T-cell Therapy. Clin Cancer Res 2020;26(23):6299–309.

24. Baur K, Heim D, Beerlage A, et al. Dasatinib for treatment of CAR T-cell therapy-related complications. J Immunother Cancer 2022;10(12). https://doi.org/10. 1136/jitc-2022-005956.

25. McNerney KO, DiNofia AM, Teachey DT, et al. Potential Role of IFNgamma Inhibition in Refractory Cytokine Release Syndrome Associated with CAR T-cell Therapy. Blood Cancer Discov 2022;3(2):90–4.

26. Shah NN, Johnson BD, Fenske TS, et al. Intrathecal chemotherapy for management of steroid-refractory CAR T-cell-associated neurotoxicity syndrome. Blood Adv 2020;4(10):2119–22.

27. Baird JH, Epstein DJ, Tamaresis JS, et al. Immune reconstitution and infectious complications following axicabtagene ciloleucel therapy for large B-cell lymphoma. Blood Adv 2021;5(1):143–55.

28. Logue JM, Zucchetti E, Bachmeier CA, et al. Immune reconstitution and associated infections following axicabtagene ciloleucel in relapsed or refractory large B-cell lymphoma. Haematologica 2021;106(4):978–86.

29. Rejeski K, Perez A, Sesques P, et al. CAR-HEMATOTOX: a model for CAR T-cell-related hematologic toxicity in relapsed/refractory large B-cell lymphoma. Blood 2021;138(24):2499–513.

30. Pennisi M, Sanchez-Escamilla M, Flynn JR, et al. Modified EASIX predicts severe cytokine release syndrome and neurotoxicity after chimeric antigen receptor T cells. Blood Adv 2021;5(17):3397–406.

31. Cohen AD, Parekh S, Santomasso BD, et al. Incidence and management of CAR-T neurotoxicity in patients with multiple myeloma treated with ciltacabtagene autoleucel in CARTITUDE studies. Blood Cancer J 2022;12(2):32.

32. Van Oekelen O, Aleman A, Upadhyaya B, et al. Neurocognitive and hypokinetic movement disorder with features of parkinsonism after BCMA-targeting CAR-T cell therapy. Nat Med 2021;27(12):2099–103.

33. Le Calvez B, Eveillard M, Decamps P, et al. Extensive myelitis with eosinophilic meningitis after Chimeric antigen receptor T cells therapy. EJHaem 2022;3(2): 533–6.

34. Beauvais D, Cozzani A, Blaise AS, et al. A potential role of preexisting inflammation in the development of acute myelopathy following CAR T-cell therapy for diffuse large B-cell lymphoma. Curr Res Transl Med 2022;70(2):103331.

35. Aghajan Y, Yu A, Jacobson CA, et al. Myelopathy Because of CAR-T-Related Neurotoxicity Treated With Siltuximab. Neurol Clin Pract 2021;11(6):e944–6.

36. Nair R, Drillet G, Lhomme F, et al. Acute leucoencephalomyelopathy and quadriparesis after CAR T-cell therapy. Haematologica 2021;106(5):1504–6.

37. Johnsrud A, Craig J, Baird J, et al. Incidence and risk factors associated with bleeding and thrombosis following chimeric antigen receptor T-cell therapy. Blood Adv 2021;5(21):4465–75.

38. Jiang H, Liu L, Guo T, et al. Improving the safety of CAR-T cell therapy by controlling CRS-related coagulopathy. Ann Hematol 2019;98(7):1721–32.

39. Fried S, Avigdor A, Bielorai B, et al. Early and late hematologic toxicity following CD19 CAR-T cells. Bone Marrow Transplant 2019;54(10):1643–50.

40. Wang J, Doran J. The Many Faces of Cytokine Release Syndrome-Related Coagulopathy. Clin Hematol Int 2021;3(1):3–12.

41. Hashmi H, Mirza AS, Darwin A, et al. Venous thromboembolism associated with CD19-directed CAR T-cell therapy in large B-cell lymphoma. Blood Adv 2020; 4(17):4086–90.

42. Shalabi H, Sachdev V, Kulshreshtha A, et al. Impact of cytokine release syndrome on cardiac function following CD19 CAR-T cell therapy in children and young adults with hematological malignancies. J Immunother Cancer 2020; 8(2). https://doi.org/10.1136/jitc-2020-001159.

43. Ganatra S, Carver JR, Hayek SS, et al. Chimeric Antigen Receptor T-Cell Therapy for Cancer and Heart: JACC Council Perspectives. J Am Coll Cardiol 2019; 74(25):3153–63.

44. Kritchevsky D, Klurfeld DM. Influence of caloric intake on experimental carcinogenesis: a review. Adv Exp Med Biol 1986;206:55–68.

45. Totzeck M, Michel L, Lin Y, et al. Cardiotoxicity from chimeric antigen receptor-T cell therapy for advanced malignancies. Eur Heart J 2022;43(20):1928–40.

46. Baik AH, Oluwole OO, Johnson DB, et al. Mechanisms of Cardiovascular Toxicities Associated With Immunotherapies. Circ Res 2021;128(11):1780–801.

47. Simbaqueba CC, Aponte MP, Kim P, et al. Cardiovascular Complications of Chimeric Antigen Receptor T-Cell Therapy: The Cytokine Release Syndrome and Associated Arrhythmias. J Immunother Precis Oncol 2020;3(3):113–20.

48. Guha A, Addison D, Jain P, et al. Cardiovascular Events Associated with Chimeric Antigen Receptor T Cell Therapy: Cross-Sectional FDA Adverse Events Reporting System Analysis. Biol Blood Marrow Transplant 2020;26(12): 2211–6.

49. Alvi RM, Frigault MJ, Fradley MG, et al. Cardiovascular Events Among Adults Treated With Chimeric Antigen Receptor T-Cells (CAR-T). J Am Coll Cardiol 2019;74(25):3099–108.

50. Penack O, Koenecke C. Complications after CD19+ CAR T-Cell Therapy. Cancers 2020;12(11). https://doi.org/10.3390/cancers12113445.

51. Wudhikarn K, Pennisi M, Garcia-Recio M, et al. DLBCL patients treated with CD19 CAR T cells experience a high burden of organ toxicities but low nonrelapse mortality. Blood Adv 2020;4(13):3024–33.

52. Holland EM, Yates B, Ling A, et al. Characterization of extramedullary disease in B-ALL and response to CAR T-cell therapy. Blood Adv 2022;6(7):2167–82.

53. Sun Z, Xie C, Liu H, et al. CD19 CAR-T Cell Therapy Induced Immunotherapy Associated Interstitial Pneumonitis: A Case Report. Front Immunol 2022;13: 778192.

54. Hill JA, Giralt S, Torgerson TR, et al. CAR-T - and a side order of IgG, to go? - Immunoglobulin replacement in patients receiving CAR-T cell therapy. Blood Rev 2019;38:100596.

55. Hill JA, Li D, Hay KA, et al. Infectious complications of CD19-targeted chimeric antigen receptor-modified T-cell immunotherapy. Blood 2018;131(1):121–30.

56. Logue JM, Peres LC, Hashmi H, et al. Early cytopenias and infections after standard of care idecabtagene vicleucel in relapsed or refractory multiple myeloma. Blood Adv 2022. https://doi.org/10.1182/bloodadvances.2022008320.

57. Mikkilineni L, Yates B, Steinberg SM, et al. Infectious complications of CAR T-cell therapy across novel antigen targets in the first 30 days. Blood Adv 2021;5(23): 5312–22.

58. Park JH, Romero FA, Taur Y, et al. Cytokine Release Syndrome Grade as a Predictive Marker for Infections in Patients With Relapsed or Refractory B-Cell Acute Lymphoblastic Leukemia Treated With Chimeric Antigen Receptor T Cells. Clin Infect Dis 2018;67(4):533–40.

59. Kennedy VE, Wong C, Huang CY, et al. Macrophage activation syndrome-like (MAS-L) manifestations following BCMA-directed CAR T cells in multiple myeloma. Blood Adv 2021;5(23):5344–8.

60. Lichtenstein DA, Schischlik F, Shao L, et al. Characterization of HLH-like manifestations as a CRS variant in patients receiving CD22 CAR T cells. Blood 2021;138(24):2469–84.

61. Hines MR, Keenan C, Maron Alfaro G, et al. Hemophagocytic lymphohistiocytosis-like toxicity (carHLH) after CD19-specific CAR T-cell therapy. Br J Haematol 2021; 194(4):701–7.

62. Strati P, Ahmed S, Kebriaei P, et al. Clinical efficacy of anakinra to mitigate CAR T-cell therapy-associated toxicity in large B-cell lymphoma. Blood Adv 2020; 4(13):3123–7.

63. Dreyzin A, Jacobsohn D, Angiolillo A, et al. Intravenous anakinra for tisagenlecleucel-related toxicities in children and young adults. Pediatr Hematol Oncol 2022;39(4):370–8.

64. Martin-Rojas RM, Gomez-Centurion I, Bailen R, et al. Hemophagocytic lympho-histiocytosis/macrophage activation syndrome (HLH/MAS) following treatment with tisagenlecleucel. Clin Case Rep 2022;10(1):e05209.

65. Porter TJ, Lazarevic A, Ziggas JE, et al. Hyperinflammatory syndrome resembling haemophagocytic lymphohistiocytosis following axicabtagene ciloleucel and brexucabtagene autoleucel. Br J Haematol 2022. https://doi.org/10.1111/bjh.18454.

66. Major A, Collins J, Craney C, et al. Management of hemophagocytic lymphohistiocytosis (HLH) associated with chimeric antigen receptor T-cell (CAR-T) therapy using anti-cytokine therapy: an illustrative case and review of the literature. Leuk Lymphoma 2021;62(7):1765–9.

67. Hashmi H, Bachmeier C, Chavez JC, et al. Haemophagocytic lymphohistiocytosis has variable time to onset following CD19 chimeric antigen receptor T cell therapy. Br J Haematol 2019;187(2):e35–8.

68. Cordeiro A, Bezerra ED, Hirayama AV, et al. Late Events after Treatment with CD19-Targeted Chimeric Antigen Receptor Modified T Cells. Biol Blood Marrow Transplant 2020;26(1):26–33.

69. Beyar-Katz O, Perry C, On YB, et al. Thrombopoietin receptor agonist for treating bone marrow aplasia following anti-CD19 CAR-T cells-single-center experience. Ann Hematol 2022;101(8):1769–76.

70. Drillet G, Lhomme F, De Guibert S, et al. Prolonged thrombocytopenia after CAR T-cell therapy: the role of thrombopoietin receptor agonists. Blood Adv 2022. https://doi.org/10.1182/bloodadvances.2022008066.

71. de Tena PS, Bailen R, Oarbeascoa G, et al. Allogeneic CD34-selected stem cell boost as salvage treatment of life-threatening infection and severe cytopenias after CAR-T cell therapy. Transfusion 2022;62(10):2143–7.

72. Mullanfiroze K, Lazareva A, Chu J, et al. CD34+-selected stem cell boost can safely improve cytopenias following CAR T-cell therapy. Blood Adv 2022;6(16):4715–8.

73. Pearson AD, Rossig C, Mackall C, et al. Paediatric Strategy Forum for medicinal product development of chimeric antigen receptor T-cells in children and adolescents with cancer: ACCELERATE in collaboration with the European Medicines Agency with participation of the Food and Drug Administration. Eur J Cancer 2022;160:112–33.

74. Fiorenza S, Turtle CJ. CAR-T Cell Therapy for Acute Myeloid Leukemia: Preclinical Rationale, Current Clinical Progress, and Barriers to Success. BioDrugs 2021;35(3):281–302.

75. Wang Y, Li H, Song X, et al. Kinetics of immune reconstitution after anti-CD19 chimeric antigen receptor T cell therapy in relapsed or refractory acute lymphoblastic leukemia patients. Int J Lab Hematol 2021;43(2):250–8.

76. Wudhikarn K, Perales MA. Infectious complications, immune reconstitution, and infection prophylaxis after CD19 chimeric antigen receptor T-cell therapy. Bone Marrow Transplant 2022;57(10):1477–88.

77. Kampouri E, Walti CS, Gauthier J, et al. Managing hypogammaglobulinemia in patients treated with CAR-T-cell therapy: key points for clinicians. Expert Rev Hematol 2022;15(4):305–20.

78. Meir J, Abid MA, Abid MB. State of the CAR-T: Risk of Infections with Chimeric Antigen Receptor T-Cell Therapy and Determinants of SARS-CoV-2 Vaccine Responses. Transplant Cell Ther 2021;27(12):973–87.

79. Kochenderfer JN, Dudley ME, Feldman SA, et al. B-cell depletion and remissions of malignancy along with cytokine-associated toxicity in a clinical trial of

anti-CD19 chimeric-antigen-receptor-transduced T cells. Blood 2012;119(12): 2709–20.

80. Arnold DE, Maude SL, Callahan CA, et al. Subcutaneous immunoglobulin replacement following CD19-specific chimeric antigen receptor T-cell therapy for B-cell acute lymphoblastic leukemia in pediatric patients. Pediatr Blood Cancer 2020;67(3):e28092.

81. Hill JA, Krantz EM, Hay KA, et al. Durable preservation of antiviral antibodies after CD19-directed chimeric antigen receptor T-cell immunotherapy. Blood Adv 2019;3(22):3590–601.

82. Walti CS, Loes AN, Shuey K, et al. Humoral immunogenicity of the seasonal influenza vaccine before and after CAR-T-cell therapy: a prospective observational study. J Immunother Cancer 2021;9(10). https://doi.org/10.1136/jitc-2021-003428.

83. Ge C, Du K, Luo M, et al. Serologic response and safety of COVID-19 vaccination in HSCT or CAR T-cell recipients: a systematic review and meta-analysis. Exp Hematol Oncol 2022;11(1):46.

84. Dhakal B, Abedin S, Fenske T, et al. Response to SARS-CoV-2 vaccination in patients after hematopoietic cell transplantation and CAR T-cell therapy. Blood 2021;138(14):1278–81.

85. Korell F, Schubert ML, Sauer T, et al. Infection Complications after Lymphodepletion and Dosing of Chimeric Antigen Receptor T (CAR-T) Cell Therapy in Patients with Relapsed/Refractory Acute Lymphoblastic Leukemia or B Cell Non-Hodgkin Lymphoma. Cancers 2021;13(7). https://doi.org/10.3390/cancers13071684.

86. Vora SB, Waghmare A, Englund JA, et al. Infectious Complications Following CD19 Chimeric Antigen Receptor T-cell Therapy for Children, Adolescents, and Young Adults. Open Forum Infect Dis 2020;7(5):ofaa121.

87. Wang M, Munoz J, Goy A, et al. Three-Year Follow-Up of KTE-X19 in Patients With Relapsed/Refractory Mantle Cell Lymphoma, Including High-Risk Subgroups, in the ZUMA-2 Study. J Clin Oncol 2022;JCO2102370. https://doi.org/10.1200/JCO.21.02370.

88. Wittmann Dayagi T, Sherman G, Bielorai B, et al. Characteristics and risk factors of infections following CD28-based CD19 CAR-T cells. Leuk Lymphoma 2021; 62(7):1692–701.

89. Wudhikarn K, Palomba ML, Pennisi M, et al. Infection during the first year in patients treated with CD19 CAR T cells for diffuse large B cell lymphoma. Blood Cancer J 2020;10(8):79.

90. Spanjaart AM, Ljungman P, de La Camara R, et al. Poor outcome of patients with COVID-19 after CAR T-cell therapy for B-cell malignancies: results of a multicenter study on behalf of the European Society for Blood and Marrow Transplantation (EBMT) Infectious Diseases Working Party and the European Hematology Association (EHA) Lymphoma Group. Leukemia 2021;35(12):3585–8.

91. Josyula S, Pont MJ, Dasgupta S, et al. Pathogen-Specific Humoral Immunity and Infections in B Cell Maturation Antigen-Directed Chimeric Antigen Receptor T Cell Therapy Recipients with Multiple Myeloma. Transplant Cell Ther 2022; 28(6):304 e1–e304 e9.

92. Wang D, Mao X, Que Y, et al. Viral infection/reactivation during long-term follow-up in multiple myeloma patients with anti-BCMA CAR therapy. Blood Cancer J 2021;11(10):168.

93. Strati P, Varma A, Adkins S, et al. Hematopoietic recovery and immune reconstitution after axicabtagene ciloleucel in patients with large B-cell lymphoma. Haematologica 2021;106(10):2667–72.

94. Thakkar A, Cui Z, Peeke SZ, et al. Patterns of leukocyte recovery predict infectious complications after CD19 CAR-T cell therapy in a real-world setting. Stem Cell Investig 2021;8:18.
95. Chakraborty R, Hill BT, Majeed A, et al. Late Effects after Chimeric Antigen Receptor T cell Therapy for Lymphoid Malignancies. Transplant Cell Ther 2021; 27(3):222–9.
96. Ruark J, Mullane E, Cleary N, et al. Patient-Reported Neuropsychiatric Outcomes of Long-Term Survivors after Chimeric Antigen Receptor T Cell Therapy. Biol Blood Marrow Transplant 2020;26(1):34–43.
97. Leahy AB, Newman H, Li Y, et al. CD19-targeted chimeric antigen receptor T-cell therapy for CNS relapsed or refractory acute lymphocytic leukaemia: a post-hoc analysis of pooled data from five clinical trials. Lancet Haematol 2021;8(10):e711–22.
98. Wang XS, Srour SA, Whisenant M, et al. Patient-Reported Symptom and Functioning Status during the First 12 Months after Chimeric Antigen Receptor T Cell Therapy for Hematologic Malignancies. Transplant Cell Ther 2021;27(11):930 e1–e930, e10.
99. Chakraborty R, Sidana S, Shah GL, et al. Patient-Reported Outcomes with Chimeric Antigen Receptor T Cell Therapy: Challenges and Opportunities. Biol Blood Marrow Transplant 2019;25(5):e155–62.
100. Chow EJ, Anderson L, Baker KS, et al. Late Effects Surveillance Recommendations among Survivors of Childhood Hematopoietic Cell Transplantation: A Children's Oncology Group Report. Biol Blood Marrow Transplant 2016;22(5): 782–95.
101. Majhail NS, Rizzo JD, Lee SJ, et al. Recommended screening and preventive practices for long-term survivors after hematopoietic cell transplantation. Bone Marrow Transplant 2012;47(3):337–41.
102. Armenian SH, Sun CL, Kawashima T, et al. Long-term health-related outcomes in survivors of childhood cancer treated with HSCT versus conventional therapy: a report from the Bone Marrow Transplant Survivor Study (BMTSS) and Childhood Cancer Survivor Study (CCSS). Blood 2011;118(5):1413–20.
103. Martin T, Lin Y, Agha M, et al. Health-related quality of life in patients given ciltacabtagene autoleucel for relapsed or refractory multiple myeloma (CARTITUDE-1): a phase 1b-2, open-label study. Lancet Haematol 2022;9(12):e897–905.
104. Shah N, Delforge M, San-Miguel J, et al. Patient experience before and after treatment with idecabtagene vicleucel (ide-cel, bb2121): qualitative analysis of patient interviews in the KarMMa trial. Leuk Res 2022;120:106921.
105. Sidana S, Dueck AC, Thanarajasingam G, et al. Longitudinal Patient Reported Outcomes with CAR-T Cell Therapy Versus Autologous and Allogeneic Stem Cell Transplant. Transplant Cell Ther 2022;28(8):473–82.
106. Kamal M, Joseph J, Greenbaum U, et al. Patient-Reported Outcomes for Cancer Patients with Hematological Malignancies Undergoing Chimeric Antigen Receptor T Cell Therapy: A Systematic Review. Transplant Cell Ther 2021;27(5): 390 e1–e390 e7.
107. Elsawy M, Chavez JC, Avivi I, et al. Patient-reported outcomes in ZUMA-7, a phase 3 study of axicabtagene ciloleucel in second-line large B-cell lymphoma. Blood 2022;140(21):2248–60.
108. Laetsch TW, Myers GD, Baruchel A, et al. Patient-reported quality of life after tisagenlecleucel infusion in children and young adults with relapsed or refractory B-cell acute lymphoblastic leukaemia: a global, single-arm, phase 2 trial. Lancet Oncol 2019;20(12):1710–8.

109. Locke FL, Ghobadi A, Jacobson CA, et al. Long-term safety and activity of axicabtagene ciloleucel in refractory large B-cell lymphoma (ZUMA-1): a single-arm, multicentre, phase 1-2 trial. Lancet Oncol 2019;20(1):31–42.
110. Hsieh EM, Myers RM, Yates B, et al. Low rate of subsequent malignant neoplasms after CD19 CAR T-cell therapy. Blood Adv 2022;6(17):5222–6.
111. Myers RM, Taraseviciute A, Steinberg SM, et al. Blinatumomab Nonresponse and High-Disease Burden Are Associated With Inferior Outcomes After CD19-CAR for B-ALL. J Clin Oncol 2022;40(9):932–44.
112. Lamble A, Myers RM, Taraseviciute A, et al. Preinfusion factors impacting relapse immunophenotype following CD19 CAR T cells. Blood Adv 2022. https://doi.org/10.1182/bloodadvances.2022007423 (In eng).
113. Schultz LM, Eaton A, Baggott C, et al. Outcomes After Nonresponse and Relapse Post-Tisagenlecleucel in Children, Adolescents, and Young Adults With B-Cell Acute Lymphoblastic Leukemia. J Clin Oncol 2022. https://doi.org/10.1200/jco.22.01076. Jco2201076. (In eng).
114. Cummins KD, Gill S. Will CAR T cell therapy have a role in AML? Promises and pitfalls. Semin Hematol 2019;56(2):155–63.
115. Linette GP, Stadtmauer EA, Maus MV, et al. Cardiovascular toxicity and titin cross-reactivity of affinity-enhanced T cells in myeloma and melanoma. Blood 2013;122(6):863–71.
116. Majzner RG, Ramakrishna S, Yeom KW, et al. GD2-CAR T cell therapy for H3K27M-mutated diffuse midline gliomas. Nature 2022;603(7903):934–41.
117. Shah NN, Fry TJ. Mechanisms of resistance to CAR T cell therapy. Nat Rev Clin Oncol 2019;16(6):372–85.
118. Winship AL, Alesi LR, Sant S, et al. Checkpoint inhibitor immunotherapy diminishes oocyte number and quality in mice. Nat Cancer 2022;3(8):1–13.
119. Roberts SA, Dougan M. Checking ovarian reserves after checkpoint blockade. Nat Cancer 2022;3(8):907–8.
120. Ligon JA, Fry A, Maher JY, et al. Fertility and CAR T-cells: Current practice and future directions. Transplant Cell Ther 2022;28(9):605 e1–e605 e8.

Mechanisms of Resistance to Chimeric Antigen Receptor T Cell Therapy

Grace A. Johnson, BS[a], Frederick L. Locke, MD[b],*

KEYWORDS

- CAR T-cell therapy • Cellular immunotherapy • Large B-cell lymphoma
- Chronic lymphocytic leukemia • Acute lymphocytic leukemia
- Tumor microenvironment

KEY POINTS

- Multiple mechanisms contribute to disease resistance to, or progression after, CAR T.
- Patients with pre-treatment immune dysregulation have worse outcomes after CAR T.
- Tumor size and CAR-T expansion are key features associated with disease resistance.
- Negative prognostic factors tied to immune dysregulation include the presence of circulating monocytic myeloid-derived suppressive cells, chronic tumor interferon-gamma signaling, and elevation of ferritin and IL-6 levels.
- T cells with a less differentiated juvenile phenotype make CAR-T cells with superior proliferative capacity.

BACKGROUND

Chimeric antigen receptor (CAR) T-cell therapy has proved effective for putting both indolent and aggressive malignancies into remissions that endure longer than former standards of care (SOC). CAR T cells directed toward the CD19 antigen have resulted in superior outcomes for relapsed/refractory large B-cell lymphoma,[1] mantle cell lymphoma,[2] marginal zone lymphoma, follicular lymphoma, and acute lymphoblastic lymhpoma.[3] CAR T directed against BCMA for multiple myeloma has additionally harbored impressive overall response rates nearing 100% for patients refractory to multiple prior lines of therapy.[4] Importantly, CAR T can lead to durable results,[5] particularly when compared to historically dismal outcomes for patients with refractory disease,[6] such as seen in the SCHOLAR-1 study for refractory DLBCL.[7] CAR T has also been tested

[a] University of South Florida Morsani College of Medicine, 560 Channelside Drive, Tampa, FL 336022, USA; [b] H. Lee Moffitt Cancer Center, Department of Blood and Marrow Transplant and Cellular Immunotherapy, 12902 USF Magnolia Drive, Suite 3057, Tampa, FL 33612, USA
* Corresponding author. H. Lee Moffitt Cancer Center, Department of Blood and Marrow Transplant and Cellular Immunotherapy, 12902 USF Magnolia Drive, Suite 3057, Tampa, FL 33612.
E-mail address: Frederick.locke@moffitt.org

Hematol Oncol Clin N Am 37 (2023) 1189–1199
https://doi.org/10.1016/j.hoc.2023.07.003
0889-8588/23/© 2023 Elsevier Inc. All rights reserved.

as the treatment of other oncologic diseases such as glioblastoma multiforme,[8] as well as rheumatologic disorders such as systemic lupus erythematosus.[9]

While CAR T has increased the likelihood of a cure for certain malignancies, CAR T is not infallible, with late and early relapses still occurring in certain high-risk groups.[6,10] Suggested contributions to CAR T resistance include high baseline disease burden, immunosuppressive tumor microenvironment, evasion through loss of targeted antigen, or defective CAR T cells.[11-15] Here, we aim to explore mechanisms of treatment failure of targeted CAR T cell therapy in an effort to understand how to remedy features that underlie progression or relapse after CAR T, organized by resistance mechanisms.

RESISTANCE MECHANISMS
Target Loss

The CD19 antigen against which many CAR T-cells are directed may be lost or down-regulated as an evasion tactic. An analysis of patients in the US Lymphoma CAR-T Consortium found that CD19 loss occurred in only 30% of relapsed patients, when measured locally by Immunohistochemistry (IHC) or flow cytometry in the standard clinical lab.[16] IHC staining of tumor from patients in a post-hoc analysis of the ZUMA-1 trial, testing CAR T as a third or later line of therapy for r/r large B-cell lymphoma, found loss of CD19 expression in only 25% of relapsed tumor samples.[13] Recent work has also shown that a more nuanced analysis of CD19 target expression by examining fresh biopsies via a quantitative flow panel, further reveals that low levels of CD19 on LBCL tumors associates with resistance.[17] Taken together, this indicates that loss of CD19 target is not necessarily the only mechanism of relapse.

Alternatively, Kazantseva and colleagues found that CD19 negative tumors have a higher proportion of TP53 mutations compared to CD19 positive tumors (81% vs 21%, $P < .001$).[14] They hypothesized that the absent CD19 expression may result from aberrant differentiation associated with TP53 mutations. Therefore, it is possible that CD19 loss may not cause relapse, rather it may reflect a more aggressive tumor from the TP53 mutation it likely bears.

Emerging data suggests CD19 expression may not be a binary feature as it relates to CAR-T efficacy. An analysis of CD19 protein by centralized IHC assessment in pre-treatment tumor biopsies from patients in the ZUMA-7 trial, which randomized CAR T in the second-line against existing SOC (chemotherapy followed by autologous transplant), found that although CAR T demonstrates event-free survival superiority regardless of CD19 expression relative to SOC, patients getting CAR-T had better event-free survival if their tumor had higher CD19 expression.[18] Similar results were seen with RNA sequencing quantitation of CD19 or B cell gene scores.

Additionally, it has been hypothesized that the CD19 negative relapses are a result of selective pressures imposed by anti-CD19 CARs.[13] CD19 can lose the binding epitope via exon splice variants or lead to truncated proteins prone to degradation via intron retention events.[19,20] Another mechanism of CD19 loss is described in patients with ALL; lineage switch. Patients with a pre-existing myeloblast population can proliferate once lymphoblasts are eradicated in ALL to allow an AML phenotypes switch.[21] Lineage switch may also occur from lymphoid to myeloid phenotypes in leukemias bearing the mixed lineage leukemia gene (MLL) on chromosome 11q23.[22,23]

Regardless of these findings, it is important to note that pre-treatment CD19-negativity does not necessarily portend resistance or relapse, as patients on ZUMA-1 could benefit despite the complete absence of CD19 by IHC.[17] It remains to be seen if bicistronic or dual CARs targeting CD19 and other B cell antigens such as CD22 could lead to improved outcomes as compared to CD19 directed CAR T cells alone, or whether sequential CAR-T cells against different targets is a viable strategy for disease control.[17]

Ineffective Chimeric Antigen Receptor T-cells

A primary mechanism of resistance is failure of the manufactured CAR-T cells to proliferate, persist, or provide adequate cytotoxicity to overcome dividing tumor cells.[24] Inadequate autologous CAR-T product is most likely to be due to dysfunctional T cells collected from the patient's blood to serve as starting material for manufacture. Features which could lead to increased de novo T cell differentiation, exhaustion, or regulatory phenotype, some of which will be discussed later, include increasing lines of therapy, tumor biology, systemic immune dysregulation, genetic features, or patient demographic features. Here we review data linking poor efficacy outcomes to de novo T cell and/or CAR-T cell differentiation, exhaustion or regulatory phenotype.

More differentiated and exhausted T cell phenotypes have decreased proliferative capacity

Ineffective CAR-T cell expansion, persistence, and killing could be caused by multiple factors. The blood level of CAR-T within the first month after infusion is critical, as the degree of expansion in vivo is linked to response. The ability of CAR-T cells to expand in vitro is sometimes referred to as their "fitness," and is also linked to treatment success.[25–27]

Fraietta and colleagues investigated molecular signatures of pre-treatment CD8 T-cells and post-treatment transduced CAR T cells that associated with good responses in patients with chronic lymphocytic leukemia (CLL).[27] Patients with higher peak expansion of CAR transgene and CAR transgene persistence during the first 6 months after infusion strongly associated with the likelihood of a complete response. These expanding, persisting cells were associated with the pre-manufacture enrichment of central memory markers $CD27^+CD45RO^-$ on CD8 T-cells.[27] T cell exhaustion marked by PD-1 expression on T-cells was inversely related to proliferative capacity, and directly related to poorer responses after infusion, particularly when co-expressed with exhaustion markers as TIM-3 and LAG-3.[27,28] Thus, T-cell activation as indicated by PD-1 expression may portend good effectiveness until exhaustion ensues, as indicated by subsequently expressing LAG-3 and TIM-3.

Similar to findings in CLL, a final axicabtagene ciloleucel CAR-T product that had a greater effector cell population with a paucity of juvenile-like cells expressing CCR7 is less likely to expand in vivo after infusion, and less likely to lead to a durable response in patients with DLBCL.[25] The presence of these cells in the final product is directly informed by the presence of these phenotypes in the blood, the same cells used as starting material for manufacture of autologous CAR-T.

Deng and colleagues characterized molecular aspects of CAR T products associated with complete responses.[28] Genes associated with CD8 T-cell activation and exhaustion such as LAG3, BATF, interferon gamma, and PD-1 were more highly expressed in patients who did not achieve complete response, while genes associated with a central memory CD8 T-cell phenotype such as CCR7, CD27, and SELL were more highly expressed in patients achieving complete response. $CCR7^+/CD27^+$ double positive CD8 T-cells were three times as high in patients with complete response, and were less expressed in patients with more severe disease (stage III/IV, higher international prognostic indicator (IPI) score of 3 to 4).[28] Intra-tumoral biopsy showed that CAR CD8s with $LAG3^+TIM3^+$ double positivity were present in a higher proportion in relapsed tumors than intra-tumoral CD8s in CAR-naïve tumors.[28] An activated yet not exhausted T cell phenotype in the pre-treatment tumor microenvironment appears important for optimal outcomes.[29] It is possible that co-inhibitory molecule blockade or allogeneic

CAR T cells may circumvent the exhaustion faced by native CAR T cells that have experienced many lines of therapy and been subjected to an inflammatory milieu which produces an exhausted, futile anti-tumor effort. However, to date, single agent immune checkpoint blockade in combination with CD19 CAR-T has not clearly improved outcomes,[30,31] and allogeneic adoptive cell therapy approaches are in early stages.[32]

Chimeric antigen receptor-T cells with T regulatory features

While exhausted circulating T cells make poor CAR T infusion products, T-cells with T regulatory (T-reg) phenotypes also appear suboptimal. CD4+ CAR T-cells that expressed FOXP3 and other T-reg phenotypic markers were associated with progressive disease. Subsequently, these T-reg-like CARs were protective against severe neurotoxicity, but had sub-optimal cytotoxicity necessary for clearing tumors.[33] Haradhvala and colleagues similarly found that high frequency of CAR T-regulatory population to be suppressive to CAR expansion and associated with non-responders, whereas CD8 expansion associates with long-term response.[34]

Chimeric antigen receptor-T expansion in vivo, persistence, and target vs. effector ratio

A high level of tumor burden before infusion, whether quantified by circulating free tumor DNA (ctDNA) or gross radiographic measurements, negatively impact event-free survival.[25,35,36] Additionally, those with higher pre-treatment disease burden are more likely to have a higher ctDNA throughout therapy despite a relative decline after infusion, and subsequently have worse prognoses.[35]

It is now well established that increased expansion of CD19 CAR-T within the first month after infusion is linked to responses to CAR-T. In addition larger tumors are less likely to be cleared with CAR-T. With axicabtagene ciloleucel for LBCL the degree which CAR-T cells could expand in relationship to tumor size was directly related to durable remissions, demonstrating the importance of target:effector ratio in patients, a concept long understood as relevant in the pre-clinical field of tumor immunology.[24–26] Similarly, ALL tumor burden in the bone marrow was associated with response to CAR-T.[16] The importance of persistence of CAR-T over time is less well established.

Data in patients with ALL treated with tisagenlecleucel shows that relapse corresponds to lack or persistence of the CAR-T, similar to that described with CLL.[16,27] In contrast, CAR persistence did not appear linked to durable remission with brexucabtagene autoleucel for ALL, and CAR transgene persistence may not be essential to maintaining durable remissions in lymphoma.[37] In a 5-year follow up of patients with follicular lymphoma and DLBCL who received tisagenlecleucel (anti-CD19 with 4-1BB costimulatory domain), CAR transgene persistence was not necessary to maintain remissions, as 50% of patients who maintained a complete response after 5 years did not have detectable levels of CAR transgene.[5] Similarly, CAR-T persistence beyond 1 month was not associated with durable remissions of LBCL following axicabtagene ciloleucel treatment.[1] Finally, Sworder, Kurtz, and others found that levels of cell-free CAR transgene did not significantly differ between patients who had treatment failure versus those with an ongoing response.[35]

These conflicting results demonstrate the importance of persistence, and the required duration of persistence, of CAR-T varies depending upon the CAR-T construct and the diagnosis.

Tumor Driven Suppressive Mechanisms

Tumor immune cell composition

The presence of infiltrative T cells, and the absence of suppressive myeloid cells, within the lymphoma microenvironment is linked to better effectiveness of CAR-T therapy. Pretreatment biopsies from patients with ZUMA-1 found that activated CD8 T-cells with PD-1$^+$/LAG$^{+/-}$/TIM-3$^-$ phenotype were most associated with good response after infusion.[29,38] Importantly fewer tumor infiltrating T cells and a more suppressive and inhospitable immune milieu increases with resistance to each subsequent line of therapy.[18]

Resistance against, and exposure to, prior lines of therapy

It is possible that CAR T outcomes may be remedied by initiating anti-CD19 CAR therapy earlier on in the treatment course. Real-world data from patients with LBCL clearly illustrates that chemotherapy resistance is associated with worse outcomes with axicabtagene ciloleucel.[39-41] Results from the ZUMA-7 clinical trial comparing second-line CAR T cell therapy to SOC platinum-based salvage therapy[42] for LBCL reveal improved progression-free survival (PFS) with axicabtagene ciloleucel compared to that seen in long-term follow up of ZUMA-1 trial[1] where CAR T was utilized as a third or later line of therapy. Further minimizing the number of prior lines of chemoimmunotherapy before CAR T may be beneficial: the ZUMA-12 trial evaluated response to CAR T when implemented in the first line after two cycles of R-CHOP. It showed very high durable responses at median follow up of 15.9 months, with 78% of patients in complete response,[43] greater than that seen in ZUMA-1 or ZUMA-7.[44] This suggests an efficacy benefit of CAR-T for less-heavily pretreated patients.

Axis of immune dysregulation and suppressive myeloid cells in the tumor and periphery

Chronic tumor-associated inflammation associates with the upregulation of checkpoint ligands on tumor, increased suppressive myeloid cells, and induction of T cell exhaustion.[45] Our group was able to demonstrate similar features in patients with LBCL with patients less likely to experience durable response after CAR-T treatment when their tumors had increased genes associated with chronic interferon stimulation.[26]

The number of circulating monocytic-myeloid-derived suppressor cells (MDSCs) associate with poor outcomes following CAR-T for LBCL.[26] These cells are stimulated by chronic inflammation and are immunosuppressive as a result of IL-10, transforming growth factor-beta (TGF-beta) production, among other tolerizing cytokines,[46] which induce T-regulatory cells and polarize macrophage predominance into an M2 phenotype–which also promotes an immune-tolerizing environment. Specifically, LBCL treated with axicabtagene ciloleucel, a pattern of chronic inflammation, poor CAR expansion, and failure to achieve durable responses was associated with elevated circulating suppressive myeloid cells and worse outcomes.[26] This finding of circulating MDSCs associated with tumor inflammation provides an explanation for the observation that pre-treatment systemic inflammation, measured by proxy via elevated IL-6, CRP, and ferritin levels, associates with decreased durable responses after CAR T.[25]

Checkpoint and stimulatory ligands on tumor

Chronic inflammation reflected by enriched interferon-stimulated gene signatures associated with tumor checkpoint ligand expression (PD-L1 and others) and exhaustion of tumor-infiltrating lymphocytes.[26] Expression of PD-L1 is determined to significantly associate with a non-durable response after CAR T.[26] This systemic inflammation is also hallmarked by elevated IL-6 and ferritin, features associated with durable response after CAR T.[25] Thus, a pre-treatment inflammatory milieu, as reflected by interferon-stimulated gene signatures and monocytic myeloid-derived suppressive cells (MMDSCs),[47] hastens tumor PD-L1 expression, which impairs anti-tumor T cell activation against the tumor, and thus underlies less durable responses (**Fig. 1**).

The balance between CAR T activation without exhaustion was studied by Romain and colleagues, with a focus on T-cell CD2 protein and tumor CD58.[48] They noted that while CD2 activates T cells, it may do so in a non-exhaustive way without PD-1-upregulation or global exhaustion. Importantly, LBCL tumor expression of CD58 serves as a co-stimulator for this activation. Thus, tumor biopsies with lower expression of CD58 were found in patients who progressed after CAR T.[48] It is possible that efforts to upregulate CD58 in tumors may improve CAR-T efficacy.

Tumor TP53 mutations

Inherent tumor features may confer resistance to CAR T cell therapy. TP53 mutations have been historically characterized to portend poor outcomes in B cell lymphomas.[49,50] Shouval and colleagues recently determined that the risk of death is 2.19 times higher (HR 95% CI 1.18–4.10) in LBCL with mutant TP53 compared to wild-type TP53 after CAR T cell therapy, and this relationship remained significant when controlling for factors typically predictive of poor outcome such as baseline LDH, performance score, age, and having primary refractory disease.[12] Additionally, the rate of survival after 1 year was 44% in patients with LBCL bearing mutant TP53 compared to 77% in those with wild-type TP53. They also found that downregulated interferon (IFN) alpha and gamma signaling was associated with TP53 mutations, suggesting that TP53 mutations may associate with impaired cytotoxic T-cell infiltration into the tumor microenvironment from downregulated IFN signaling.[11,12]

Impaired death receptor signaling

CAR T-cell cytotoxicity mediated by the perforin/granzyme pathway or death receptor ligation is essential to tumor eradication.[51] Singh and colleagues demonstrated that disruptions of FADD (Fas-associated death domain) and BID (BH3 interacting-domain death agonist) proteins involved in FAS-FASL downstream signaling to enact apoptosis, are associated with CAR T treatment failure, yet maintain susceptibility to chemotherapy. Additionally, when co-cultured with death signaling pathway knock-outs, the CAR T-cells were seen to develop increased expression of exhaustion or dysfunction markers such as TIM3 and CTLA4, and produced less interferon-gamma. This was correlated clinically, in that death receptor pathways in non-responding ALL patient tumors had significantly lower death receptor gene signatures.[52]

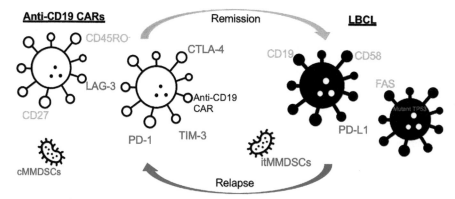

Fig. 1. Cell markers and tumor microenvironment features associating with remission (green font) and relapse (red font) after CAR T therapy. CAR, chimeric antigen receptor; cMMDSC, circulating monocytic myeloid-derived suppressor cells; itMMDSC, intra-tumor monocytic myeloid-derived suppressor cells; LBCL, large B-cell lymphoma; MMDSC, monocytic myeloid-derived suppressor cells.

SUMMARY

CAR T cell therapy is effective at eradicating relapsed or refractory disease in some patients; however, treatment failure remains an obstacle. While CD19 antigen loss in a relapsed tumor is one mechanism of resistance, it is not the sole route of tumor escape. Additional mechanisms are at play such as the corruption of de novo T cells that are used to make autologous CAR-T, or the CAR-T themselves after adoptive transfer, by a chronic inflammatory tumor environment that grooms them to express exhaustion markers impairing their activation and cytotoxicity against the tumor. High levels of pre-treatment inflammation, tumor interferon gene expression, checkpoint ligand expression, and monocytic myeloid-derived immunosuppressive cells associate with impaired CAR T expansion, impaired intratumor T-cell infiltration, and thus underlie progressive disease.[25,26] Large tumors also pose problems as CAR-T cells must expand to eradicate these tumors and achieve effective target:effector ratios. Ineffective CARs may be a result of pre-treatment exhausted CD8 T cells, such that their transduction products are equally as expressing of PD1, TIM3, or CTLA4. Or, these worn-out characteristics may be acquired from interaction with tumors bearing impaired death receptor pathways, such that persistent antigen exposure inducing checkpoint marker upregulation and that blunts the CAR cytotoxic effect. While a problem of pre-treatment exhausted T cells might be circumvented by allogeneic CAR T products, this effort might be foiled by tumors that resist apoptosis. Efforts to incorporate genomic characterization of the tumors into risk-stratifying scoring systems, such as TP53 mutation status, FADD or other downstream Fas signaling pathway proteins, are warranted allowing the prioritization of these patients for experimental therapies. Initiating CAR T cell therapy earlier on in the treatment course may also precede the development of an inflammatory environment that underlies a suboptimal tumor microenvironment and impairs tumor-effector cell interactions. While great strides have been achieved in getting effective responses with CAR T cell therapy, there is great opportunity to enhance the efficacy of these therapies by further exploration of the mechanisms of resistance including systemic immune dysregulation, the tumor microenvironment, and how it is influenced by tumor genomics, and CAR T exhaustion.

CLINICS CARE POINTS

Bulleted list of evidence-based pearls and pitfalls relevant to the point of care.

- Co-inhibitory molecule blockade or allogenic CAR T-cells may overcome exhausting-mediated treatment failure, however remain investigational.
- Earlier implementation of CAR T therapy may contribute to improved responses.
- Tumor and systemic immune dysregulation is associated with worse clinical outcomes, and is clinically marked by elevated CRP and ferritin.

DISCLOSURES

F.L.L. performed a consulting/advisory role for Allogene, Amgen, bluebird bio, BMS, Calibr, Cellular Biomedicine Group, Cowen, ecoR1, Emerging Therapy Solutions Gerson Lehman Group, GammaDelta Therapeutics, Iovance, Janssen, Kite, Legend Biotech, Novartis, Umoja, and Wugen; received research funding from Allogene, BMS, United States, Kite, and Novartis, Switzerland; and the institution holds patents, royalties, other intellectual property from several patents in author's name (unlicensed) in the field of cellular immunotherapy. The remaining authors have no disclosures.

REFERENCES

1. Locke FL, Ghobadi A, Jacobson CA, et al. Long-term safety and activity of axicabtagene ciloleucel in refractory large B-cell lymphoma (ZUMA-1): a single-arm, multicentre, phase 1-2 trial. Lancet Oncol 2019;20(1):31–42.

2. Wang M, Munoz J, Goy A, et al. KTE-X19 CAR T-Cell Therapy in Relapsed or Refractory Mantle-Cell Lymphoma. N Engl J Med 2020;382(14):1331–42.

3. Jacobson CA, Chavez JC, Sehgal AR, et al. Axicabtagene ciloleucel in relapsed or refractory indolent non-Hodgkin lymphoma (ZUMA-5): a single-arm, multicentre, phase 2 trial. Lancet Oncol 2022;23(1):91–103.

4. Berdeja JG, Madduri D, Usmani SZ, et al. Ciltacabtagene autoleucel, a B-cell maturation antigen-directed chimeric antigen receptor T-cell therapy in patients with relapsed or refractory multiple myeloma (CARTITUDE-1): a phase 1b/2 open-label study. Lancet 2021;398(10297):314–24.

5. Chong EA, Ruella M, Schuster SJ. Five-Year Outcomes for Refractory B-Cell Lymphomas with CAR T-Cell Therapy. N Engl J Med 2021;384(7):673–4.

6. Costa LJ, Maddocks K, Epperla N, et al. Diffuse large B-cell lymphoma with primary treatment failure: Ultra-high risk features and benchmarking for experimental therapies. Am J Hematol 2017;92(2):161–70.

7. Crump M, Neelapu SS, Farooq U, et al. Outcomes in refractory diffuse large B-cell lymphoma: results from the international SCHOLAR-1 study. Blood 2017; 130(16):1800–8.

8. Brown CE, Alizadeh D, Starr R, et al. Regression of Glioblastoma after Chimeric Antigen Receptor T-Cell Therapy. N Engl J Med 2016;375(26):2561–9.

9. Mackensen A, Müller F, Mougiakakos D, et al. Anti-CD19 CAR T cell therapy for refractory systemic lupus erythematosus. Nat Med 2022;28(10):2124–32.

10. Perez A, Johnson G, Patel K, et al. Primary progression during frontline CIT associates with decreased efficacy of subsequent CD19 CAR T-cell therapy in LBCL. Blood Adv 2022;6(13):3970–3 (In eng).

11. Gao J, Shi LZ, Zhao H, et al. Loss of IFN-γ Pathway Genes in Tumor Cells as a Mechanism of Resistance to Anti-CTLA-4 Therapy. Cell 2016;167(2):397–404.e9 (In eng).

12. Shouval R, Alarcon Tomas A, Fein JA, et al. Impact of TP53 Genomic Alterations in Large B-Cell Lymphoma Treated With CD19-Chimeric Antigen Receptor T-Cell Therapy. J Clin Oncol 2022;40(4):369–81 (In eng).

13. Plaks V, Rossi JM, Chou J, et al. CD19 target evasion as a mechanism of relapse in large B-cell lymphoma treated with axicabtagene ciloleucel. Blood 2021;138(12): 1081–5.

14. Kazantseva M, Hung NA, Mehta S, et al. Tumor protein 53 mutations are enriched in diffuse large B-cell lymphoma with irregular CD19 marker expression. Sci Rep 2017;7(1):1566 (In eng).

15. Brown CE, Mackall CL. CAR T cell therapy: inroads to response and resistance. Nat Rev Immunol 2019;19(2):73–4.

16. Spiegel JY, Dahiya S, Jain MD, et al. Outcomes of patients with large B-cell lymphoma progressing after axicabtagene ciloleucel therapy. Blood 2021;137(13): 1832–5.

17. Spiegel JY, Patel S, Muffly L, et al. CAR T cells with dual targeting of CD19 and CD22 in adult patients with recurrent or refractory B cell malignancies: a phase 1 trial. Nat Med 2021;27(8):1419–31.

18. Locke FL, Chou J, Vardhanabhuti S, et al. Association of pretreatment (preTx) tumor characteristics and clinical outcomes following second-line (2L) axicabtagene ciloleucel (axi-cel) versus standard of care (SOC) in patients (pts) with relapsed/refractory (R/R) large B-cell lymphoma (LBCL). J Clin Oncol 2022; 40(16_suppl):7565.

19. Sotillo E, Barrett DM, Black KL, et al. Convergence of Acquired Mutations and Alternative Splicing of CD19 Enables Resistance to CART-19 Immunotherapy. Cancer Discov 2015;5(12):1282–95 (Research Support, N.I.H., Extramural. Research Support, Non-U.S. Gov't) (In eng). DOI: .CD-15-1020.

20. Asnani M, Hayer KE, Naqvi AS, et al. Retention of CD19 intron 2 contributes to CART-19 resistance in leukemias with subclonal frameshift mutations in CD19. Leukemia 2020;34(4):1202–7.

21. Rossi JG, Bernasconi AR, Alonso CN, et al. Lineage switch in childhood acute leukemia: an unusual event with poor outcome. Am J Hematol 2012;87(9): 890–7 (In eng).

22. Gardner R, Wu D, Cherian S, et al. Acquisition of a CD19-negative myeloid phenotype allows immune escape of MLL-rearranged B-ALL from CD19 CAR-T-cell therapy. Blood 2016;127(20):2406–10 (Case Reports) (In eng).

23. Locke FL, Davila ML. Chimeric antigen receptor T cells get passed by leukemia. Transl Cancer Res 2016;S315–7. https://tcr.amegroups.com/article/view/8530.

24. Kimmel GJ, Locke FL, Altrock PM. The roles of T cell competition and stochastic extinction events in chimeric antigen receptor T cell therapy. Proc Biol Sci 2021; 288(1947):20210229.

25. Locke FL, Rossi JM, Neelapu SS, et al. Tumor burden, inflammation, and product attributes determine outcomes of axicabtagene ciloleucel in large B-cell lymphoma. Blood Adv 2020;4(19):4898–911.

26. Jain MD, Zhao H, Wang X, et al. Tumor interferon signaling and suppressive myeloid cells are associated with CAR T-cell failure in large B-cell lymphoma. Blood 2021;137(19):2621–33.

27. Fraietta JA, Lacey SF, Orlando EJ, et al. Determinants of response and resistance to CD19 chimeric antigen receptor (CAR) T cell therapy of chronic lymphocytic leukemia. Nat Med 2018;24(5):563–71.

28. Deng Q, Han G, Puebla-Osorio N, et al. Characteristics of anti-CD19 CAR T cell infusion products associated with efficacy and toxicity in patients with large B cell lymphomas. Nat Med 2020;26(12):1878–87.

29. Scholler N, Perbost R, Locke FL, et al. Tumor immune contexture is a determinant of anti-CD19 CAR T cell efficacy in large B cell lymphoma. Nat Med 2022;28(9): 1872–82.

30. Jacobson CA, Locke FL, Miklos DB, et al. End of Phase 1 Results from Zuma-6: Axicabtagene Ciloleucel (Axi-Cel) in Combination with Atezolizumab for the Treatment of Patients with Refractory Diffuse Large B Cell Lymphoma. Blood 2018; 132(Supplement 1):4192.

31. Chong EA, Svoboda J, Dwivedy Nasta S, et al. Sequential Anti-CD19 Directed Chimeric Antigen Receptor Modified T-Cell Therapy (CART19) and PD-1 Blockade with Pembrolizumab in Patients with Relapsed or Refractory B-Cell Non-Hodgkin Lymphomas. Blood 2018;132(Supplement 1):4198.

32. Locke FL, Lekakis LJ, Eradat H, et al. Phase 1 results with anti-CD19 allogeneic CAR T ALLO-501/501A in relapsed/refractory large B-cell lymphoma (r/r LBCL). J Clin Oncol 2023;41(16_suppl):2517.

33. Good Z, Spiegel JY, Sahaf B, et al. Post-infusion CAR TReg cells identify patients resistant to CD19-CAR therapy. Nat Med 2022;28(9):1860–71.

34. Haradhvala NJ, Leick MB, Maurer K, et al. Distinct cellular dynamics associated with response to CAR-T therapy for refractory B cell lymphoma. Nat Med 2022; 28(9):1848–59.

35. Sworder BJ, Kurtz DM, Alig SK, et al. Determinants of resistance to engineered T cell therapies targeting CD19 in large B cell lymphomas. Cancer Cell 2023; 41(1):210–25.e5.

36. Kurtz DM, Scherer F, Jin MC, et al. Circulating Tumor DNA Measurements As Early Outcome Predictors in Diffuse Large B-Cell Lymphoma. J Clin Oncol 2018;36(28):2845–53.

37. Shah BD, Ghobadi A, Oluwole OO, et al. KTE-X19 for relapsed or refractory adult B-cell acute lymphoblastic leukaemia: phase 2 results of the single-arm, open-label, multicentre ZUMA-3 study. Lancet 2021;398(10299):491–502.

38. Galon J, Scholler N, Perbost R, et al. Tumor microenvironment associated with increased pretreatment density of activated PD-1+ LAG-3+/− TIM-3− CD8+ T cells facilitates clinical response to axicabtagene ciloleucel (axi-cel) in patients (pts) with large B-cell lymphoma. J Clin Oncol 2020;38(15_suppl):3022.

39. Nastoupil LJ, Jain MD, Feng L, et al. Standard-of-Care Axicabtagene Ciloleucel for Relapsed or Refractory Large B-Cell Lymphoma: Results From the US Lymphoma CAR T Consortium. J Clin Oncol 2020;38(27):3119–28.

40. Jacobson CA, Hunter BD, Redd R, et al. Axicabtagene Ciloleucel in the Non-Trial Setting: Outcomes and Correlates of Response, Resistance, and Toxicity. J Clin Oncol 2020;38(27):3095–106.

41. Jacobson CA, Locke FL, Ma L, et al. Real-World Evidence of Axicabtagene Ciloleucel for the Treatment of Large B Cell Lymphoma in the United States. Transplant Cell Ther 2022;28(9):581 e1–e581 e8.

42. Locke FL, Miklos DB, Jacobson CA, et al. Axicabtagene Ciloleucel as Second-Line Therapy for Large B-Cell Lymphoma. N Engl J Med 2021;386(7):640–54.

43. Neelapu SS, Dickinson M, Munoz J, et al. Axicabtagene ciloleucel as first-line therapy in high-risk large B-cell lymphoma: the phase 2 ZUMA-12 trial. Nat Med 2022;28(4):735–42.

44. Neelapu SS, Locke FL, Bartlett NL, et al. Axicabtagene Ciloleucel CAR T-Cell Therapy in Refractory Large B-Cell Lymphoma. N Engl J Med 2017;377(26): 2531–44 (In eng).

45. Benci JL, Xu B, Qiu Y, et al. Tumor Interferon Signaling Regulates a Multigenic Resistance Program to Immune Checkpoint Blockade. Cell 2016;167(6):1540–1554 e12.

46. Liu Z, Zhou Z, Dang Q, et al. Immunosuppression in tumor immune microenvironment and its optimization from CAR-T cell therapy. Theranostics 2022;12(14): 6273–90 (In eng).

47. DeNardo DG, Ruffell B. Macrophages as regulators of tumour immunity and immunotherapy. Nat Rev Immunol 2019;19(6):369–82 (In eng).

48. Romain G, Strati P, Rezvan A, et al. Multidimensional single-cell analysis identifies a role for CD2-CD58 interactions in clinical antitumor T cell responses. J Clin Investig 2022;132(17). https://doi.org/10.1172/JCI159402.

49. Leroy K, Haioun C, Lepage E, et al. p53 gene mutations are associated with poor survival in low and low-intermediate risk diffuse large B-cell lymphomas. Ann Oncol 2002;13(7):1108–15 (In eng).

50. Xu-Monette ZY, Wu L, Visco C, et al. Mutational profile and prognostic significance of TP53 in diffuse large B-cell lymphoma patients treated with R-CHOP: report from an International DLBCL Rituximab-CHOP Consortium Program Study. Blood 2012;120(19):3986–96 (In eng).
51. Lemoine J, Ruella M, Houot R. Overcoming Intrinsic Resistance of Cancer Cells to CAR T-Cell Killing. Clin Cancer Res 2021;27(23):6298–306.
52. Singh N, Lee YG, Shestova O, et al. Impaired Death Receptor Signaling in Leukemia Causes Antigen-Independent Resistance by Inducing CAR T-cell Dysfunction. Cancer Discov 2020;10(4):552–67.

The Role of Chimeric Antigen Receptor T-Cell Therapy in the Era of Bispecific Antibodies

Karthik Nath, MD[a], Sham Mailankody, MD[a,b,c],
Saad Z. Usmani, MD, MBA, FACP[a,b,c,d],*

KEYWORDS

- CAR T-cell therapy • Bispecific antibodies • Immunotherapeutic agents
- Multiple myeloma

KEY POINTS

- Chimeric antigen receptor (CAR) T-cell therapy and bispecific antibodies have led to significant advancements in the management of relapsed/refractory blood cancers with several FDA approved products for multiple myeloma, non-Hodgkin lymphoma and B-cell lymphoblastic leukemia.
- In the absence of head-to-head comparisons of CAR T-cell therapy versus bispecific antibodies, treatment selection is personalized and needs to balance the toxicity and efficacy of each product.
- The community eagerly awaits ongoing multicenter studies to determine where in the treatment paradigm T-cell engaging therapies are best utilized, and if their earlier use may enhance their curative potential.

INTRODUCTION

T-cell redirecting therapies, which include chimeric antigen receptor (CAR) T-cell therapy and bispecific antibodies, have revolutionized the management of blood cancers. There are now several US Food and Drug Administration (FDA) approved CAR T-cell therapies for relapsed/refractory (r/r) multiple myeloma (MM), non-Hodgkin lymphoma, and B-cell lymphoblastic leukemia (B-ALL).[1–9] Despite the high response rates and durability in a subset of patients, the use of autologous CAR T-cell therapy can be challenging. This is especially the case for patients with rapidly progressive disease where a

[a] Cellular Therapy Service, Department of Medicine, Memorial Sloan Kettering Cancer Center, New York, NY, USA; [b] Myeloma Service, Department of Medicine, Memorial Sloan Kettering Cancer Center, New York, NY, USA; [c] Department of Medicine, Weill Cornell Medical College, New York, NY, USA; [d] Adult Bone Marrow Transplant Service, Memorial Sloan Kettering Cancer Center, New York, NY, USA
* Corresponding author. 530 East 74th Street, Room 20-228, New York, NY 10021.
E-mail address: usmanis@mskcc.org

Hematol Oncol Clin N Am 37 (2023) 1201–1214
https://doi.org/10.1016/j.hoc.2023.05.011
0889-8588/23/© 2023 Elsevier Inc. All rights reserved.

delay of several weeks for product manufacture is often unacceptable. Limitations in the availability of manufacturing slots and potential geographic and resourcing constraints often compound delays to accessing commercial products. Off-the-shelf bispecific antibodies, some of which were recently FDA approved, appear to have similar efficacy to CAR T-cell therapy and offer a readily accessible therapeutic option.[10–12] However, bispecific antibodies often require a continuous administration schedule and can be associated with high rates of infection. In the absence of head-to-head comparisons between CAR T-cell therapy and bispecific antibodies, clinicians will need to decide between the optimal sequencing of bispecific agents and CAR T-cell therapies.[13] Such decisions are often guided by availability, differing logistics and safety profiles. What is certain is that T-cell redirecting therapies have dramatically increased the treatment armamentarium and continue to improve outcomes for our patients. Ongoing studies of combination approaches and the use of T-cell redirecting therapies in earlier lines of treatment are eagerly awaited. An increased understanding of the predictive biomarkers and mechanisms of resistance to these novel class of agents offers exciting avenues for research and should be pursued. This review summarizes the role of CAR T-cell therapy in the era of bispecific antibodies with a particular focus on MM.

DISCUSSION
Background–Chimeric Antigen Receptor T-Cell Therapy

CAR T-cell therapy represents a pivotal advancement in the field of immunotherapy. This personalized approach involves apheresis of peripheral blood T cells which are then transferred to a Good Manufacturing Practice facility where they undergo in vitro activation and genetic modification to encode a CAR, and subsequent expansion of CAR-expressing T cells. Autologous CAR-T cells are then reinfused into a patient after they receive mandatory lymphodepleting chemotherapy. FDA approved CAR constructs are second generation, composed of an extracellular antigen-binding domain, transmembrane domain, and intracellular costimulatory and CD3 signaling domains. Each product has important differences including the antigen-binding domain, costimulatory domains (CD28 or 4-1BB), gene-transfer technique, and product manufacturing times. In addition to the logistical challenges of CAR manufacturing and administration, specific immune-mediated toxicities of cytokine release syndrome (CRS) and immune effector cell-associated neurotoxicity syndrome (ICANS) means that sites administering CAR-T cells require a robust clinical infrastructure for the management of such complications.[14]

In addition to improving efficacy, identifying resistance mechanisms, and reducing toxicity, the development of efficient manufacturing techniques is vital, particularly for the significant number of patients who have rapid progression of disease.[15] In this regard, translational insights have led to the investigation of off-the-shelf allogeneic and inducible pluripotent stem cells derived CAR-T cells.[16]

CAR T-cell therapy is being brought forward in the treatment armamentarium. Three prospective phase 3 clinical trials were conducted to define the optimal second-line treatment for large B-cell lymphoma. Two of these studies (ZUMA-7 and TRANS-FORM) demonstrated significant improvements in outcomes with CARs and led to the FDA approval of CD19 CARs in the second line.[6,9,17] The phase 3 KarMMA-3 and CARTITUDE-4 studies are asking similar questions in MM (NCT03651128; NCT04181827).[18]

Background–Bispecific Antibodies

Bispecific antibodies are off-the-shelf antibody molecules with at least 2 arms, one with binding specificity for a tumor antigen and the other typically for an activation receptor on endogenous T-cell surfaces (eg, CD3). The first FDA approved bispecific antibody was blinatumomab, which targets CD19 and is used for the treatment of r/r B-ALL.[12] Since then, there has been a dramatic advancement with a diverse family of antibody constructs, particularly in lymphoid cancers and MM. This therapeutic class is not only limited to blood cancers but is also being studied in solid tumors and noncancer indications (eg, hemophilia A).[19] After engagement of a bispecific antibody to a tumor antigen on a malignant cell, and CD3 on the T-cell, the proximity of the 2 cells leads to T-cell and immune activation, which in turn leads to tumor cell death.

Unlike blinatumomab, which has a short half-life requiring continuous infusion, novel full-length bispecific antibodies share pharmacokinetic characteristics with monoclonal antibodies and can be dosed less frequently. The FDA recently approved teclistamab (once-weekly subcutaneous administration after step-up dosing), a CD3-BCMA (B-cell maturation antigen) bispecific antibody in October 2022 for patients with r/r MM, and soon after, mosunetuzumab, the first-in-class CD3-CD20 bispecific antibody for r/r follicular lymphoma.[10,11] Both these therapies are administered until progression of disease. Although high-grade immune-mediated toxicities are uncommon, patients are usually admitted for close monitoring during initiation of therapy.

There is no doubt that bispecific antibodies have demonstrated remarkable single-agent activity. Of great curiosity is whether adjunctive pharmaceutical interventions could enhance the therapeutic efficacy of these agents. Furthermore, some bispecific antibodies in development have a trivalent design to induce greater tumor lysis such as glofitamab, a CD3-CD20 bispecific with 2 CD20 binding sites (2:1 configuration).[20] Preclinical data also demonstrate that RG6234, a novel 2:1 GPRC5D (G protein-coupled receptor, class-C, group-5, member-D) T-cell bispecific in MM, has superior T-cell activation and myeloma cell depletion.[21]

Bispecific Antibodies in the Context of Chimeric Antigen Receptor T-Cell Therapy

CAR T-cell therapy is appealing given as it is a one-time treatment. However, a critical advantage of bispecific antibodies is their off-the-shelf availability, obviating any concern for long processing times and potential manufacturing failures. The lack of lymphodepleting chemotherapy, which is mandatory with CAR T-cell therapy, also avoids the adverse effects from cytotoxic chemotherapy.

Regarding safety profiles, immune-mediated toxicities of CRS and ICANS are described in both treatments. However, the pathogenesis of ICANS with bispecifics may be distinct to CAR T-cell therapy. CAR T-cells are known to traffic to the cerebrospinal fluid but IgG-like bispecific antibodies are not expected to cross the blood-brain barrier, and accordingly, neurological adverse events are less common, and typically self-resolving.[22] Treatment with bispecific antibodies also allows for the administration of small to intermediate "priming" doses prior to the full dose of the therapy, which may help mitigate toxicities, and regular dosing provides the option of dose interruptions for toxicity. Regarding CRS and ICANS, there remains concern that nonspecific immune suppression with corticosteroids may impact CAR T-cell expansion, but this is not a concern for bispecific antibodies.[23] Infection rates after bispecific antibodies in MM is significantly higher than with CAR T-cell therapy and underscores the need for comprehensive infection prophylaxis protocols—opportunistic infections including cytomegalovirus infection have also been reported.[13,24] The higher incidence of infections may relate to ongoing B-cell aplasia and hypogammaglobulinemia from continuous therapy, differences in the number of prior lines of therapy between recipients of CAR T-cell therapy and bispecific antibodies, and the potential for bispecific antibodies to activate immunosuppressive regulatory T cells.

Lenalidomide is reported to fortify the T-cell immune synapse via downregulation of immune inhibitor ligands, and the potential synergy of bispecific antibodies with lenalidomide is being tested in MM.[25,26] In addition to combination strategies, studying both classes of T-cell engaging therapies in earlier lines is ongoing. Enrichment of immunophenotypically naive T cells has shown to enhance both the persistence and efficacy of CAR T-cell manufactured products and preservation of naive T-cell subsets can be accomplished by limiting immune-suppressive therapies from multiple lines of treatment. Another obvious question remains: where in the context of therapeutic sequencing should CAR T-cell versus bispecific antibody therapies be considered? No accepted standard approach exists–decisions are often guided by availability and logistics. Nonetheless, in patients with MM who relapse after CAR T-cell therapy, we have shown that subsequent treatment with bispecific antibodies appears to maintain pronounced clinical activity.[27]

Finally, the cost of anticancer drugs continues to increase in the United States, and it is critical to partner with the biopharmaceutical industry to ensure cost-effectiveness of cellular therapies. Technological innovations have led to place-of-care manufacturing of CAR T-cell therapy which may be a fiscally prudent and sustainable model, particularly in financially constrained regions.[28]

T-Cell Redirecting Therapies in Multiple Myeloma

There are a range of modern immune-based therapies for MM, some of which are in development and others are FDA approved (**Fig. 1**). The remainder of this review will summarize CAR T-cell therapies and bispecific antibodies in MM. Readers can review **Table 1** and **Table 2** which summarizes selected CAR T-cell and bispecific antibody studies in multiple myeloma.

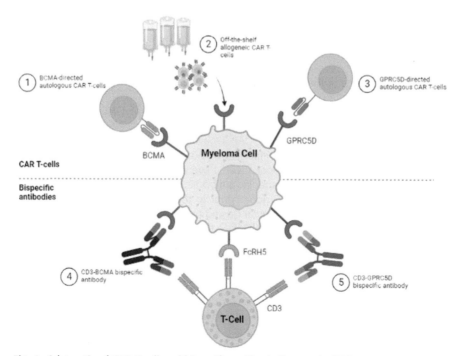

Fig. 1. Schematic of CAR T-cell and bispecific antibody therapy in MM.

Table 1

Conceptual overview of selected chimeric antigen receptor T-cell therapy studies in multiple myeloma with available results

Setting	Trial ID	Report Format	Phase	Study	Drug(s)	CAR Target	N.	ORR (CR), %	DOR, mo	PFS, mo	CRS, %	Neurotoxicity, %
≥ fourth line	NCT03361748	Paper	II	KarMMA	Ide-cel	BCMA	128	73 (33)	10.7	8.8	84	18
	NCT03548207	Paper	I/II	CARTITUDE-1	Cilta-cel	BCMA	97	98 (83)	NR	NR	95	21
	NCT04555551	Paper	I	-	MCARH109	GPRC5D	17	71 (35)	7.8	NA	88	6
	NCT04674813	Abstract	I	-	CC-95266	GPRC5D	33	90 (47)	NR	NA	64	6
	NCT05016778	Paper	I	POLARIS	OriCAR-017	GPRC5D	9	100 (60)	NA	NR	100	0
	NCT04093596	Paper	I	UNIVERSAL	ALLO-715	BCMA	43	56	8.3	NA	56	14
2–4 prior lines	NCT03651128	Paper	III	KarMMA-3	Ide-cel vs standard regimens	BCMA	386	71 (39) vs 42 (5)	14.8 vs 9.7	13.3 vs 4.4	88	15
2nd line - early relapse after ASCT	NCT03601078	Abstract	II	KarMMA-2 cohort 2A		BCMA	37	84 (46)	15.7	11.4	83	22
1–3 prior lines	NCT04181827	-	III	CARTITUDE-4	Cilta-cel vs PVd or DPd	BCMA	-	-	-	-	-	-
1st line after VRd induction - not intended for ASCT	NCT04923893	-	III	CARTITUDE-5	Cilta-cel vs Rd	BCMA	-	-	-	-	-	-
1st line after D-VRd induction	NCT05257083	-	III	CARTITUDE-6	Cilta-cel vs ASCT	BCMA	-	-	-	-	-	-

Reported abstract data refer to the time of their presentation.

Abbreviations: –, not reported; ASCT, autologous stem cell transplant; BCMA, B-cell maturation antigen; CAR, chimeric antigen receptor; cilta-cel, ciltacabtagene autoleucel; CRS, cytokine release syndrome; DPd, daratumumab-pomalidomide-dexamethasone; GPRC5D, G protein-coupled receptor, class-C, group-5, member-D; ide-cel, idecabtagene vicleucel; MM, multiple myeloma; N, number; NA, not available; NR, not reached; ORR, overall response rate; PFS, progression-free survival; PVd, pomalidomide-bortezomib-dexamethasone; Rd, lenalidomide-dexamethasone; VRd, bortezomib-lenalidomide-dexamethasone.

Table 2
Conceptual overview of selected bispecific antibody studies in multiple myeloma with available results

Setting	Trial ID	Report Format	Phase	Study	Drug(s)	Bispecific Target	N.	ORR (CR), %	DOR, mo	PFS, mo	CRS, %	Neurotoxicity, %
≥ fourth line	NCT04557098	Paper	I-II	MajesTEC-1	Teclistamab	BCMA: CD3	165	63 (39)	18.4	11.3	72	14
≥ fourth line	NCT03486067	Abstract	I	-	Alnuctamab	BCMA: CD3	68[a]	53 (23)	NR	NR	53	3
1–3 prior lines	NCT04722146	Abstract	Ib	MajesTEC-2	Tec-Dara-Len	BCMA: CD3	32	94 (55)	NA	NA	81	0
RRMM	NCT03399799	Paper	I	MonumenTAL1	Talquetamab	GPRC5D: CD3	74[a]	64–70	7.8–10.2	NA	78	7
RRMM	NCT04649359	Abstract	2	MagnetisMM-1	Elrantamab	BCMA: CD3	123	61 (28)	NR	NR	58	3
RRMM	NCT04557150	Abstract	I	-	RG6234	GPRC5D: CD3	57[a]	64 (26)	12.5	NA	79	2
RRMM	NCT03275103	Abstract	I	-	Cevostamab	FcRH5: CD3	18	100 (64)	NA	NA	NA	NA

Reported abstract data refer to the time of their presentation.

Abbreviations: -, not reported; BCMA, B-cell maturation antigen; CRS, cytokine release syndrome; Dara, daratumumab; DOR, duration of response; FcRH5, Fc receptor-homolog 5; GPRC5D, G protein-coupled receptor, class-C, group-5, member-D; len, lenalidomide; MM, multiple myeloma; N, number; NA, not available; NR, not reached; ORR, overall response rate; PFS, progression-free survival; RRMM, relapsed/refractory multiple myeloma.

[a] Data indicated for subcutaneous route of administration.

B-Cell Maturation Antigen-Directed Chimeric Antigen Receptor T-Cell Therapy for Multiple Myeloma

In the absence of modern immunotherapeutic strategies, patients with triple-class exposed MM had limited treatment options. The LocoMMotion trial prospectively enrolled patients with triple-class exposed r/r MM after greater than or equal 3 prior lines of therapy and demonstrated that only 20% of patients responded to their next line of therapy, and the MAMMOTH study reported that the median overall survival of triple-class refractory disease is only 9 months.[29,30] As such, the increasing availability of BCMA-directed CAR T-cell therapy is changing the natural history of triple-class exposed r/r MM.

BCMA, a member of the TNF superfamily, has a favorable expression pattern as a CAR target given its expression on myeloma cells, and otherwise, limited expression on nonmalignant plasma cells and small B-cell subsets.[31] Idecabtagene vicleucel (ide-cel) is the first FDA approved BCMA-directed autologous CAR T-cell therapy for triple-class exposed r/r MM after greater than 3 prior lines of therapy.[1] Ide-cel has a 4-1BB costimulatory domain and uses a lentivirus vector for CAR delivery, and the pivotal phase KarMMA trial reported a 73% response with ide-cel ($\geq$ complete response, CR 33%). But the median time from leukapheresis to product availability was 33 days and this can be challenging in patients with rapid disease progression, often necessitating bridging therapy between apheresis and CAR infusion. Among patients with a CR, the median progression-free survival was 20.2 months. Patients who received the highest target dose (450×10^6) of CAR-positive T cells appeared to have a higher frequency and depth of response. Immune-mediated toxicities with ide-cel were mostly low grade.

A recent multicenter analysis from 11 US sites reported outcomes of standard of care ide-cel in a real-world population.[32] Of the 196 leukapheresed patients, there were 17 patients who did not proceed to cell infusion due to manufacturing failure (n = 5) or disease progression (n = 12). Despite 75% of treated patients being ineligible for the KarMMA inclusion criteria, the efficacy and safety profile of ide-cel in this real-world cohort were comparable to the KarMMA study. Prior use of BCMA-targeted therapy, high-risk cytogenetics, poor performance status, and younger patient age were associated with an inferior progression-free survival.

Ciltacabtagene autoleucel (cilta-cel) is the second FDA approved CAR T-cell therapy for the treatment of triple-class exposed patients with r/r MM after greater than 3 prior lines of therapy.[2] The median time from receipt of apheresis material to release of this product was 29 days. The updated 2-year results from CARTITUDE-1 demonstrated an extremely favorable overall response rate (ORR) of 97.9% (82.5% stringent CR), which is unprecedented in this patient population.[33] Median overall survival was not reached at 27-month follow-up with a progression-free survival of 55% at 27 months. The cilta-cel construct has 2 BCMA-targeting domains and whether this contributes to its high efficacy warrants consideration. The investigators report a high rate of second primary malignancies which is likely reflective of the heavily pretreated nature of the patient population.

Unique Toxicities of Chimeric Antigen Receptor T-Cell Therapy in Multiple Myeloma

CAR-T cells are known to traffic to the cerebrospinal fluid. This is relevant not only in the context of ICANS but also because there have been reports of late-onset, progressive movement disorders after receipt of BCMA-directed CAR T-cell therapy which may relate to on-target, off-tumor effects in the central nervous system.[34] On postmortem analysis in one such patient, BCMA was found to be expressed within the basal ganglia.[35] Similarly, there have been 2 cases of late-onset cerebellar toxicity in patients who received the highest dose level of MCARH109, a GPRC5D CAR.[36] Whether this relates to possible low-level expression of GPRC5D within the inferior olivary nucleus of the brainstem requires additional study.[36]

Real-world data have also highlighted protracted high-grade cytopenias in a subset of patients. The rate of grade greater than or equal 3 neutropenia persisting beyond 30 days was 60%, anemia 38%, and thrombocytopenia 59% after ide-cel.[32] Another retrospective analysis of patients treated with BCMA-directed CAR T-cell therapy found that approximately one-third had persistent grade greater than or equal 3 cytopenias at 4 months post CAR T-cell infusion.[37]

Finally, one of the biggest hurdles with CAR T-cell therapy is limited manufacturing slot availability. Presently, the median waitlist for commercial BCMA-directed CAR T-cell therapy in the United States is approximately 6 months, and approximately a quarter of patients die whilst waiting for treatment.[38]

Novel Chimeric Antigen Receptor T-Cell Therapies in Multiple Myeloma

An effective allogeneic CAR product can overcome limitations of lengthy manufacturing times and slot availability. In this regard, Mailankody and colleagues reported interim results from the phase I UNIVERSAL trial of ALLO-715, a first-in-class "off-the-shelf" allogeneic anti-BCMA CAR T-cell therapy.[16] Patients are lymphodepleted with fludarabine, cyclophosphamide and ALLO-647 (an anti-CD52 antibody), which in turn eradicates CD52-expressing host immune cells and reduces the risk of a host-versus-graft reaction. The ALLO-715 CAR product has knockout of CD52 to allow for cell expansion and persistence in the context of ALLO-647. Interim data from the UNIVERSAL trial suggest that allogeneic CAR T-cell therapy is safe and efficacious, but longer-term data are awaited to determine durability. Importantly, no patient required bridging therapy. Part-B of the UNIVERSAL trial incorporates a gamma secretase inhibitor (nirogacestat) with ALLO-715 with the aim of preserving myeloma cell expression of BCMA to reduce antigen escape.[39]

Given a downregulation of BCMA expression has been observed in some patients who relapse post CAR T-cell therapy another strategy is to target an alternative antigen.[40] We recently reported that GPRC5D-directed CAR T-cell therapy (MCARH109) is safe and an effective novel immunotherapeutic strategy in MM. Early results of GPRC5D CARs from other groups are also promising.[41] Notably, on-target, off-tumor skin, tongue, and nail toxicities from GPRC5D CAR T-cell therapy appear to be lower than with GPRC5D bispecific antibodies, and differences in the pharmacokinetics and dosing schedules between the 2 drug classes may be contributing. Clinical studies of dual antigen targeting of both BCMA and GPRC5D are ongoing (NCT05431608; NCT05325801).

Cell manufacture with NEX-T technology is designed to shorten the manufacturing times and improve the potency and phenotypic attributes of the autologous CAR-T cells. BMS-986354, a BCMA-directed CAR T-cell therapy, is manufactured using NEX-T, and interim results of the ongoing CC-98633-MM-001 trial demonstrated an excellent ORR of 98% with this product.[42]

BCMA-directed CAR-T cells are being studied in earlier treatment lines. Interim results from the KarMMa-2 Cohort 2A study reported a favorable clinical risk–benefit profile of ide-cel in the second line for a clinically high-risk patient population.[43] CARTITUDE-5 and CARTITUDE-6 are investigating the incorporation of cilta-cel as part of frontline therapy in MM (NCT04923893; NCT05257083). The outcomes of these upfront studies of CAR T-cell therapy are eagerly awaited and could dramatically alter the current treatment paradigm of patients with multiple myeloma. Indeed, the phase 3 KarMMa-3 trial demonstrated that ide-cel significantly prolonged progression-free survival as compared with standard regimens in triple-class exposed r/r MM.[18]

BISPECIFIC ANTIBODIES IN MULTIPLE MYELOMA
Teclistamab

Teclistamab is a bispecific IgG4 antibody with dual binding sites for CD3 and BCMA. The pivotal MajesTEC-1 phase I–II clinical trial studied teclistamab in patients with triple-class exposed MM, after ≥ 3 prior lines of therapy and established a new standard of care for r/r MM with recent FDA approval.[10] Patients with prior exposure to BCMA-targeting therapies were excluded. Enrolled patients were treated with once-weekly subcutaneous teclistamab (preceded by 2 step-up doses), and patients required hospitalization and premedication with glucocorticoids to mitigate immune-mediated toxicities. There was substantial clinical activity with teclistamab with a 63% ORR (39% CR) and median response duration of 18.4 months. Notably, 7% of patients died from COVID-19 infection and this may relate to immune deficiencies from BCMA expression on normal plasma cells and necessitates infection prophylaxis and close monitoring of immune functions.

Correlative analyses have demonstrated that achievement of a higher clinical response with teclistamab is associated with higher naïve CD8+ T cells and lower expression T-cell exhaustion markers, supporting the study of teclistamab in earlier lines where patients are expected to have a more favorable immune profile.[44] Combination strategies of teclistamab and other anti-myeloma drugs are also being explored in earlier lines and include a phase 3 randomized trial that will compare teclistamab-daratumumab-lenalidomide versus daratumumab-lenalidomide-dexamethasone in newly diagnosed MM (MajesTEC-7).[45]

Talquetamab

Talquetamab is a bispecific antibody that binds to CD3 on T cells and GPRC5D on myeloma cells. The ongoing phase I MonumenTAL trial of talquetamab in r/r MM is composed of a dose-escalation and dose-expansion phase and the pivotal phase 2 portion enrolled patients with ≥ 3 prior lines of therapy and included those with prior exposure to CAR T-cell or bispecific antibodies.[46] Despite the high-risk characteristics of enrolled patients, the ORR was 64% to 70% and the median duration of response was 7.8 to 10.2 months. Within the subset of patients who had a prior T-cell redirecting therapy (71% prior CAR T-cell therapy, 35% prior bispecific antibody), the ORR was still promising at 63% with a median duration of response of 13 months.

Given the expression of GPRC5D on the skin and nail folds, low-grade and reversible skin- and nail-related changes were seen in some patients. The rate of grade 3 to 4 infections was less than 20% and the rate of COVID-19 infection was approximately 10%. RG6234 is another GPRC5D-CD3 bispecific with a 2:1 configuration that is also being studied.[47]

Cevostamab

Cevostamab is a bispecific antibody that targets Fc receptor-homolog 5 (FcRH5) on myeloma cells and CD3 on T cells. FcRH5 is expressed across the B-cell lineage with the highest expression on plasma cells and near ubiquitous expression on myeloma cells.[48] Cevostamab has an intravenous route of administration (3-weekly cycle), and preliminary results from the GO39775 phase 1 study of this agent are promising.[49] Given the crucial role of IL-6 in mediating CRS, an important study arm is investigation of pretreatment tocilizumab (an IL-6 receptor blocking antibody) to mitigate CRS.[50] Despite higher rates of neutropenia, the rate of CRS in patients who received tocilizumab was only 39% compared with 91% in patients who did not receive tocilizumab ($P < 0.001$), without any difference in response rates. Further investigation of prophylactic tocilizumab with bispecific antibodies is appealing, especially in the setting of their outpatient initiation.

Elranatamab

Elranatamab is a humanized bispecific antibody targeting BCMA on myeloma cells and CD3 on T cells. Interim results from the ongoing phase I, first-in-human MagnetisMM-1 trial of patients who received subcutaneous elranatamab monotherapy (weekly or every-other-week) have been presented.[51] Patients received a median of 5 prior lines of therapy, including prior BCMA-targeted therapies (antibody drug conjugates [15%] and CAR T-cell therapy [16%]). The ORR was 64% (38% $\geq$ CR) with 54% of patients exposed to a prior BCMA-targeted therapy achieving a response. Grade 3 and 4 infections occurred in 22% and 6% of patients, respectively.

SUMMARY

CAR T-cell therapy and bispecific antibodies have no doubt revolutionized the treatment of blood cancers. Together, these therapies are allowing for the median overall survival of our patients to improve. Yet, many questions remain. If we are to fully harness their therapeutic potential much work needs to be done—from improving access, defining optimal sequencing and adjunctive pharmaceutical agents, minimizing toxicity, and identifying resistance mechanisms and predictive biomarkers. In closing, the biggest question remains—can novel immunotherapeutic strategies cure blood cancers such as MM? That we can now plausibly ask such questions suggests that the future is bright for MM.

CLINICS CARE POINTS

- Envisioning a randomized controlled study that compares CAR T-cell therapy to bispecific antibodies is difficult. Treatment selection is often personalized, taking into consideration unique patient and disease characteristics, toxicity profiles, and logistics and access to therapy. It is hoped that emerging data will help identify the optimal sequencing of these agents, resistance mechanisms, and pretherapy biomarkers of response.

- Translational insights are leading to ongoing advancements in the drug development of T-cell engaging therapies. This includes the identification of novel target antigens and off-the-shelf CAR T-cell products. However, much work remains to be done to mitigate the treatment-related toxicities.

- Considering the therapeutic efficacy of CAR T-cell therapy and bispecific antibodies, should such therapies be brought more proximal in our treatment armamentarium–particularly given as earlier use may preserve naïve T cells, which are the optimal substrates of these treatments? We look forward to results of ongoing multicenter clinical trials that are asking such questions.

DISCLOSURE

K. Nath, S. Mailankody, and S. Usmani gratefully acknowledge the US National Cancer Institute Cancer Center Support Grant (P30 CA008748) to Memorial Sloan Kettering Cancer Center. S. Mailankody has acted as a consultant of Evicore, Janssen, Legend

Biotech and Optum Oncology, receives honoraria from MJH Life sciences, Physician Education Resource and Plexus Education, and acknowledges research funding from Allogene Therapeutics Bristol Myers Squibb, United States, Fate Therapeutics, Janssen Oncology, Juno Therapeutics, United States and Takeda Oncology, United States. S. Usmani reports grants/personal fees from Amgen, United States, Celgene, United States, Sanofi, United States, Seattle Genetics, United States, Janssen, United States, Takeda, United States, SkylineDx, Netherlands, Merck, United States, and GSK, grant funding from Bristol Myers Squibb and Pharmacyclics, United States; and personal fees from AbbVie, MundiPharma, Gilead, Genentech, and Oncopeptides. The figure was created using biorender.com.

REFERENCES

1. Munshi NC, Anderson LD, Shah N, et al. Idecabtagene Vicleucel in Relapsed and Refractory Multiple Myeloma. N Engl J Med 2021;384(8):705–16.
2. Berdeja JG, Madduri D, Usmani SZ, et al. Ciltacabtagene autoleucel, a B-cell maturation antigen-directed chimeric antigen receptor T-cell therapy in patients with relapsed or refractory multiple myeloma (CARTITUDE-1): a phase 1b/2 open-label study. Lancet 2021;398(10297):314–24.
3. Neelapu SS, Locke FL, Bartlett NL, et al. Axicabtagene Ciloleucel CAR T-Cell Therapy in Refractory Large B-Cell Lymphoma. N Engl J Med 2017;377(26):2531–44.
4. Schuster SJ, Bishop MR, Tam CS, et al. Tisagenlecleucel in Adult Relapsed or Refractory Diffuse Large B-Cell Lymphoma. N Engl J Med 2018;380(1):45–56.
5. Abramson JS, Palomba ML, Gordon LI, et al. Lisocabtagene maraleucel for patients with relapsed or refractory large B-cell lymphomas (TRANSCEND NHL 001): a multicentre seamless design study. Lancet 2020;396(10254):839–52.
6. Kamdar M, Solomon SR, Arnason J, et al. Lisocabtagene maraleucel versus standard of care with salvage chemotherapy followed by autologous stem cell transplantation as second-line treatment in patients with relapsed or refractory large B-cell lymphoma (TRANSFORM): results from an interim analysis of an open-label, randomised, phase 3 trial. Lancet 2022;399(10343):2294–308.
7. Wang M, Munoz J, Goy A, et al. KTE-X19 CAR T-Cell Therapy in Relapsed or Refractory Mantle-Cell Lymphoma. N Engl J Med 2020;382(14):1331–42.
8. Shah BD, Ghobadi A, Oluwole OO, et al. KTE-X19 for relapsed or refractory adult B-cell acute lymphoblastic leukaemia: phase 2 results of the single-arm, open-label, multicentre ZUMA-3 study. Lancet 2021;398(10299):491–502.
9. Locke FL, Miklos DB, Jacobson CA, et al. Axicabtagene Ciloleucel as Second-Line Therapy for Large B-Cell Lymphoma. N Engl J Med 2021;386(7):640–54.
10. Moreau P, Garfall AL, van de Donk NWCJ, et al. Teclistamab in Relapsed or Refractory Multiple Myeloma. N Engl J Med 2022;387(6):495–505.
11. Budde LE, Sehn LH, Matasar M, et al. Safety and efficacy of mosunetuzumab, a bispecific antibody, in patients with relapsed or refractory follicular lymphoma: a single-arm, multicentre, phase 2 study. Lancet Oncol 2022;23(8):1055–65.
12. Kantarjian H, Stein A, Gökbuget N, et al. Blinatumomab versus Chemotherapy for Advanced Acute Lymphoblastic Leukemia. N Engl J Med 2017;376(9):836–47.
13. Cliff ERS, Reynolds G, Popat R, et al. Acknowledging Infection Risk in Bispecific Antibody Trials in the Treatment of Multiple Myeloma. J Clin Oncol 2023;22:02197.
14. Lee DW, Santomasso BD, Locke FL, et al. ASTCT Consensus Grading for Cytokine Release Syndrome and Neurologic Toxicity Associated with Immune Effector Cells. Biol Blood Marrow Transplant 2019;25(4):625–38.

15. Al Hadidi S, Szabo A, Esselmann J, et al. Clinical outcome of patients with relapsed refractory multiple myeloma listed for BCMA directed commercial CAR-T therapy. Bone Marrow Transplant 2022. https://doi.org/10.1038/s41409-022-01905-1.

16. Mailankody S, Matous JV, Chhabra S, et al. Allogeneic BCMA-targeting CAR T cells in relapsed/refractory multiple myeloma: phase 1 UNIVERSAL trial interim results. Nat Med 2023. https://doi.org/10.1038/s41591-022-02182-7.

17. Bishop MR, Dickinson M, Purtill D, et al. Second-Line Tisagenlecleucel or Standard Care in Aggressive B-Cell Lymphoma. N Engl J Med 2021;386(7):629–39.

18. Rodriguez-Otero P, Ailawadhi S, Arnulf B, et al. Ide-cel or Standard Regimens in Relapsed and Refractory Multiple Myeloma. N Engl J Med 2023. https://doi.org/10.1056/NEJMoa2213614.

19. Esfandiari A, Cassidy S, Webster RM. Bispecific antibodies in oncology. Nat Rev Drug Discov 2022;21(6):411–2.

20. Dickinson MJ, Carlo-Stella C, Morschhauser F, et al. Glofitamab for Relapsed or Refractory Diffuse Large B-Cell Lymphoma. N Engl J Med 2022;387(24):2220–31.

21. Dekhtiarenko I, Lelios I, Attig J, et al. Intravenous and Subcutaneous Administration of RG6234, a Novel GPRC5DxCD3 T-Cell Engaging Bispecific Antibody, Is Highly Active in Patients with Relapsed/Refractory Multiple Myeloma (RRMM): Biomarker Results from a Phase I Study. Blood 2022;140(Supplement 1):10137–9.

22. Falchi L, Vardhana SA, Salles GA. Bispecific antibodies for the treatment of B-cell lymphoma: Promises, unknowns and opportunities. Blood 2022;2021011994, blood.

23. Strati P, Ahmed S, Furqan F, et al. Prognostic impact of corticosteroids on efficacy of chimeric antigen receptor T-cell therapy in large B-cell lymphoma. Blood 2021; 137(23):3272–6.

24. Mohan M, Nagavally S, Dhakal B, et al. Risk of infections with B-cell maturation antigen-directed immunotherapy in multiple myeloma. Blood Advances 2022; 6(8):2466–70.

25. Ramsay AG, Clear AJ, Fatah R, et al. Multiple inhibitory ligands induce impaired T-cell immunologic synapse function in chronic lymphocytic leukemia that can be blocked with lenalidomide: establishing a reversible immune evasion mechanism in human cancer. Blood 2012;120(7):1412–21.

26. Zamagni E, Boccadoro M, Spencer A, et al. MajesTEC-4 (EMN30): A Phase 3 Trial of Teclistamab + Lenalidomide Versus Lenalidomide Alone As Maintenance Therapy Following Autologous Stem Cell Transplantation in Patients with Newly Diagnosed Multiple Myeloma. Blood 2022;140(Supplement 1):7289–91.

27. Van Oekelen O, Nath K, Mouhieddine TH, et al. Interventions and outcomes of multiple myeloma patients receiving salvage treatment after BCMA-directed CAR T therapy. Blood 2022;2022017848, blood.

28. Palani HK, Arunachalam AK, Yasar M, et al. Decentralized manufacturing of anti CD19 CAR-T cells using CliniMACS Prodigy®: real-world experience and cost analysis in India. Bone Marrow Transplant 2022. https://doi.org/10.1038/s41409-022-01866-5.

29. Mateos M-V, Weisel K, De Stefano V, et al. LocoMMotion: a prospective, non-interventional, multinational study of real-life current standards of care in patients with relapsed and/or refractory multiple myeloma. Leukemia 2022;36(5):1371–6.

30. Gandhi UH, Cornell RF, Lakshman A, et al. Outcomes of patients with multiple myeloma refractory to CD38-targeted monoclonal antibody therapy. Leukemia 2019;33(9):2266–75.

31. Tai Y-T, Anderson KC. Targeting B-cell maturation antigen in multiple myeloma. Immunotherapy 2015;7(11):1187–99.

32. Hansen DK, Sidana S, Peres LC, et al. Idecabtagene Vicleucel for Relapsed/Refractory Multiple Myeloma: Real-World Experience From the Myeloma CAR T Consortium. J Clin Oncol 2023;22:01365.

33. Martin T, Usmani SZ, Berdeja JG, et al. Ciltacabtagene Autoleucel, an Anti–B-cell Maturation Antigen Chimeric Antigen Receptor T-Cell Therapy, for Relapsed/Refractory Multiple Myeloma: CARTITUDE-1 2-Year Follow-Up. J Clin Oncol 2022;22:00842.

34. Cohen AD, Parekh S, Santomasso BD, et al. Incidence and management of CAR-T neurotoxicity in patients with multiple myeloma treated with ciltacabtagene autoleucel in CARTITUDE studies. Blood Cancer J 2022;12(2):32.

35. Van Oekelen O, Aleman A, Upadhyaya B, et al. Neurocognitive and hypokinetic movement disorder with features of parkinsonism after BCMA-targeting CAR-T cell therapy. Nat Med 2021;27(12):2099–103.

36. Mailankody S, Devlin SM, Landa J, et al. GPRC5D-Targeted CAR T Cells for Myeloma. N Engl J Med 2022;387(13):1196–206.

37. Zhuang TZ, Rupji M, Santapuram PR, et al. Real-World Analysis of Cytopenias after Chimeric Antigen Receptor T-Cell Therapy: A Comparison of BCMA and CD19 Based Outcomes. Blood 2022;140(Supplement 1):12133–4.

38. Kourelis T, Bansal R, Berdeja J, et al. Ethical challenges with multiple myeloma BCMA CAR-T slot allocation: a multi-institution experience. Transplantation and cellular therapy 2023. https://doi.org/10.1016/j.jtct.2023.01.012.

39. Shearer T, Williams RL Jr, Johnson M, et al. Pharmacodynamic Effects of Nirogacestat, a Gamma Secretase Inhibitor, on B-Cell Maturation Antigen in Healthy Participants. Blood 2022;140(Supplement 1):3080–1.

40. Smith EL, Harrington K, Staehr M, et al. GPRC5D is a target for the immunotherapy of multiple myeloma with rationally designed CAR T cells. Sci Transl Med 2019;11(485):eaau7746.

41. Zhang M, Wei G, Zhou L, et al. GPRC5D CAR T cells (OriCAR-017) in patients with relapsed or refractory multiple myeloma (POLARIS): a first-in-human, single-centre, single-arm, phase 1 trial. Lancet Haematology 2023;10(2):e107–16.

42. Costa LJ, Kumar SK, Atrash S, et al. Results from the First Phase 1 Clinical Study of the B-Cell Maturation Antigen (BCMA) Nex T Chimeric Antigen Receptor (CAR) T Cell Therapy CC-98633/BMS-986354 in Patients (pts) with Relapsed/Refractory Multiple Myeloma (RRMM). Blood 2022;140(Supplement 1):1360–2.

43. Usmani S, Patel K, Hari P, et al. KarMMa-2 Cohort 2a: Efficacy and Safety of Idecabtagene Vicleucel in Clinical High-Risk Multiple Myeloma Patients with Early Relapse after Frontline Autologous Stem Cell Transplantation. Blood 2022;140(Supplement 1):875–7.

44. Cortes-Selva D, Casneuf T, Vishwamitra D, et al. Teclistamab, a B-Cell Maturation Antigen (BCMA) x CD3 Bispecific Antibody, in Patients with Relapsed/Refractory Multiple Myeloma (RRMM): Correlative Analyses from MajesTEC-1. Blood 2022;140(Supplement 1):241–3.

45. Krishnan AY, Manier S, Terpos E, et al. MajesTEC-7: A Phase 3, Randomized Study of Teclistamab + Daratumumab + Lenalidomide (Tec-DR) Versus Daratumumab + Lenalidomide + Dexamethasone (DRd) in Patients with Newly Diagnosed Multiple Myeloma Who Are Either Ineligible or Not Intended for Autologous Stem Cell Transplant. Blood 2022;140(Supplement 1):10148–9.

46. Chari A, Minnema MC, Berdeja JG, et al. Talquetamab, a T-Cell–Redirecting GPRC5D Bispecific Antibody for Multiple Myeloma. N Engl J Med 2022;387(24): 2232–44.

47. Carlo-Stella C, Mazza R, Manier S, et al. RG6234, a GPRC5DxCD3 T-Cell Engaging Bispecific Antibody, Is Highly Active in Patients (pts) with Relapsed/Refractory Multiple Myeloma (RRMM): Updated Intravenous (IV) and First Subcutaneous (SC) Results from a Phase I Dose-Escalation Study. Blood 2022; 140(Supplement 1):397–9.

48. Li J, Stagg NJ, Johnston J, et al. Membrane-Proximal Epitope Facilitates Efficient T Cell Synapse Formation by Anti-FcRH5/CD3 and Is a Requirement for Myeloma Cell Killing. Cancer Cell 2017;31(3):383–95.

49. Lesokhin AM, Richter J, Trudel S, et al. Enduring Responses after 1-Year, Fixed-Duration Cevostamab Therapy in Patients with Relapsed/Refractory Multiple Myeloma: Early Experience from a Phase I Study. Blood 2022;140(Supplement 1):4415–7.

50. Trudel S, Bahlis NJ, Spencer A, et al. Pretreatment with Tocilizumab Prior to the CD3 Bispecific Cevostamab in Patients with Relapsed/Refractory Multiple Myeloma (RRMM) Showed a Marked Reduction in Cytokine Release Syndrome Incidence and Severity. Blood 2022;140(Supplement 1):1363–5.

51. Raje N, Bahlis NJ, Costello C, et al. Elranatamab, a BCMA Targeted T-Cell Engaging Bispecific Antibody, Induces Durable Clinical and Molecular Responses for Patients with Relapsed or Refractory Multiple Myeloma. Blood 2022;140(Supplement 1): 388–90.

The Future of Chimeric Antigen Receptor T Cell Therapy

Eric L. Smith, MD, PhD

KEYWORDS

- Chimeric antigen receptor • CAR • CAR T cell therapy • Adoptive cellular therapy
- Cellular therapy

KEY POINTS

The future of CAR T cell therapies will include:

- Improved durable responses in B/plasma cell malignancies including in earlier lines of treatment.
- Expansion of efficacy to T-cell, myeloid, and solid malignancies.
- Enhanced manufacturing and delivery to address the expanded patient population.

INTRODUCTION

CAR T cell therapy of B- and plasma cell malignancies has demonstrated unprecedented efficacy for heavily pre-treated patients. Trials with CD19-[1-3] and BCMA-[4,5] targeted therapies resulted in FDA approvals across B-cell ALL, non-Hodgkin lymphomas, and multiple myeloma. Additional targets such as CD22[6] and GPRC5D[7,8] further show outstanding clinical results in earlier phase studies solidifying that CAR T cell therapy will continue to be a pillar of oncology care for these cancers. As our field passes the 10-year milestone from the first published reports of high clinical activity in adult[9] and pediatric[10] B-ALL (2013) it continues to evolve and advance at a more rapid pace than ever. The next 10 years will address key challenges in the field including: improving the cure rate for B cell malignancies; expansion of efficacy to additional histologies such as AML and solid tumors; and an overhaul in how adoptive cellular therapy is manufactured and delivered.

DISCUSSION

Improving the Cure Rate for B Cell Malignancies

It cannot be overstated the dramatic advance CAR T cell therapies have been for patients with multiply relapsed B/plasma cell malignancies, adding years of quality

Dana-Farber Cancer Institute, 450 Brookline Avenue, Boston, MA 02215, USA
E-mail address: EricL_Smith@dfci.harvard.edu

Hematol Oncol Clin N Am 37 (2023) 1215–1219
https://doi.org/10.1016/j.hoc.2023.06.005
0889-8588/23/© 2023 Elsevier Inc. All rights reserved.

life to patients with otherwise limited therapeutic options. Despite this, truly durable responses–cures, occur in fewer than half of patients with B-cell ALL/NHL and far fewer still in MM. The coming years will see an increasingly higher percent of patients cured. At least two near term advances will drive this improvement: multi-targeted approaches and moving these therapies to earlier lines of treatment. "Antigen escape" is a major mechanism of relapse for CD19-targeted malignancies. While the percent varies by disease, CAR construct, and trial, in one study of pediatric B-ALL 94% (15/16; 6 relapses unknown antigen status) have been attributed to antigen escape.[3] In MM while frank genetic perturbations are less frequent, there is evidence from MM cells identified while patients are in response that a BCMA-low/negative reservoir contributes to BCMA-positive relapse.[11,12] Trials are ongoing exploring simultaneous targeting through a variety of manufacturing approaches including pooled products ("CARpool"), viral co-transduction, and engineering of bicistronic and tandem CAR vectors. Ongoing combinations include CD19/CD22, CD19/CD20, and even CD19/CD20/CD22 for B cell malignancies and BCMA/GPRC5D and BCMA/CD19, among others for MM. One can reasonably expect that in the near-term antigen escape relapses will be mitigated with some of these approaches.

Treatment in the earlier disease setting will be another near-term major advance. We know that as B/plasma cell malignancies are treated and relapse they become more highly proliferative and evolve a more immunosuppressive tumor microenvironment. In parallel, as T cells are exposed to additional lines of therapy, they become less fit and less likely to clear large burdens of disease. Trials are already reporting on CAR T cell therapies in earlier disease settings such as NHL[13,14] and MM.[15] Additional trials are enrolling in all stages of these malignancies and, if successful in the upfront setting, hold the promise of replacing or delaying years of multi-agent small molecule, antibody, and cytotoxic chemotherapies for some patients.

Expansion of Efficacy to Additional Histologies

Holding the field back from impacting cancers more broadly including with blood cancers beyond B/plasma cell malignancies and solid tumors are major challenges of: (1) limited target antigens with acceptable ubiquitous tumor expression and lack of on-target/off-tumor potential toxicity; and (2) suppressive and/or T cell exclusive tumor microenvironments.

For hematologic malignancies additional antigens are being made accessible by advances in genetic engineering allowing the alteration of healthy cell expression. For example, ex vivo engineering of T cells to CRISPR out potential T cell leukemia/lymphoma targets such as CD7,[16,17] or limited fratricide seen targeting CD5[18] opens the door to utilizing CAR T cells to treat T cell malignancies. In AML where target antigen expression largely overlaps with healthy hematopoietic stems cells (HSCs), CAR T cell therapy is either being used as a bridge to allo-transplant or targets on HSCs are being modified ex vivo by knock-out or minimal binding epitope engineering via base editors prior to CAR T cell administration to spare transplanted HSCs.[19,20]

In solid tumors antigen heterogeneity is the predominate target-based challenge, and the suppressive TME limits efficacy. Here, CAR product developers are designing and evaluating approaches to overcome aspects of the TME and recruit and activate endogenous TCR-based immunity. Only through the activation of endogenous immunity (epitope spread) can one feasibly approach inducing cure. Pre-clinical evidence of so called "armored CAR" designs, where a second gene, such as a gene encoding a cytokine, pro-inflammatory ligand, or secreted antibody fragment is included within the CAR vector show promising signs of increasing efficacy in solid tumors. For example, IL12[21] and anti-PD1[22] secreting CARs have been shown to induce efficacy in syngeneic immunocompetent solid tumor models. Synthetic and chimeric cytokine circuits such as orthogonal IL2 receptor triggering IL9 intracellular signaling or GM-CSF secretion triggering intracellular IL18 signaling are further enhancing the potential efficacy of CAR T cell therapies relevant to solid tumors.[23,24] To enhance safety, secretion of cytokines (or other payload) may be engineered to be inducible. In a recent example inducible IL2 secretion from a circuit independent to the CAR uniquely enhanced both safety and migration of CAR T cells and efficacy into a solid tumor model.[25] Further, given the recent renewed promise of cancer vaccinees for solid tumors, including mRNA injections that encode for cytokines, co-stimulatory ligands, or target antigen outside the suppressive TME one could also foresee combinations with this approach and CAR T cell therapies inducing responses in solid tumors.[26,27] As these approaches transition to the clinic we will gain important insights into the translatability of these pre-clinical results to patients.

Manufacturing

If the field is ever to develop a highly effective CAR T cell therapy approach for solid tumors where hundreds of thousands of patients per year may benefit, single patient week-plus long autologous manufacturing would be unlikely to keep up with demand from physicians and patients. Recently several groups have validated the pre-clinical observation that rapid manufacturing preserves CAR T cells in a more naïve state and affords similar efficacy from magnitudes higher doses of longer manufactured cells.[28] Many groups are also evaluating off-the-shelf approaches. These take many forms including with NK cells from induced pluripotent stem cells, healthy donors, or cord blood. T cells, which unlike NK cells, carry the risk of GvHD, require genetic engineering to remove the TCR. To prevent host-vs-allo T cell rejection, these products are being further engineered to prevent expression of MHC class I and II and, as is then subsequently required, to inhibit endogenous NK mediated cytotoxicity towards the adoptive cellular therapy. While several off-the-shelf approaches are already being evaluated in the clinic with some demonstration of efficacy,[29] it is unclear if the robust expansion of autologous CAR T cell therapies will be matched by these approaches. Another strategy that is not quite as far along is in situ genetic modification. This can be accomplished via targeting nucleic acid containing nanoparticles to T cells.[30,31] While many questions remain around the feasibility and efficacy of such off-the-shelf approaches, should the efficacy of autologous CAR T cell therapies be replicated, this would be transformative for the field.

SUMMARY

In conclusion, the field of CAR T cell therapy is in the first inning of a nine-inning engagement. CAR T cell therapies for B/plasma cell malignancies has already been transformative for patients with heavily pretreated disease. This proof-of-concept for the potential CAR T cell therapies may hold in other malignancies has patients and physicians excitedly awaiting the next generation of advances in the field. Advances in CAR design, understanding and addressing how to target challenging antigens, and the interaction between the CAR T cells and the solid tumor microenvironment will lead to unlocking the potential in additional cancer histologies. Concomitant with this expansion to additional malignancies that is to come, advances in manufacturing will be needed to unleash the maximum benefit as CAR T cell therapy becomes an ever increasingly used therapeutic modality to eradicate cancer.

FUNDING

NIH (K08CA241400), Parker Institute for Cancer Immunotherapy, Massachusets Life Sciences Center, the Mathers Foundation, Wellcome/Leap R3, and the International Myeloma Society.

CONFLICT OF INTEREST

IP licensed to BMS, Sanofi; SAB: Chimeric Therapeutics; BMS; Sanofi; Consultant: Chroma Medicine; Clade Therapeutics; ONK; Eureka Therapeutics; ImmuneBridge; GC Cell; Sana Biotech.

REFERENCES

1. Schuster SJ, Svoboda J, Chong EA, et al. Chimeric Antigen Receptor T Cells in Refractory B-Cell Lymphomas. N Engl J Med 2017;377(26):2545–54.
2. Neelapu SS, Locke FL, Bartlett NL, et al. Axicabtagene ciloleucel CAR T-cell therapy in refractory large B-cell lymphoma. N Engl J Med 2017;377:2531–44.
3. Maude SL, Laetsch TW, Buechner J, et al. Tisagenlecleucel in children and young adults with B-Cell lymphoblastic leukemia. N Engl J Med 2018;378:439–48.
4. Munshi NC, Anderson LD Jr, Shah N, et al. Idecabtagene Vicleucel in Relapsed and Refractory Multiple Myeloma. N Engl J Med 2021;384(8):705–16.
5. Berdeja JG, Madduri D, Usmani SZ, et al. Ciltacabtagene autoleucel, a B-cell maturation antigen-directed chimeric antigen receptor T-cell therapy in patients with relapsed or refractory multiple myeloma (CARTITUDE-1): a phase 1b/2 open-label study. Lancet 2021;398(10297):314–24.
6. Fry TJ, Shah NN, Orentas RJ, et al. CD22-targeted CAR T cells induce remission in B-ALL that is naive or resistant to CD19-targeted CAR immunotherapy. Nat Med 2017;24:20–8.
7. Mailankody S, Devlin SM, Landa J, et al. GPRC5D-Targeted CAR T Cells for Myeloma. N Engl J Med 2022;387:1196–206.
8. Smith EL, Harrington K, Staehr M, et al. GPRC5D is a target for the immunotherapy of multiple myeloma with rationally designed CAR T cells. Sci Transl Med 2019;11:eaau7746.
9. Brentjens RJ, Davila ML, Riviere I, et al. CD19-targeted T cells rapidly induce molecular remissions in adults with chemotherapy-refractory acute lymphoblastic leukemia. Sci Transl Med 2013;5(177). https://doi.org/10.1126/scitranslmed.3005930.
10. Grupp SA, Kalos M, Barrett D, et al. Chimeric antigen receptor–modified T cells for acute lymphoid leukemia. N Engl J Med 2013;368(16). https://doi.org/10.1056/nejmoa1215134.
11. Brudno JN, Maric I, Hartman SD, et al. T cells genetically modified to express an anti-B-cell maturation antigen chimeric antigen receptor cause remissions of poor-prognosis relapsed multiple myeloma. J Clin Oncol 2018. https://doi.org/10.1200/JCO.2018.77.8084. JCO2018778084.
12. Cohen AD, Garfall AL, Stadtmauer EA, et al. B cell maturation antigen–specific CAR T cells are clinically active in multiple myeloma. J Clin Invest 2019. https://doi.org/10.1172/JCI126397.
13. Locke FL, Miklos DB, Jacobson CA, et al. Axicabtagene ciloleucel as second-line therapy for large B-cell lymphoma. N Engl J Med 2022;386(7). https://doi.org/10.1056/nejmoa2116133.

14. Sehgal A, Hoda D, Riedell PA, et al. Lisocabtagene maraleucel as second-line therapy in adults with relapsed or refractory large B-cell lymphoma who were not intended for haematopoietic stem cell transplantation (PILOT): an open-label, phase 2 study. Lancet Oncol 2022;23:1066–77.
15. Rodriguez-Otero P, Ailawadhi S, Arnulf B, et al. Ide-cel or standard regimens in relapsed and refractory multiple myeloma. N Engl J Med 2023;388:1002–14.
16. Gomes-Silva D, Srinivasan M, Sharma S, et al. CD7-edited T cells expressing a CD7-specific CAR for the therapy of T-cell malignancies. Blood 2017;130:285–96.
17. Cooper ML, Choi J, Staser K, et al. An 'off-the-shelf' fratricide-resistant CAR-T for the treatment of T cell hematologic malignancies. Leukemia 2018;32:1970–83.
18. Mamonkin M, Rouce RH, Tashiro H, et al. A T-cell-directed chimeric antigen receptor for the selective treatment of T-cell malignancies. Blood 2015;126:983–92.
19. Kim MY, Yu KR, Kenderian SS, et al. Genetic Inactivation of CD33 in hematopoietic stem cells to enable CAR T cell immunotherapy for acute myeloid leukemia. Cell 2018;173:1439–53.e19.
20. Borot F, Wang H, Ma Y, et al. Gene-edited stem cells enable CD33-directed immune therapy for myeloid malignancies. Proc Natl Acad Sci U S A 2019;116: 11978–87.
21. Pegram HJ, Lee JC, Hayman EG, et al. Tumor-targeted T cells modified to secrete IL-12 eradicate systemic tumors without need for prior conditioning. Blood 2012; 119:4133–41.
22. Rafiq S, Yeku OO, Jackson HJ, et al. Targeted delivery of a PD-1-blocking scFv by CAR-T cells enhances anti-tumor efficacy in vivo. Nat Biotechnol 2018;36(9): 847–56.
23. Lange S, Sand LGL, Bell M, et al. A Chimeric GM-CSF/IL18 Receptor to Sustain CAR T-cell Function. Cancer Discov 2021;11:1661–71.
24. Kalbasi A, Siurala M, Su LL, et al. Potentiating adoptive cell therapy using synthetic IL-9 receptors. Nature 2022;607(7918):360–5.
25. Allen GM, Frankel NW, Reddy NR, et al. Synthetic cytokine circuits that drive T cells into immune-excluded tumors. Science 2022;378(6625). https://doi.org/10.1126/SCIENCE.ABA1624.
26. Hewitt SL, Bai A, Bailey D, et al. Durable anticancer immunity from intratumoral administration of IL-23, IL-36γ, and OX40L mRNAs. Sci Transl Med 2019;11.
27. Reinhard K, Rengstl B, Oehm P, et al. An RNA vaccine drives expansion and efficacy of claudin-CAR-T cells against solid tumors. Science 2020;367(6476): 446–53.
28. Ghassemi S, Durgin JS, Nunez-Cruz S, et al. Rapid manufacturing of non-activated potent CAR T cells. Nat Biomed Eng 2022;6(2):118–28.
29. Mailankody S, Matous JV, Chhabra S, et al. Allogeneic BCMA-targeting CAR T cells in relapsed/refractory multiple myeloma: phase 1 UNIVERSAL trial interim results. Nat Med 2023;29(2):422–9.
30. Smith TT, Stephan SB, Moffett HF, et al. In situ programming of leukaemia-specific T cells using synthetic DNA nanocarriers. Nat Nanotechnol 2017;12(8):813–22.
31. Rurik JG, Tombácz I, Yadegari A, et al. T cells produced in vivo to treat cardiac injury. Science 2022;375(6576):91–6.